The New Neurotology

Pedro Luiz Mangabeira Albernaz
Francisco Zuma e Maia • Sergio Carmona
Renato Valério Rodrigues Cal • Guillermo Zalazar

The New Neurotology

A Comprehensive Clinical Guide

Springer

Pedro Luiz Mangabeira Albernaz
Department of Otolaryngology
Albert Einstein Hospital
São Paulo, São Paulo
Brazil

Francisco Zuma e Maia
Otology / Neurotology
Clínica Maia
Canoas, Rio Grande do Sul
Brazil

Sergio Carmona
Neurotology
Fundación San Lucas para la Neurociencia
Rosário, Santa Fé
Argentina

Renato Valério Rodrigues Cal
Curso de Medicina
Centro Universitário do Pará
Belém, Pará
Brazil

Guillermo Zalazar
Department of Neurology in Hospital de San Luis
Fundación San Lucas para la Neurociencia
Rosario, Santa Fé
Argentina

ISBN 978-3-030-11282-0 ISBN 978-3-030-11283-7 (eBook)
https://doi.org/10.1007/978-3-030-11283-7

Library of Congress Control Number: 2019935147

This Springer imprint is published by the registered company Springer Nature Switzerland AG
The registered company address is: Gewerbestrasse 11, 6330 Cham, Switzerland

My very special thanks to Jorge Kattah, who accepted the invitation to write the foreword to our book.

—Pedro Luiz Mangabeira Albernaz

Foreword

The New Neurotology is a multiple-author book written both for new learners of this subject and for specialists alike. The authors from Brazil, Pedro Luiz Mangabeira Albernaz, M.D.; Francisco Carlos Zuma e Maia, M.D.; and Renato Valerio Cal, M.D., and from Argentina, Sergio Carmona, M.D., and Guillermo Salazar, M.D., known specialists in the field, bridged neurology, audiology, and vestibular medicine to deliver a very comprehensive text, in English, highlighting the most important concepts in neurotology practice. The writing style is appealing, explaining difficult concepts with clarity. An additional positive aspect of this book is the historical context in each chapter; to the reader, knowledge of the slow pace of neurotology through the twentieth century is a strong motivating experience; even though advances are tangible, there is still need for a better understanding and management of the most common illnesses in neurotology. The 1914 Nobel Prize for Medicine awarded to Robert Bárány, M.D., for the major breakthrough understanding of clinical vestibular pathophysiology and implementation of routine testing of the vestibular apparatus, which are still in use today, marked the beginning of the modern era of neurotology. The authors describe the impact of recent technologic advances in physiology, imaging, surgery, and the introduction of video recording of eye movements in the different chapters.

The contributing otologists and neurologists who coauthored this book, worldwide known for their expertise and teaching ability, provide an easy transition from basic physiology and anatomy concepts to clinical syndrome pathophysiology and management. The positional vertigo and acute vestibular sections provide the state-of-the-art presentation and management of continuous and episodic triggered vertigo. A basic summary of auditory testing to complement this book's focus in vestibular function is excellent and particularly helpful to neurologists in this field. The summary of surgical options for the management of these disorders likewise offers clear understanding. A chapter describing alterations of glucose metabolism in the inner ear outlines arguments in favor of additional investigation.

In summary, the authors' scope in this book is broad and will generate enthusiastic acceptance. I foresee a copy of this text in each neurotologist's and medical school's library. The global enthusiasm for neurotology will likely stimulate the pace of discovery to resolve the most basic unresolved questions.

Jorge C. Kattah
University of Illinois College of Medicine
Peoria, IL, USA

Preface

Neurotology is a medical discipline devoted to the interface between otolaryngology and neurology, exploring the clinical evaluation and management of the sensorineural systems of hearing and equilibrium and its related research. It deals with all aspects of the auditory and vestibular sense organs and its central nervous system pathways, including auditory sensations and perception, the neurophysiology of balance, including special tests, auditory and vestibular electrical responses, congenital and acquired hearing problems related to both the ear and central nervous system, cochlear and vestibular implantation, and all aspects of the vestibular system. The advent of new surgical techniques related to the temporal bone and its vicinities led to the expansion of the specialty to include facial nerve disorders, intracranial complications of ear diseases, and pathological processes of the skull base.

Neurotology is mainly concerned with two important functions: hearing and equilibrium. Hearing is the basis of speech, language, and communication. Diseases of the vestibular system are frequent in the population, and many new medications and rehabilitation methods have been developed, and several diagnostic tools and surgical procedures have been developed or perfected. The vestibular sense organs and their central pathways have also become important in the area of space medicine, since astronauts have to deal with different gravities and accelerations in their travels.

The term *labyrinth* was coined by Galen when, in his dissections, he found so many complex structures in the inner ear. It was surmised that parts of these structures were auditory, but the others remained a mystery for many centuries. This is understandable, for the vestibular organs are related to gravity and accelerations, and gravity was only discovered by Isaac Newton in 1687. The symptom vertigo was known, but it was considered as a type of central nervous system disorder until Prosper Menière, in 1861, published his observations that demonstrated that the sensation of vertigo originated in the vestibular organs. Menière's clinical reasoning on describing his case was certainly influenced by his knowledge of the work of a French neurophysiologist, Jean Pierre Flourens, who had performed experiments in the semicircular canals of pigeons and was the first scientist to conclude that the vestibular system was related to balance and was not a part of the auditory system, as it was believed at the time. The name *Menière's disease* is still given to the vestibular disorder that he described, which affects both the auditory and vestibular sense organs.

The systematic clinical study of the vestibular system was established by Robert Bárány, who won the Nobel Prize for Medicine in 1914 for his work. In 1961, Georg von Békésy won the Nobel Prize for his enormous contribution to hearing physiology. In 1926, Georges Portmann, in France, proposed a surgical technique for Menière's disease, of decompression of the endolymphatic sac, thus pioneering surgical neurotology. He based his technique on the concept advanced by Knapp that Menière's disease might be due to an increased pressure in the labyrinth, comparable to glaucoma in the eye. Endolymphatic hydrops as the underlying pathology of Menière's disease, however, was only identified in 1938 by Hallpike and Cairns. Many other investigators, throughout the years, contributed to the progress of the specialty.

The surgical era of neurotology began with the techniques created or perfected by William F. House, who standardized the approaches to the internal auditory meatus through the middle cranial fossa and through the labyrinth. These techniques made it possible to decompress the facial nerve in all of its intratemporal portions and became extensively used procedures for the removal of vestibular schwannomas, meningiomas of the cerebellopontine angle, and glomus tumors. He also perfected Portmann's endolymphatic sac operation and pioneered cochlear implants.

My personal involvement with neurotology started in Saint Louis, Missouri, when I met Dr. José Santiago Riesco MacClure, a physician from Chile who created two neurotology clinics in the United States: the one in Saint Louis and a second in Chicago, Illinois. Many American neurotologists were his disciples.

Riesco once told me that when Dr. Alfonso Asenjo, an eminent neurosurgeon, founded his Institute of Neurosurgery in Santiago, Chile, in 1939, he and his colleague, Dr. César Fernandez, were invited to become the neurotologists of the institute. At that time, Riesco and Fernandez shared an otolaryngology clinic in Santiago.

Neither of them knew anything about neurotology, so they acquired some books and studied very hard. They were called to the institute to see patients and wrote their reports.

One day, Riesco finished his office earlier than usual and decided to go to the institute's clinical discussion, which he seldom attended. The meeting had already started, and nobody saw him entering the room. As they were discussing a patient, one of the physicians inquired: "What does the neurotological report say?" Another doctor read the report: "They say that the patient has a cerebellar tumor." And the first physician said: "Then the patient must have a frontal lobe tumor." And everybody laughed.

Riesco left the room as quietly as he had arrived and called his associate: "Fernandez, we are the clowns of the Institute."

They put their books aside and began to follow the patients, observe the operations to see the precise location of the lesions, and gradually acquired the knowledge that they had not succeeded in getting from books.

In Saint Louis, he gave us a series of lectures based on his own experience. To this day, I believe that these are the only lectures worth listening; I have no interest in hearing a lecturer who limits himself to quote papers or books, because I can read them myself. And we got together to see patients and to perform electronystagmography, which was, at that time, a new way of recording eye movements. Besides teaching me neurotology, he also taught me to think. For that was what we did, analyzing the data from each patient to reach a diagnostic conclusion.

Before I went to Saint Louis, both Riesco and Fernandez spent some time in the Research Department of the Central Institute for the Deaf. For many years, this department was conducted by Dr. Rafael Lorente de Nó; when this eminent neurophysiologist moved to the NIH laboratories in Bethesda, Maryland, he was replaced by the equally eminent Dr. Hallowell Davis, my professor of neurophysiology, the father of electrical response audiometry. Riesco went back to his clinical practice in Santiago, where he stayed, except for his years as visiting professor in Saint Louis and in Chicago. Fernandez, on his way back to Chile, decided to make a brief stop in Mexico City to work with another important neurophysiologist, Prof. Arturo Rosenblueth. The brief sojourn extended to 2 years, and then he received an invitation from Dr. John R. Lindsay to join the Department of Otolaryngology of the University of Chicago. So it happened that Fernandez never went back to Chile, except to visit his relatives. He was an extraordinary researcher, with enormous contributions to the field of neurotology. And he was also a good friend. It is interesting to add that he spoke English with a marked Spanish accent. And I have a distinct feeling that he could no longer speak Spanish; he only spoke English, even to Riesco.

Along the many medical meetings that I attended, I met many people who added knowledge to the discipline of neurotology, like Profs. George Greiner, from Strasbourg; Leonard B. W. Jongkees, from Amsterdam; Peter C. R. Pfaltz, from Basel; Brian F. McCabe, from Iowa City; Wallace Rubin, from New Orleans; Kenneth H. Brookler, from New York City; Vicente Honrubia, from Los Angeles; and many others. I did not have the opportunity to meet C.S. Hallpike, but I met Dr. Dix, for she attended several of my first meetings of the Collegium Amicitiae Sacrum.

Another important neurotologist in my life was Nils Henriksson, who worked in the University of Lund in Sweden. He was a disciple of Jongkees and also worked with Cesar Fernandez in Chicago. I visited him in Lund and he also came to São Paulo to visit me.

Claus-Frenz Claussen was also an important neurotologist who, in 1974, founded the Neurootological and Equilibriometric Society (NES) in Bad Kissingen, a small German town. One of the cofounders of NES was Prof. Juan Manuel Tato, from Buenos Aires. In one of the NES meetings, I received a special homage and was saluted by Wallace Rubin.

The later portion of the twentieth century and the present times brought many important changes to neurotology. There were many new contributions to neurotology, brought by researchers like Michael Halmagyi and Ian Curthoys, from Sydney; David Newman-Toker and David Zee, from Baltimore; Jorge Kattah, from Peoria;

Michael Strupp and Thomas Brandt, from Germany; Herman Kingma, from Holland; and many others. It must be mentioned that Halmagyi, Curthoys, Newman-Toker, Zee, Strupp, Brandt, and Kingma are neurologists, and Kattah is a neuro-ophthalmologist, demonstrating how interdisciplinary is our medical specialty. And I am grateful to my friends Francisco Zuma e Maia, from Porto Alegre; Sergio Carmona, from Rosario (Argentina); and Renato Cal, from Belém, who help me in the pursuit of the new neurotology. We live in an age of changes, and neurotology is also definitely experiencing a phase of intense progress.

This book is essentially dedicated to the study of the vestibular system. Vestibular disorders are frequent and can be severely incapacitating. The development of vestibular tests has always been a challenge, in view of the intimate interaction between the vestibular system and other sensory systems, mainly the visual and somatosensory systems. Unlike other systems, which rely on one individualized primary cortical area, the vestibular system sends information to many different central nervous system centers, which also receive signals from other sensory systems. Tests that depend on the subjective sensations that result from different movements are thoroughly unreliable.

Most of the present-day vestibular tests rely on the vestibulo-ocular reflex (VOR). Caloric and rotational tests, first described by Bárány, have been employed for many years. New tests have been gradually added, including simple tests that can be performed at the patient's "bedside" and that do not require a complex equipment. Vestibular myogenic electrical responses are among the new technologies that added information regarding the function of the saccule and utricle.

This book revises the old and new techniques involved in diagnosing and treating vestibular disorders. The information presented here is mostly available in medical journals related to otology, neurology, and other specialties, but since these publications are found in many different journals, they are often difficult to be obtained.

We hope that this book will become a practical reference for all physicians interested in neurotology.

São Paulo, São Paulo, Brazil — Pedro Luiz Mangabeira Albernaz
Canoas, Rio Grande do Sul, Brazil — Francisco Zuma e Maia
Rosário, Santa Fé, Argentina — Sergio Carmona
Belém, Pará, Brazil — Renato Valério Rodrigues Cal
Rosario, Santa Fé, Argentina — Guillermo Zalazar

Contents

Anatomy and Clinical Physiology of the Organs of Equilibrium 1
Hair Cells ... 2
Otoliths ... 2
The Human Labyrinth ... 4
The Vestibular System ... 6
The Semicircular Canals ... 7
The Saccule and Utricle ... 10
The Endolymphatic Sac and Duct ... 12
The Vestibular Nerves ... 13
The Central Vestibular Pathways ... 13
Operational Model of the Vestibular System ... 14
The Physiology of the Vestibular System ... 17
The Eyes ... 27
The Cerebellum ... 33
Sensorial Convergence ... 34
References ... 35

The Role of Clinical History in Neurotology ... 39
References ... 41

An Introduction to Vestibular Disorders ... 43
Structural Defects ... 43
The Perilymphatic Space ... 44
The Endolymphatic Space ... 44
Receptor Cells ... 45
Cupulae and Semicircular Ducts ... 46
Maculae and Otolithic Membranes ... 46
The Vestibular Nerves ... 47
The Central Vestibular Disorders ... 47
References ... 48

The Bedside Tests: Practical Key Strategies to the Diagnosis of Vestibular and Oculomotor Disorders 49
The First Practical Key Strategy: Understanding the Six Eye Movements. 49
The Second Practical Key Strategy: The Essential Knowledge of Anatomy and Physiology of the Vestibulo-Ocular Reflex (VOR) and the Brainstem Centers for Triggering and Controlling Eye Movements 50
The Third Practical Key Strategy: A Detailed Patient History 53
The Fourth Practical Key Strategy: Systematic Clinical Bedside Examination. 54
Static Observation of the Two Systems. 54
Head Tilt 54
Subjective Visual Vertical (SVV) 54
Spontaneous Nystagmus. 54
Examination of the Eye Movements with the Head Still (Without the Participation of the Vestibular System). 55
Ocular Alignment: The Cover Test 55
Spontaneous Nystagmus Pattern with and Without Fixation (Frenzel Lenses to Remove Fixation) and Gaze-Evoked Nystagmus. 56
Saccades 57
Smooth Pursuit 57
Vergence 58
Optokinetic Nystagmus. 58
Stimulation of the Vestibular System (Without Participation of the Vision) 58
Positional Test. 58
Vibration-Induced Nystagmus 58
Head-Shaking Nystagmus (HSN) and Head-Shaking Tilt Suppression (HSTS). 59
Hyperventilation-Induced Nystagmus 59
Valsalva-Induced Nystagmus 59
Tullio's Phenomenon 60
Stimulation of the Vestibular System (with Participation of the Vision) 60
Dynamic Visual Acuity 60
Visually Enhanced Vestibular Ocular Reflex (VVOR) 60
Vestibulo-Ocular Reflex Suppression (VORS). 61
Head Impulse Test. 61
Examination of the Vestibulospinal Reflex 61
The HINTS Protocol. 61
References. 62

Clinical Evaluation of the Vestibular System: The Vestibular Laboratory Tests 65
Electronystagmography and Videonystagmography 66
The Vestibular Tests 66
Spontaneous Nystagmus 67
Gaze Nystagmus 67
Smooth Pursuit 68
Saccade Tests 68
Optokinetic Test 69
Dynamic Positional Tests 69
Rotatory Chairs 70
Caloric Tests 71
The Video Head Impulse Test: vHIT 73
Vestibular-Evoked Myogenic Potentials: VEMPs 73
Comments 75
References 75

The Video Head Impulse Test (vHIT) 79
Vestibulo-Ocular Reflex (VOR) 80
Corrective Saccades 81
Equipment 82
Examination 82
vHIT Parameters 83
Gain 83
Corrective Saccades 83
Clinical Applications 84
vHIT Artifacts 85
The SHIMP Test 86
Conclusion 86
References 86

The Role of Audiology in Neurotology 89
Basic Audiological Tests 90
Thresholds 90
Discrimination 93
Recruitment of Loudness 94
Adaptation 95
Immittance Tests 95
Otoacoustic Emissions 96
Electrical Response Audiometry 96
Electrocochleography 97
Auditory Brainstem Responses (ABR) 99
Middle Latency Responses (MLR) 100

Cortical Electrical Response Audiometry . . . 101
P_{300} . . . 101
Evoked Responses to Electrical Stimulation . . . 102
Neurotological Aspects of Audiological Diagnosis . . . 103
Normal Hearing . . . 103
Middle Ear Mechanical Hearing Loss . . . 103
Inner Ear Mechanical Loss . . . 103
Sudden Sensorineural Hearing Loss . . . 104
Progressive Sensorineural Hearing Loss . . . 104
Mixed Hearing Loss . . . 109
The Role of Audiology in Differential Diagnosis . . . 109
Final Comments . . . 111
References . . . 111

The Vestibular Syndromes . . . 115
Episodic Spontaneous Syndromes . . . 115
Menière's Disease . . . 116
Vestibular Migraine . . . 116
Cerebellar Transient Ischemic Attacks . . . 116
Other Episodic Spontaneous Peripheral Vestibular Disorders . . . 118
Other Episodic Spontaneous Central Vestibular Disorders . . . 118
Episodic Positional Syndromes . . . 119
Orthostatic Hypotension . . . 119
Benign Paroxysmal Positional Vertigo (BPPV) . . . 119
Central Paroxysmal Positional Vertigo . . . 120
Acute Vestibular Syndromes . . . 121
Unilateral Peripheral Acute Vestibular Syndrome . . . 121
Bilateral Peripheral Acute Vestibular Syndrome . . . 122
Central Acute Vestibular Syndromes . . . 122
Ototoxicity . . . 124
Cranial Trauma . . . 125
Wernicke's Encephalopathy . . . 125
Truncal Ataxia in Acute Vestibular Syndrome . . . 125
Chronic Vestibular Syndromes . . . 127
Bilateral Peripheral Vestibular Syndrome . . . 127
Vestibular Paroxysmia . . . 128
Persistent Postural-Perceptual Dizziness . . . 128
References . . . 129

Menière's Disease . . . 133
Pathology . . . 134
Etiology . . . 135
Symptoms and Signs . . . 136
Clinical History . . . 136
Hearing Loss . . . 137
Vertigo . . . 139

Imaging . . . 140
Bilateral and Unilateral Cases . . . 140
Treatment . . . 140
Vertigo Episodes . . . 140
Treatment Between Attacks of Vertigo . . . 141
Final Comments . . . 141
References . . . 141

Vestibular Migraine . . . 143
Clinical Picture . . . 143
Migraine and Hearing Symptoms . . . 144
Pathophysiology . . . 144
Diagnosis . . . 145
Differential Diagnosis . . . 146
Treatment . . . 146
Symptomatic Treatment . . . 147
Prophylactic Treatment . . . 147
Benign Paroxysmal Vertigo of Childhood and Benign Paroxysmal Torticollis of Childhood . . . 147
Clinical Picture . . . 148
Natural History . . . 148
Pathophysiology . . . 148
Treatment . . . 148
Motion Sickness . . . 148
References . . . 149

Benign Paroxysmal Positional Vertigo . . . 151
Posterior Semicircular Canal BPPV (PSC BPPV) . . . 153
Epley's Maneuver . . . 156
Semont's Maneuver . . . 157
Apogeotropic Variant of PSC BPPV . . . 159
Lateral Semicircular Canal BPPV (LSC BPPV) . . . 159
Anterior Semicircular Canal BPPV (ASC BPPV) . . . 168
Atypical Paroxysmal Positional Vertigo . . . 169
Atypical Lateral Canal BPPV . . . 170
Atypical Posterior Canal BPPV . . . 171
Vestibular Neuritis with Positional Nystagmus . . . 171
Comments . . . 171
References . . . 172

Bilateral Vestibulopathy . . . 175
Epidemiology . . . 176
Differential Diagnosis . . . 176
Ototoxicity . . . 176
Sequential Vestibular Loss . . . 177
Autoimmune Inner Ear Disease . . . 177

Primary Cerebellar Atrophy 177
Otosclerosis 177
Bone Dysplasias 177
Other Diseases Related to Vestibular Disorders 178
Diagnostic Criteria 178
Diagnostic Criteria for Bilateral Vestibulopathy 178
Diagnostic Criteria for Probable Bilateral Vestibulopathy 179
References 179

Ataxia 181
Introduction 181
Signs and Symptoms 181
Cerebellar Ataxia 182
Gait and Posture Alteration 182
Limb Ataxia 182
Dysarthria and Bulbar Symptoms 183
Visual Symptoms and Oculomotor Findings 183
Sensory Ataxia 183
Semiologic Maneuvers 183
Maneuvers for Static Ataxia 184
Maneuvers for Dynamic Ataxia 184
Etiology 185
Alcoholic Cerebellar Degeneration 185
Toxic Ataxia 187
Paraneoplastic Cerebellar Degeneration 187
Autoimmune Ataxia 187
Ataxia Related to Anti-GAD Antibodies 187
Ataxia Related to Hashimoto's Encephalopathy 188
Multiple System Atrophy (MSA) 188
Vitamin Deficiency 188
Idiopathic Late-Onset Cerebellar Ataxia (ILOCA) 189
Episodic Ataxia 189
Infections 189
Mitochondrial Diseases 190
Spinocerebellar Ataxia 190
Autosomal Recessive Ataxia 190
References 190

Functional Vestibular Disorders 193
Medications for Hypertension 193
Alcohol 193
Toxic Substances 194
Metabolic and Endocrinal Disorders 194
Other Medications 195
References 195

Glucose, Insulin, and Inner Ear Pathology 197
Symptoms 200
Findings. 201
Audiological Tests. 201
Vestibular Examination. 201
Glucose and Insulin Assays 202
Menière's Disease and Disorders of Carbohydrate Metabolism. 204
Discussion. 204
Conclusions. 209
References. 209

Surgical Treatment of Vestibular Disorders 213
Surgery for Menière's Disease 213
Labyrinthectomy 213
Endolymphatic Fistulas. 214
Endolymphatic Sac Operations. 215
Nerve Sections 215
Transtympanic Treatments 216
Surgery for Perilymphatic Fistulas 216
Surgery for Benign Paroxysmal Positional Vertigo 217
The Perilymphatic Hypertension Syndrome. 218
Surgery for Dehiscence of the Superior Semicircular Canal 218
Vascular Loops 219
Vestibular Schwannomas 219
Vestibular Implants 220
Final Comments 220
References. 221

Index. 225

Anatomy and Clinical Physiology of the Organs of Equilibrium

Valsalva, in his *De Aure Humana Tractatus*, an extensive otological handbook published in 1704, divided the ear in three parts: the external ear, the middle ear, and the inner ear. This division has been maintained to this date.

This chapter will be limited to the inner ear, discussing its anatomy from a physiological point of view, with emphasis on the low-frequency receptors that constitute the vestibular organs. Some anatomical details will be omitted for the sake of brevity.

The inner ear is also known as the *labyrinth*, a name given by Galen in the second century AD when he was performing anatomical studies of the skull. The complexity of the anatomy led him to compare this area to the Cretan labyrinth of Greek mythology, where people got lost and could not escape.

By the end of the eighteenth century, the anatomy of the inner ear had been extensively studied, but it was believed to be related to hearing. The notion that a part of the system had to do with to balance was achieved only in the nineteenth century [1]. Although the word *labyrinth* designates the whole inner ear, it is often used to name only the balance structures, also called *vestibular organs*.

Hallowell Davis [2], in his study of "a sensory system in evolution," mentions that throughout the zoological scale, there is always a sensory system that relies on one type of sensory cell, the hair cell. In all vertebrates, this sensory system has a common embryonal origin, and the afferent stimuli are taken to bulbar centers by a cranial nerve from VII to X.

The peripheral receptors may present three different configurations: the labyrinth, the lateral line, and the cochlea. The labyrinth exists in practically all multicellular organisms capable of movement, beginning with the coelenterates. The lateral line is important in fishes and amphibians but disappears in the terrestrial animals and in birds. The acoustic part of the system, although present in amphibians and fishes, is particularly associated with the terrestrial habitat.

A brief review of the essential components of the labyrinth will precede the description of the human inner ear.

P. L. M. Albernaz et al., *The New Neurotology*,
https://doi.org/10.1007/978-3-030-11283-7_1

Hair Cells

Cells with cilia are common in nature. The flagellum presented by many protozoa is a common type of cilium. This kind of cilium, however, is not a sensory structure but a means of locomotion. Similar kinocilia are also common in the respiratory tracts of all air-breathing vertebrates.

The cilia of the inner ear cells, however, are totally different. They are specialized components of sensory receptors and have a passive mechanical function. They are organized in such a fashion that only movements in specific directions cause deformities of the membrane from which they emerge.

The inner ear hair cells are located in a conglomerate of supporting cells. Each cell has approximately 100 stereocilia. The cells of the vestibular portion also have one kinocilium, with a different kind of structure. During the morphogenesis of the hair bundle, the kinocilium is at the center of the apical surface of the hair cell, surrounded by microvilli; afterward, it moves to the cell periphery, dictating the orientation of the hair bundle. As the kinocilium moves, the microvilli begin to elongate and form stereocilia [3].

The cochlear hair cells do not have kinocilia. They have only *basal bodies*, which are remainders of kinocilia that have regressed once the hair bundle has matured. The movement of the hair bundle, as a result of endolymph flow, will cause potassium channels on the stereocilia to open. This is mostly due to the pulling force that the stereocilium exerts on its neighboring stereocilia via interconnecting links that hold them together, and this leads to the depolarization of the hair cell.

The kinocilia of the crista ampullaris of the semicircular ducts, as well as those of the sensory maculae of the utricle and saccule, remain active throughout life. During the movements of the body, the hair cell is depolarized when the stereocilia move toward the kinocilium. The depolarization of the hair cell causes neurotransmitters to be released and an increase in firing frequency of the nerve fibers. When the stereocilia tilt away from the kinocilium, the hair cell is hyperpolarized, decreasing the amount of neurotransmitter released, which decreases the firing frequency of the vestibular nerves (Fig. 1).

Otoliths

The most primitive of the vestibular organs is the *statocyst*, a sensory receptor present in some aquatic invertebrates, which evolved to form the utricular and saccular maculae of the vertebrates.

The statocyst (as the utricle and saccule) responds to gravity, helping the animal to maintain an erect posture (Fig. 2). An *otolith*, with a density higher than that of

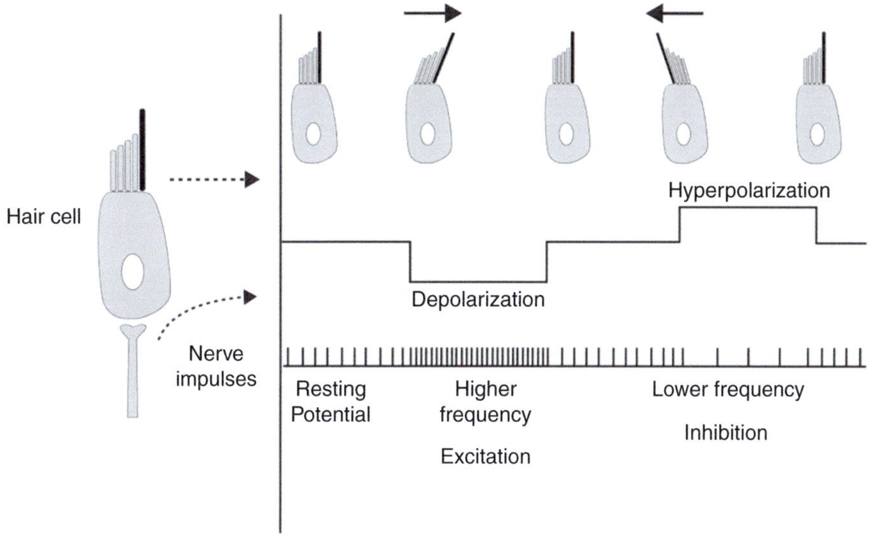

Fig. 1 Hyperpolarization and depolarization of vestibular hair cells

Fig. 2 A schematic drawing of a statocyst. (From Wikimedia Commons)

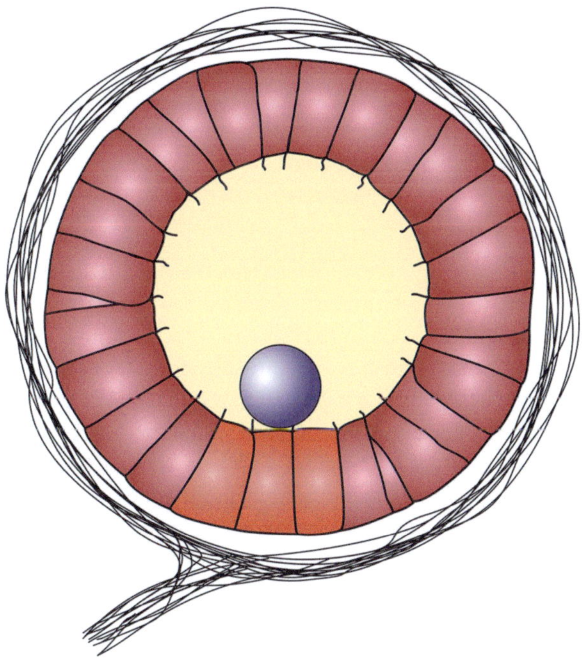

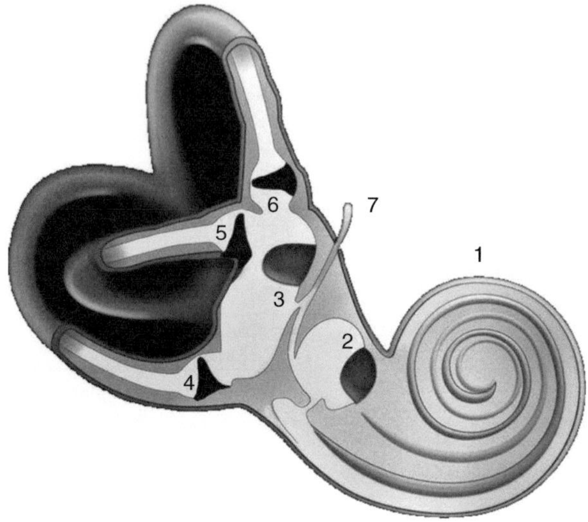

Fig. 3 A schematic view of the labyrinth. 1, cochlea; 2, saccule; 3, utricle; 4, ampulla of the posterior semicircular canal; 5, ampulla of the lateral semicircular canal; 6, ampulla of the anterior semicircular canal; 7, endolymphatic duct. (Adapted from Wikimedia Commons)

water, is loose in a cavity lined with hair cells. In invertebrates, the otolith is often a grain of sand; in vertebrates, it is usually made of calcium carbonate in contact with a gelatinous semi-viscous structure that dampens and limits its movements. The gravity-induced movements of the otolith flex the cilia and hyperpolarize or depolarize the hair cells, according to their orientation (Fig. 3).

The Human Labyrinth

Figure 1 shows a schematic view of the inner ear, which comprises the part dedicated to hearing, the *cochlea*, and the part dedicated to balance that includes the *saccule*, the *utricle*, and the *semicircular canals*.

The whole system is enclosed in very hard bone – the hardest in the body – called the *otic capsule*. Inside the bony labyrinth, there is a membranous labyrinth.

The cochlea is a spiral canal that winds 2½ turns around a *modiolus*. An osseous lamina spirals around the modiolus and incompletely subdivides the spiral canal in two different parts, the *scala vestibuli*, which connects to the oval window, and the *scala tympani*, which connects with the round window. The two scalae join at the tip of the cochlea through a canal called *helicotrema*. In addition to the scala vestibuli and the scala tympani, there is a smaller triangular space, the *scala media*, or *cochlear duct*, which is separated from the scala vestibuli by a thin membrane, *Reissner's membrane*.

The scala vestibuli and the scala tympani, as well as the semicircular canals, are filled with *perilymph*, a fluid with a composition very similar to that of cerebrospinal fluid, being rich in sodium and having a small concentration of potassium. The concentration of protein in perilymph is a little higher than that of the spinal fluid, but this is probably due to a more reduced circulation. The spinal fluid in the area of the cauda equina also has a higher protein content than that of other levels.

The portions of the membranous labyrinth that are inside the semicircular canals are called *semicircular ducts*. Each of the ducts has in one of its endings an enlarged area, the *ampulla*, that contains sensory cells.

The cochlear duct, the semicircular ducts, the saccule, and the utricle contain *endolymph*, a fluid that has a high content of potassium and a low content of sodium. In fact, endolymph is the only extracellular fluid that is rich in potassium, being similar to the intracellular fluids. Endolymph is produced by the *stria vascularis*, an area of intense metabolic activity located in the superior portion of the spiral ligament.

Figure 4 shows us a detailed drawing of the first turn of a guinea pig's cochlea. The human cochlea is very similar to this. Figure 5 shows the organ of Corti alone.

It will be noted that a *basilar membrane*, inserted in the osseous spiral lamina, completes the division between the scala tympani and the scala media. On the lateral side, it ends in a *spiral ligament*. On top of the basilar membrane is the organ of Corti, a complex structure that contains one row of inner hair cells and three rows

Fig. 4 First turn of a guinea pig's cochlea

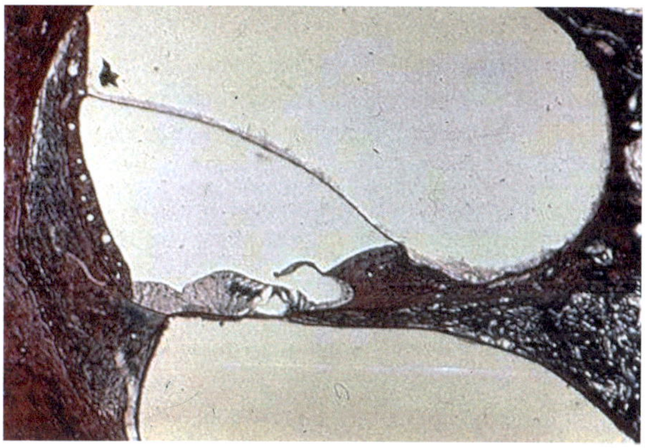

Fig. 5 The organ of Corti. 1,2,3 – the rows of external hair cells; I – the row of inner hair cells

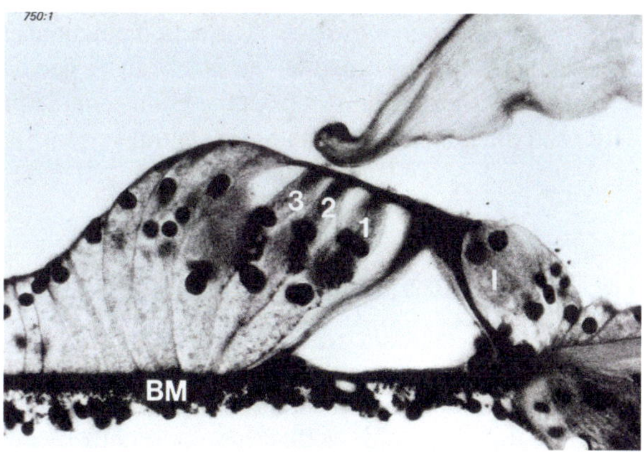

of external hair cells, located on each side of the rods that constitute the tunnel of Corti. The fluid inside the tunnel of Corti is perilymph.

The total number of hair cells is approximately 19,000, of which 3500 are inner hair cells. The inner hair cells are the true mechanoreceptors that send signals to the cochlear nuclei in the brainstem; the outer hair cells are charged with the task of refining the signals, creating conditions for better hearing discrimination.

The human cochlea is a highly specialized sensory organ, with a complex neurophysiology. This specialization is intimately associated with the acquisition of language. In spite of the fact that some inner ear disorders affect both the hearing and the balance organs, a more detailed study of the cochlear physiology will not be included in this chapter.

It is important, however, to mention the electrical activity of the cochlea, since important clinical information can be obtained by recording the cochlear potentials.

Several electrical responses can be recorded. They were extensively studied by neurophysiologists before the advent of the clinical tests of auditory electrical responses in man.

Endocochlear potential This is a direct current potential of 80 mV present in the endolymph of the cochlea, described by Békésy in 1952 [4]. It is not present in the endolymph of the vestibular organs, although no discontinuity or electrical barrier can be demonstrated [5, 6]. Patients with atrophy of the stria vascularis usually present flat hearing losses [7], and it has been experimentally demonstrated that the atrophy of the stria reduces the endocochlear potential [8].

Cochlear microphonics Discovered by Wever and Bray in 1930 [9], they are alternate potentials that exactly reproduce the waveforms that reach the ear, so that researchers at that time felt that the cochlea worked as a microphone. These potentials rise from the external hair cells and are probably a result of their contractions. They can be recorded by means of electrocochleography (ECochG).

Summating potentials Discovered by Davis in 1950 [10], they probably result from depolarization of the inner hair cells. They can also be recorded by ECochG.

Acoustic nerve action potentials The action potentials that result from the cochlear stimulation can be recorded at the level of the cochlea by ECochG and also by recording electrical responses from the brainstem (auditory brainstem responses, or ABR) and other areas of the auditory central system.

The Vestibular System

In terms of evolution, the labyrinth is much older than the cochlea, but its function remained unknown for many centuries. Several factors contributed to this, including the circumstance that these hair cells respond to gravity and accelerations, phenomena that were totally unknown before Newton's researches in the seventeenth century.

Jean Pierre Flourens, a French pioneer in the field of neurophysiology, was the first investigator that dissociated the semicircular canals from the sensation of hearing. In 1824, he described the effects of destroying the semicircular canals of pigeons, showing how the loss of each of the ducts affected the postural equilibrium and the ability to flight, but not hearing [11].

Flourens, however, did not realize that his pigeons had vertigo. The realization that disorders of the vestibular system caused vertigo came somewhat later with Prosper Menière in 1861, and the first hypotheses about vestibular function were elaborated by Friedrich Goltz in 1870, followed by Josef Breuer and Ernst Mach in 1874.

The Semicircular Canals

Each inner ear has three semicircular canals, one in each spatial plan, each perpendicular to the others. They are named *lateral*, *anterior*, and *posterior semicircular canals*. The portions of the membranous labyrinth that are inside the semicircular canals are called *semicircular ducts*. The ducts are filled with endolymph; the spaces between the duct and the bony canals are filled with perilymph. Each of the ducts has in one of its endings an enlarged area, the *ampulla*, that contains a structure called *cupula ampullaris*, where the cilia of the sensory cells are immersed. Figure 6 shows a schematic drawing of the ampulla and cupula. A part of the superior and posterior canal (the sides opposed to the ampullae) is fused (*crus commune*).

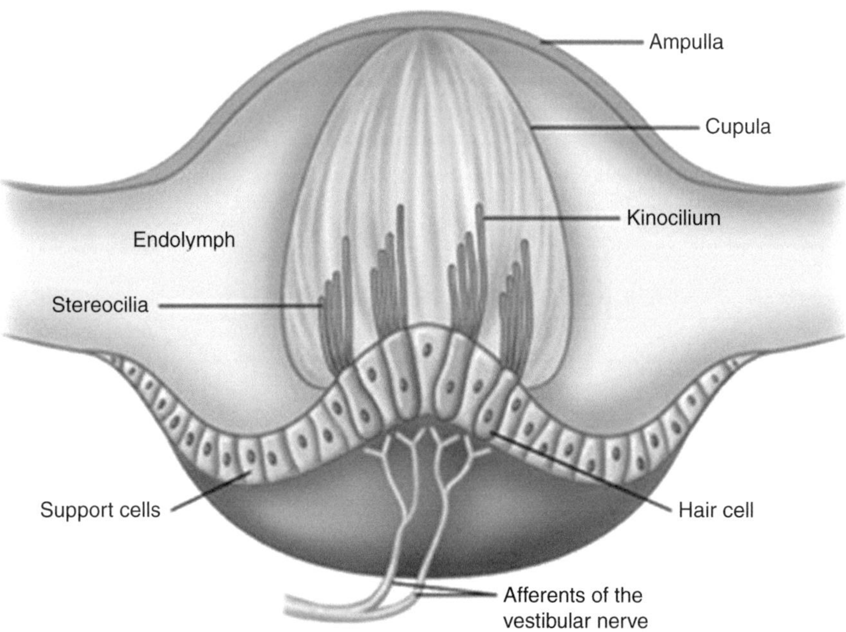

Fig. 6 Schematic drawing of the ampulla and cupula

The spatial arrangement of the canals allows them to detect rotation of the head in three directions: horizontal, vertical, and rotatory. The lateral semicircular canal maintains a 30° angle in relation to the horizontal plane. The anterior and posterior canals maintain an angle of 90° with the lateral canal and with each other. The anterior canal on each side of the head, therefore, is at the same plane of the posterior canal of the other side. In other words, the six semicircular canals act in synergic pairs: one pair consists of the two lateral canals, another one consists of the left anterior and the right posterior canal, and the third pair consists of the right anterior and left posterior canals. As a consequence of their spatial disposition, it is easy to understand that any type of head movement will stimulate at least one pair of canals (Fig. 7).

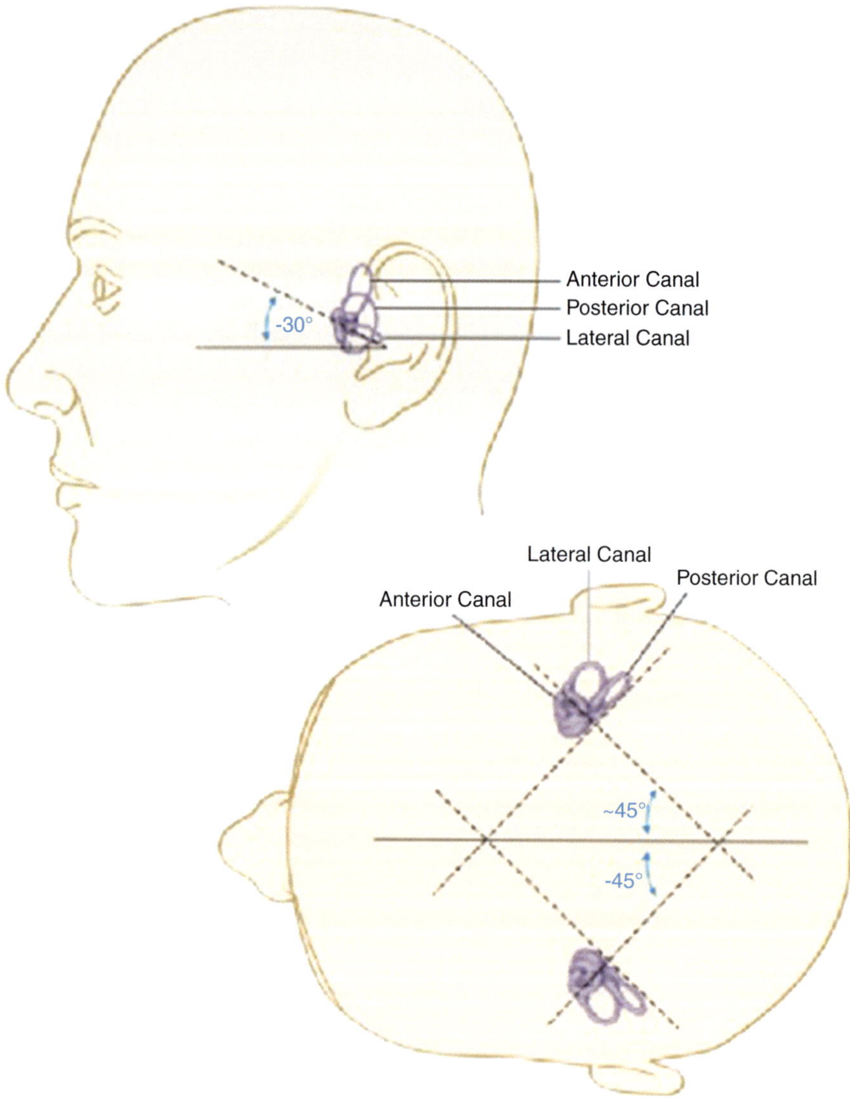

Fig. 7 Spatial orientation of the semicircular canals

The vestibular hair cells are different from the cochlear hair cells. While the latter have only rudimentary kinocilia and a much larger number of stereocilia, each vestibular cell has one well-developed kinocilium and a not so large number of stereocilia. While the cochlear cells respond to frequencies from 16 to 16,000 hertz, the vestibular hair cells respond mainly to frequencies of 0–15 Hz.

The kinocilia establish the direction of the mechanical sensitivity. Ewald, in 1892 [12], demonstrated that for the lateral canals, the endolymph displacement toward the ampulla causes a greater response than the displacement in the opposite direction; for the vertical canals, the reverse is true, the greater responses are caused by displacement away from the ampulla. These principles (Ewald's laws) agree with the position of the kinocilia in the hair cells and are of clinical importance in finding the affected side in some vestibular disorders.

The head movements cause inertial movements of the endolymph inside the ducts, stimulating the hair cells. Figure 8 shows the endolymph movements in a semicircular canal following a head movement. The same sort of movement occurs in the anterior and posterior canals in response to different head movements. The displacement of the cupula always occurs in the opposite direction of the head movements.

Figure 9 shows a schematic drawing of the vestibular hair cells. The type I cell is amphora shaped, while the type II cell is cylindrical. The type II cell has several afferent and efferent nerve endings, while the type I has only one large afferent nerve ending and a small number of efferent ones. These cells are intermingled in the cristae, but the type I is predominant at the tip of the crista, and the type II is the most frequent cell on both sides of the crista.

Figure 10 shows the polarization and depolarization of the hair cells. In the guinea pig, the vestibular nerve fibers have a resting discharge of about 12 pulses per second. When the endolymph flow moves the stereocilia in the direction of the kinocilium, the number of pulses increases; when it moves the stereocilia in the opposite direction, the number of pulses decreases. The number of pulses of the

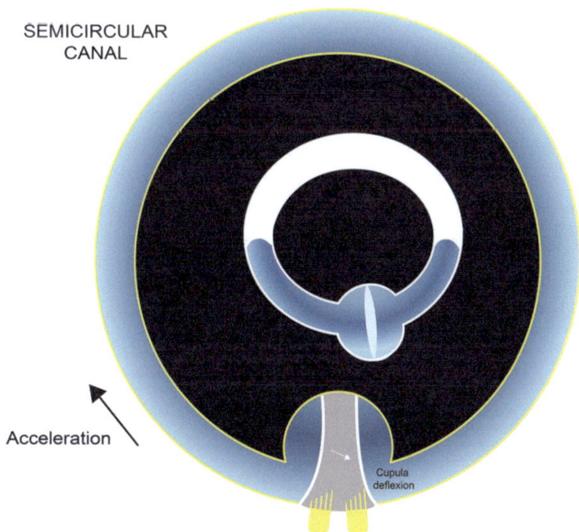

Fig. 8 Schematic representation of a semicircular canal following a head movement; the deflection of the cupula goes to the opposite side of the head movement. (Adapted from Herman Kingma [13])

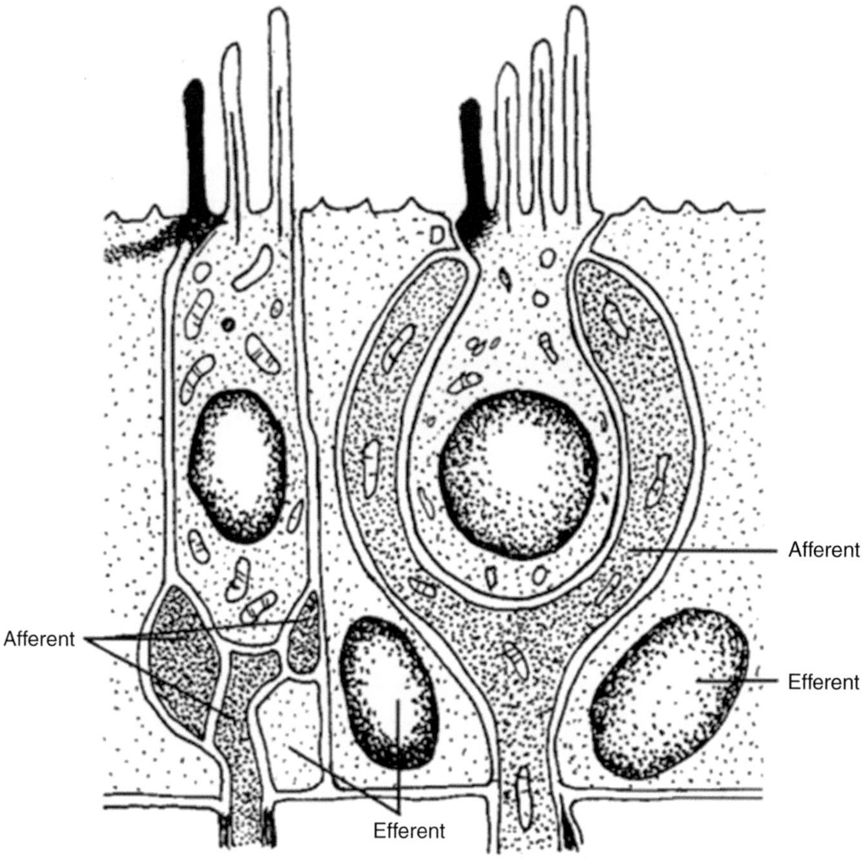

Fig. 9 The sensory cells of the vestibular organs. Type I (on the right side) has only one large afferent nerve ending that surrounds the cell almost completely; type II has several nerve endings. Both cells have efferent nerve endings, but they are less numerous in the type I cells

resting potential in the human labyrinthine fiber is unknown, but César Fernández (personal communication) found it to be 100 in the squirrel monkey, so it should be at least 100 in human beings.

The Saccule and Utricle

The saccule is a flattened sac that lies in a spherical recess on the medial wall of the vestibule. The utricle is an oval-shaped tube lying superior to the saccule on the medial wall of the vestibule. The three semicircular canals communicate with the utricle via five openings, one of which is formed by the nonampulated ends of the anterior and posterior canals (*crus commune*).

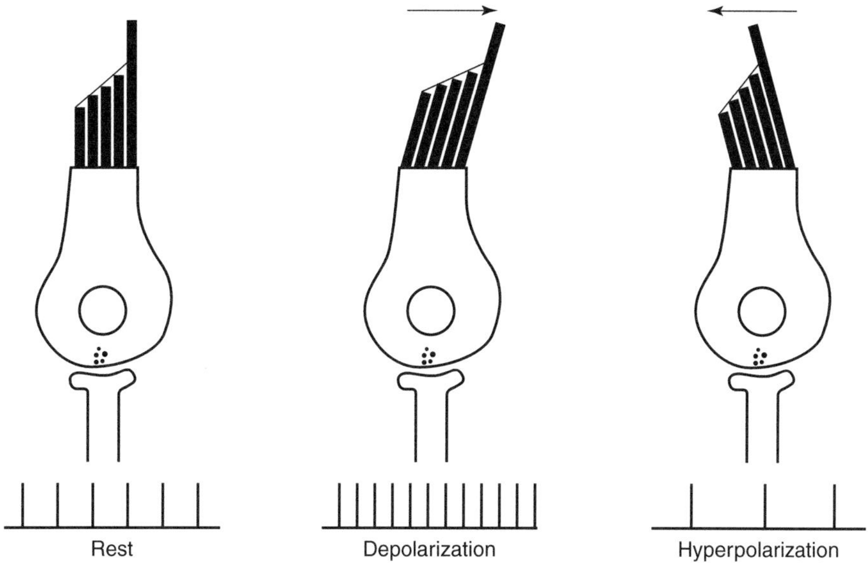

Fig. 10 Action potentials of the hair cells of the semicircular canals. The displacement of the cilia toward the kinocilium results in depolarization. The inverse movement results in hyperpolarization

The otolith organs detect linear acceleration of the head in three directions: horizontal, vertical, and fore and aft; they also detect static head tilt – the position of the head with respect to gravity.

The sensory cells of the saccule and utricle are located in structures called *maculae*, which are similar but located in different spatial planes. The macula of the utricle lies approximately in the horizontal plane, whereas the macula of the saccule lies approximately in the vertical plane.

Figure 11 shows the structure of the maculae. Each one has a basilar membrane that holds the hair cells. The cilia of the hair cells are imbedded in a gelatinous substance, the *otolithic membrane* that, in the upper part, is attached to small crystals of calcium carbonate, the *otoliths* or *otoconia*. When the head is tilted, the otoliths deform the gelatinous mass and bend the cilia on the hair cells, resulting in a receptor potential that will reach the vestibular nerve. Basically, the maculae inform the central nervous system of linear accelerations and of the head position; the nonlinear accelerations stimulate the semicircular canals.

Testing the saccular and utricular function used to require sophisticated linear acceleration devices that existed only in some research centers. Recently, it was found that linear acceleration is not the only way that otolithic receptors can be stimulated but that sound and vibration are effective otolithic stimuli [14].

In fact, both the saccular and utricular maculae have specialized areas, called striolae. The striola receptors are predominantly amphora-shaped type I receptors and have short stiff hair bundles, loosely attached to the overlying otolithic membrane. The cilia of these cells are shorter and are not tightly linked to the otolithic

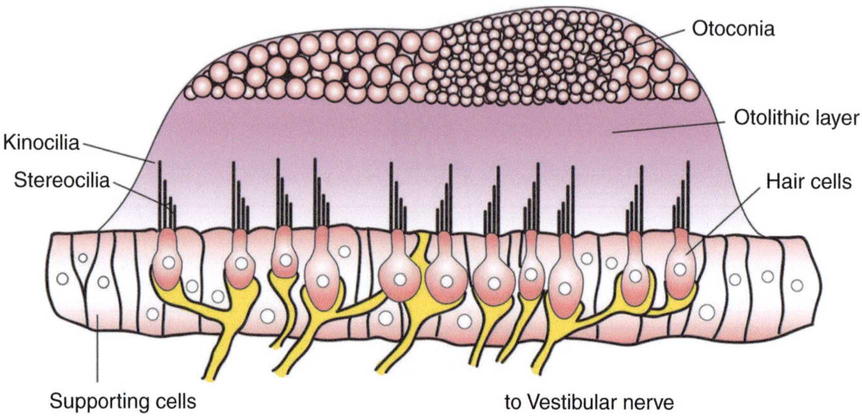

Fig. 11 Schematic drawing of the utricular macula

membrane; therefore, they deflect more easily when there is an endolymph displacement. There is also physiological evidence, from recordings of primary otolithic afferent neurons originating from striola type I receptors, that have irregular resting discharge and are activated by air- and bone-conducted sounds.

The stimulation of the striolae is believed to account for the muscular electric responses elicited by sounds that involve the function of the saccule (cervical vestibular evoked myogenic potentials – cVEMP) or the utricle (ocular vestibular evoked myogenic potentials – oVEMP).

Several circumstances may cause detachment of otoliths from the otolithic membrane, and this may cause a deposit of inorganic material in the cupula of one of the semicircular canals (cupulolithiasis [15]) or in one of the ducts (ductolithiasis [16]), the consequence of which is a disorder called *benign paroxystic positional vertigo*.

The Endolymphatic Sac and Duct

The endolymphatic sac lies within the layers of the dura mater of the posterior fossa, on the posterior surface of the petrous bone. It is connected to the endolymphatic system by the endolymphatic duct, which lies in a bony canal called *vestibular aqueduct*.

The endolymphatic sac is a pressure-adjusting system for the endolymph.

Endolymphatic hypertension, or *endolymphatic hydrops*, can be caused, among other things, by Menière's disease, tertiary syphilis, and congenital cochlear defects, such as Mondini's dysplasia. Surgery of the endolymphatic sac is often performed in patients with endolymphatic hydrops.

The endolymphatic duct may be congenitally enlarged, giving rise to cochlear and vestibular symptoms.

The Vestibular Nerves

Inside the temporal bone, there are two vestibular nerves.

The *superior vestibular nerve* receives fibers from the cristae of the anterior and lateral semicircular canals, from the macula of the utricle and from a small antero-superior portion of the macula of the saccule.

The *inferior vestibular nerve* receives fibers from the cristae of the posterior semicircular canal and from the larger part of the macula of the saccule.

The fibers from each of these nerves lead to the vestibular ganglion that is divided in two portions, one for each nerve. Medial to the ganglion cells, the nerves merge into a single trunk that goes to the brainstem.

The Central Vestibular Pathways

The phylogenesis of the central nervous system indicates that it evolved by adding successive elements. The primitive vertebrates had an equally primitive nervous system, with a limited number of nerve fibers, and the velocity of the stimuli was low. From an organizational point of view, however, the system was well structured.

The *reticular formation* is a persistent remainder of this primitive organization.

Newer systems were added to the primitive systems, as a supplement, without eliminating the function of the early ones. The new systems have nerve fibers of larger diameters and provide faster conduction, thus allowing better discriminations and better measurement capabilities [17]. The thresholds of the new systems may not be lower, but the difference limina are smaller.

The cochlear system is relatively new, reaching its full development only in the mammals. The labyrinthine system, however, is older and has fewer large diameter fibers. It should be noted that the type I vestibular hair cells belong to the new vestibular system.

Figure 12 shows schematically the "new" central pathways of the vestibular system. Like the auditory system, there are several parallel connections to the reticular formation. Most of the available information, however, relates to the semicircular canals; the knowledge of the pathways that arise from the utricle and saccule is still incomplete.

The vestibular nerve fibers connect to the vestibular nuclei on the floor of the IV ventricle. There are four main nuclei – superior, medial, lateral, and inferior – but there are seven other smaller cell groups interconnected with them.

Table 1, adapted from Vidal et al. [18], shows the main functions of the different nuclei and their afferents and efferents in the rat. Most probably, this arrangement is similar in most of the mammals.

The vestibular nuclei contact the oculomotor centers (nuclei of the III, IV, and VI cranial nerves) through the *medial longitudinal fasciculus* and also reach centers in the neck and along the spinal cord (*vestibulospinal tracts*).

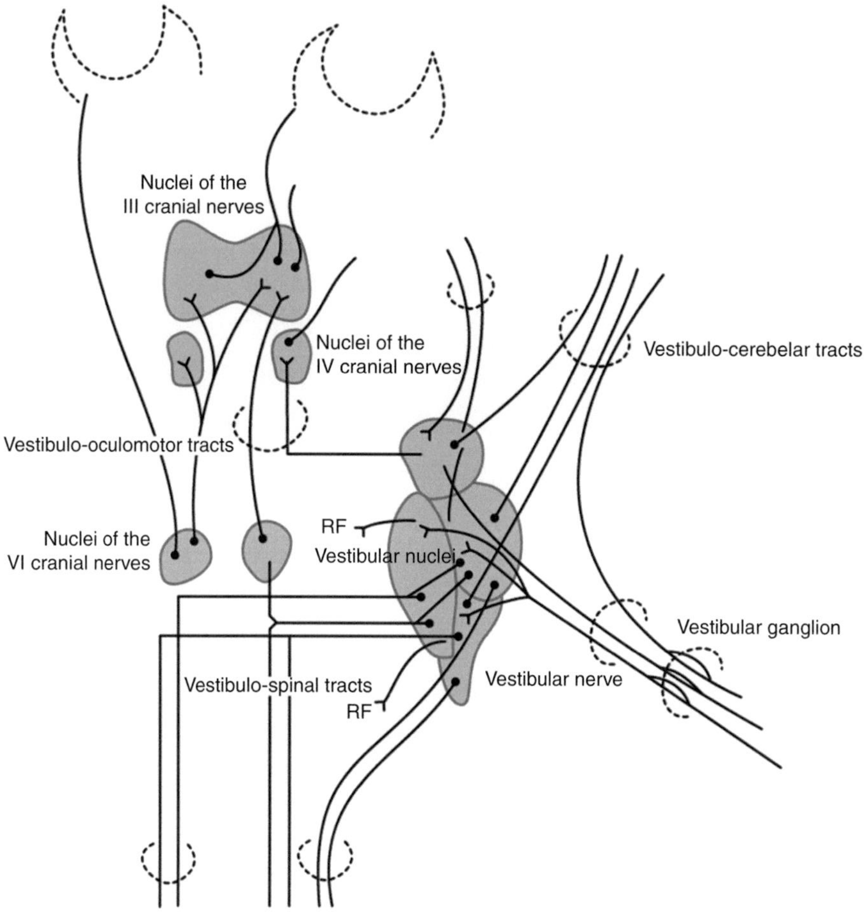

Fig. 12 Central vestibular pathways. This scheme does not include the parallel tracts through the reticular formation

The vestibular system is extensively controlled by the cerebellum, which sends fibers to all of the vestibular nuclei.

Figures 13 and 14 show schematically the afferent and efferent connections of the vestibular nuclei [19].

Operational Model of the Vestibular System

The maintenance of the body equilibrium depends fundamentally on three systems: the eyes, the proprioceptive receptors, and the vestibular organs.

The proprioceptive mechanisms involve sensory receptors located in muscles and tendons and in the fibrous capsules of joints. These receptors register mechani-

Table 1 Functions and afferents and efferents of the vestibular nuclei

Nuclei	Afferents	Efferents
Superior vestibular nucleus *Control of eye movements*	Cristae and flocculus – central Utricle, saccule Nodulus Uvula Fastigial nucleus – periphery	Ipsi- and contralateral medial longitudinal fasciculus Oculomotor nucleus Trochlear nucleus Thalamus Pontine reticular formation Flocculus
Lateral vestibular nucleus *Control of posture*	Utricle and saccule Vermis Fastigial nucleus – caudal-dorsal Cervical and lumbar spine- – rostro-dorsal Cervical and upper thorax-ventral	Cervical cord – rostro-ventral Caudal superior nucleus Caudal lateral nucleus
Medial vestibular nucleus *Stabilization of gaze and posture in the horizontal plane*	Cristae – dorso-rostral Otolith organs – ventromedial Flocculus Caudal vermis Fastigial nucleus Cervical spine Cerebral cortex – caudal	Oculomotor nuclei – via ascending medial longitudinal fascicles Cervical anterior cord via medial vestibulo spinal tract
Inferior vestibular nucleus *Integration of vestibular spinal and cerebellar messages for posture control*	Cristae – central Utricle and saccule – periphery Flocculus Nodulus Uvula Medial cerebellar nuclei Cervical and lumbar – via dorsal spinocerebellar tract Contralateral medial nucleus	Cerebellar cortex Deep cerebellar nuclei (fastigial nucleus) Cervical spine Reticular formation Contralateral vestibular nuclei

cal vibrations, and the information is sent to the vestibular nuclei. From these nuclei, there are afferent connections to the thalamus and the cortex, generating information regarding to spatial orientation and perception of movement.

Sound is also a type of vibratory information, mainly perceived by the cochlea, but also reaches the saccule and the utricle. Some patients with vestibular disorders have episodes of vertigo when submitted to intense sounds (Tullio's phenomenon).

The visual information completes the perception of movement, but this information is of a different kind. It is basically electromagnetic and is elaborated at a different level. It is, however, related to the vestibular nuclei and proprioceptive stimuli, establishing a sensorial convergence [20].

It is well known, clinically, that in order to maintain the body balance, at least two of these systems must be normal. It has been shown [21] that there are tracts

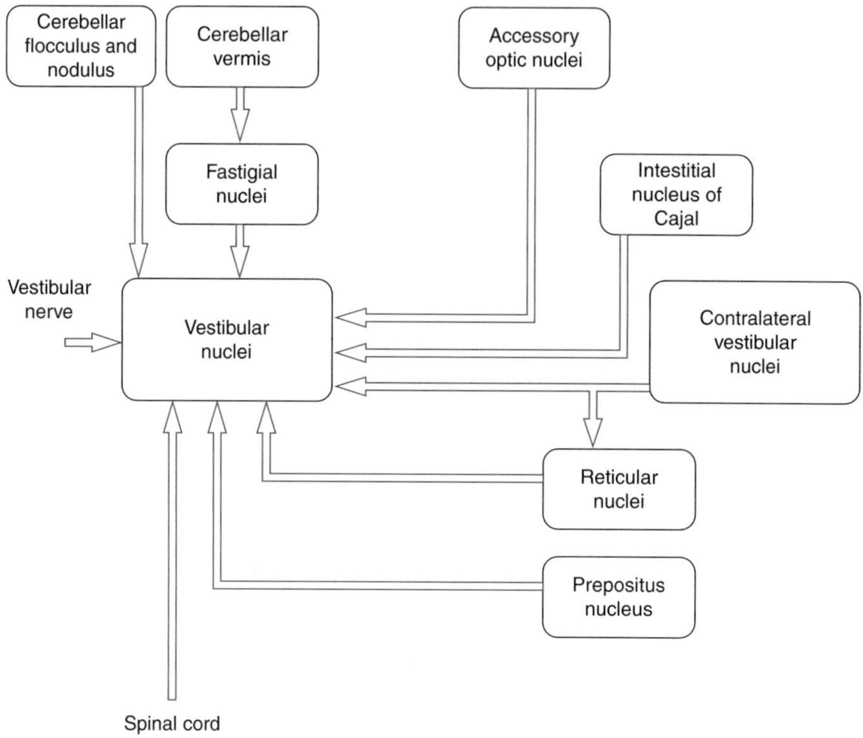

Fig. 13 Afferent connections of the vestibular nuclei. (Adapted from Lysakowski et al. [19])

that connect both the oculomotor centers and the areas of the brain that process proprioceptive information to the vestibular nuclei. These nuclei, therefore, are the integrators of the body balance system.

The vestibular system has three main functions:

1. To inform the central nervous system of the position and movements of the head and the body. This implies on correcting the eye movements to keep them in harmony with the body movements, stabilizing the gaze and ensuring a clear vision during head movements. This is accomplished by means of a vestibulo-ocular reflex (VOR), a reflex that involves three neurons and generates eye movements according to the vestibular organs. The VOR latencies (approximately 15 ms) are much smaller than those of the ocular movements of visual origin (approximately 70 ms). Actually, the vestibular acceleration sensors are able to detect head movements much sooner than the visual system can detect changes in the retinal image [22].

There are, in fact, three different types of VORs [23]:

(a) The rotational VOR (R-VOR), related to angular accelerations, mediated by the semicircular canals

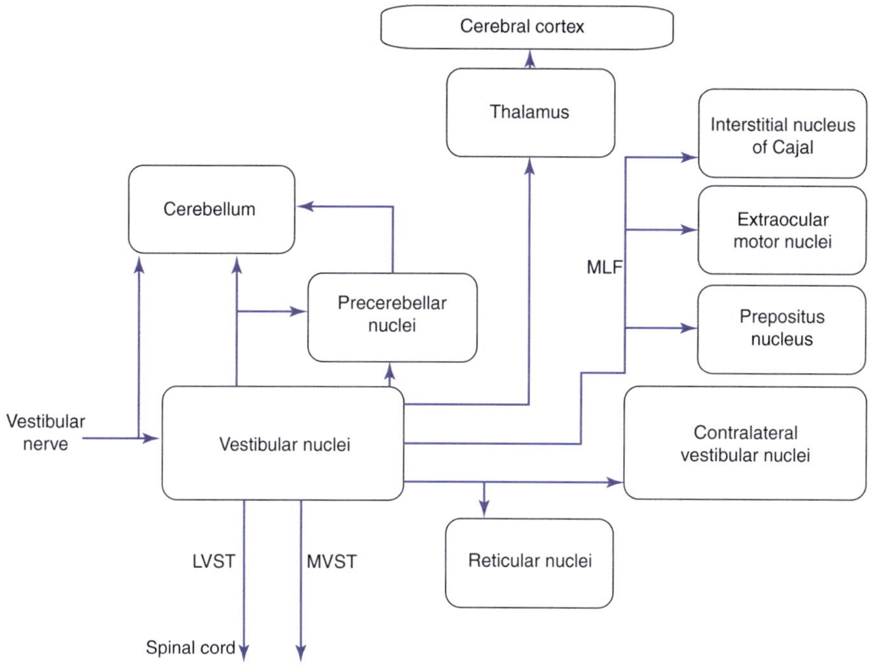

Fig. 14 Efferent connections of the vestibular nuclei. MLF = medial longitudinal fasciculus; LVST = lateral vestibulospinal tract; MVST = medial vestibulospinal tract. (Adapted from Lysakowski et al. [19])

(b) The translational VOR (T-VOR), related to linear accelerations – otolith-mediated, responding to inertial and gravitational forces
(c) Ocular counterroll (OCR), related to static head tilt

2. To adjust muscular activity and body position. This is accomplished by the vestibulospinal reflexes (VSR) that stabilize the head in relation to the trunk and the space in general, maintaining the erect posture. Vestibular stimuli activate the muscles of the neck, arms, and legs in different patterns, in order to avoid falls.
3. To allow perception of motion and spatial orientation.

The vestibular and visual functions will be discussed separately. The vestibular-cerebellar relations are an important part of the system and will also be taken in consideration.

The Physiology of the Vestibular System

The following topics illustrate the most important physiological principles of the vestibular system.

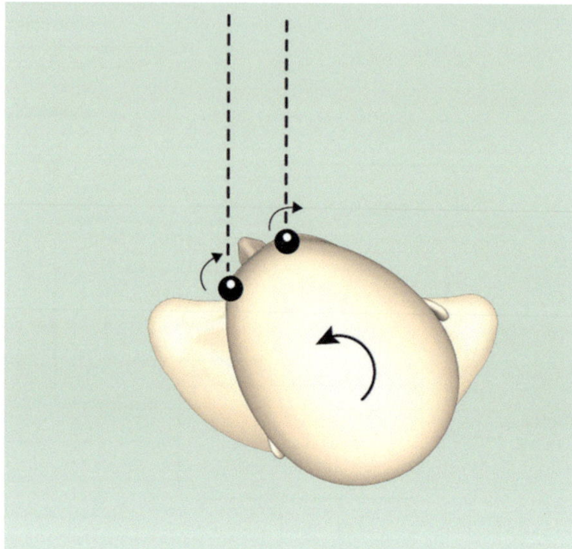

Fig. 15 The rotational vestibulo-ocular reflex (R-VOR) produces eye movements that compensate for the head movements

Head Rotation

When the head rotates with a certain speed and direction, the eyes have to rotate at the same speed, but in the reverse direction. In order to maintain a steady gaze during the head's rotation, the *rotational vestibulo-ocular reflex* (R-VOR) produces ocular movements that compensate for the head's movement (Fig. 15).

There are two important aspects in this reflex. The first is *gain* – a relation between the speed of the head and the speed of the eyes. The second is *phase* – the amount of time between the start of the head movement and that of the movement of the eyes.

The sensory receptors of the three semicircular canals at each side of the head are responsible for the capture of the angular accelerations of the head, including mass inertia, asymmetrical sensitivity, and specific stimulation frequency.

Mechanical Factors that Affect the Function of the Semicircular Canals

The main factors that affect the function of the semicircular canals are:

1. Endolymph viscosity: it exerts an influence on the gain and reduces the phase changes in low frequencies.
2. Elasticity of the cupula ampullaris: affects the VOR responses in low frequencies.
3. Mass: normally the density of endolymph and that of the cupula ampullaris are the same; mass increases, such as the presence of otoliths in the vestibular ducts (benign paroxysmal postural vertigo), or the ingestion of large amounts of alcohol will increase the endolymph's density in relation to that of the cupula.

Stimulus Frequencies

The frequencies of the head movements correspond to different amplitudes of cupular deflection, will stimulate different receptor cells, and may cause phase changes. Accelerations in the direction of the canal with frequencies between 0.1 and 10 Hz are linked to head movement's speeds; those below 0.1 Hz are related to the head's accelerations.

Resting Potentials

When the head of a normal individual is not moving, the right and left vestibular nerves and the corresponding nuclei maintain a resting potential, as seen in Fig. 10.

Horizontal Head Rotation

When the head moves in the horizontal plane to the right side, there is an increase in the activity of the ipsilateral labyrinth (excitation) and a reduction in the activity of the contralateral labyrinth (inhibition). These activity changes are interpreted by the brain as a head movement and generate precise compensatory eye movements (slow phase of the R-VOR).

In other words, when the head rotates to the right, the eyes rotate to the left. The speed of head movement is relied to vestibular nuclei by the right and left vestibular nerves. The message of the vestibular nuclei uses two paths to reach the oculomotor nuclei: a direct (new) path, through the medial longitudinal tract, and an indirect (old) path, through the reticular formation (Fig. 14).

The direct new path involves the type I neurons of the right vestibular nuclei. Its axons cross the midline and join the medial longitudinal tract, activating the motor neurons of the lateral rectus muscle (left abducens nerve – VI), which, in turn, by means of the afferent neurons of the oculomotor nerve (III), activate the motor neurons of the right medial rectus, generating a conjugate eye movement to the left. The speed of the eye movements is determined by this reflex [24].

The old path, through the reticular formation, acts like an integrating system to the left abducens nerve (VI), determining the position of the eyes.

Eye Movements

There are four types of physiological eye movements intimately related to the vestibular system: the *smooth pursuit*, the *ocular counterroll*, the *saccade*, and the *nystagmus*.

Smooth Pursuit

The smooth pursuit eye movements allow the eyes to closely follow a moving object. It is one of the two ways that make the voluntary shift gaze possible; the other one are the *saccadic eye movements*. The smooth pursuit movements are different from the ones induced by the vestibulo-ocular reflex, which only occur during head movements to stabilize the gaze on a stationary object.

The pursuit of targets moving with velocities greater than 30°/s requires catch-up saccades.

Ocular Counterroll

This is a low gain vestigial reflex that plays a major role in pathology [23]. It is a response to a static head tilt (Fig. 16).

Saccades

A *saccade* is a quick, simultaneous movement of both eyes between two or more phases of fixation in the same direction.

Saccades are the fastest eye movements – they reach 500 degrees per second – and have a very short duration, less than 10 ms. They constitute a mechanism for fixation and for rapid eye movements.

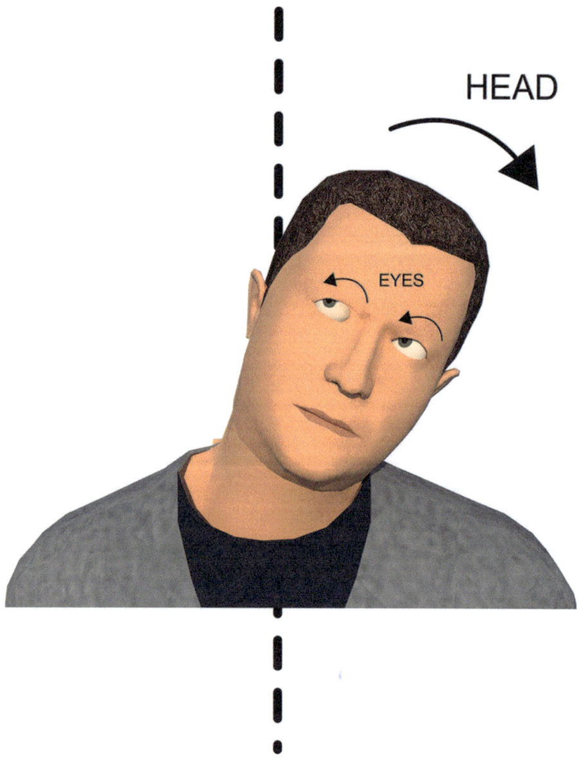

Fig. 16 Static head tilt and ocular counterrolling. (Adapted from Zee [23])

Human beings do not fix their eyes when looking at objects. The eyes move to areas surrounding the objects in order to obtain more information. That demands several saccadic movements interspersed with stops. The speed of the saccades cannot be voluntarily controlled; the eyes move as fast as they can. And there is no vision during the saccadic movements.

The human fovea is very small but plays an important role in analyzing objects. The saccadic movements make it possible for the eyes to see small objects with better resolution. The system depends, however, on the way that the input is generated. If the sensory input is due to involuntary head movements, corrective reflexes are initiated. If the same vestibular sensory input is generated by a voluntary head movement, the reflexes are suppressed. The suppression probably originates from cerebellar control of the transmission of information from the vestibular sensors to the various outputs [25].

The saccadic movement requires a *pulse* – a sudden activity of brainstem neurons that reach the agonist extraocular muscles. When the eyes reach the new position, a *step* – a new level of tonic innervation – is required, in order to keep the eyes in this position. These reflexes apply to both horizontal and vertical saccades, but the neural substrates that control the pulses different from those that control the steps. For horizontal saccades, the excitatory pulse neurons are located in the paramedian pontine reticular formation; the step integrators are the medial vestibular nucleus and the nucleus prepositus hypoglossi in the medulla. For vertical saccades, the excitatory pulse neurons are in the rostral interstitial nucleus of the medial longitudinal fasciculus, and the neural integrator is the interstitial nucleus of Cajal, also in the midbrain [26]. A special group of cells, the *omnipause neurons*, fire continuously, inhibiting the pulse neurons, except during the saccades, in order to ensure the stability of the saccadic system [27]. The omnipause neurons for both horizontal and vertical saccades are located in the raphe interpositus, in the caudal pons. In addition to brainstem saccadic generators, higher-level structures including the frontal and parietal lobes, as well as the substantia nigra reticulata and superior colliculi, also play critical roles in saccade generation [26].

Nystagmus

Nystagmus is an involuntary eye movement that is part of the vestibulo-ocular reflex (VOR). It is characterized by a *slow phase*, which is a smooth pursuit movement in one direction and a *fast phase* – a saccadic movement – in the opposite direction.

All of these physiological movements may occur in pathological conditions, usually with special characteristics.

The peripheral origin of the nystagmus was well established by Ewald [12] in 1892. In 1928, however, Lorente de Nó made observations regarding a different origin for the fast phase [28]. His observations were a consequence of a communication by Bárány of a patient with a brainstem lesion in whom the vestibular stimulation produced a conjugate deviation of the eyes but did not present a fast phase.

McCabe [29], in 1965, confirmed Lorente de Nó's idea, demonstrating that partial destructions of the vestibular nuclei affected the slow phase but had little influence on the fast phase. He concluded that the fast phase originates from the medulla oblongata area of the reticular formation. On the other hand, the destruction of this area changed the fast phase and did alter the speed of the slow phase.

It is interesting to quote the experiments conducted by Bechterew [30]. The destruction of one of the peripheral vestibular organs of a cat determines a spontaneous nystagmus with the fast phase beating to the normal side. This nystagmus gradually disappears, and the cat regains his normal equilibrium. He named this phenomenon *compensation*. The destruction of the other labyrinth also compensates after a lapse of time.

Bechterew, however, made no observations about the disequilibrium that results from bilateral destruction of the peripheral vestibular organs; he only verified that his animals did not have nystagmus.

On the other hand, the unilateral destruction of the vestibular nuclei causes a nystagmus that will not compensate.

The Bechterew experiment demonstrates that the slow phase of the nystagmus may originate from the vestibular nuclei.

Memory

The vestibular system incorporates several memory mechanisms that store the sensation of speed related to VOR and to the *optokinetic nystagmus*, the nystagmus that is seen when an individual follows a moving object with his eyes. These sub-systems adjust the saccadic eye movements in order to compensate, to a certain extent, the limitations of the semicircular canals responses to low-frequency stimuli. As a result of these memory mechanisms, the post-rotational nystagmus time is increased, delaying the return of the cupula to the original position. These systems are also active when a visual stimulus is suddenly interrupted.

These extended times of movement perception arise from specific areas of the central nervous system: the vestibular nuclei and the nucleus prepositus hypoglossi, which is located in the caudal pons and upper medulla oblongata. This nucleus is a part of the horizontal gaze-holding system, functioning as a neural integrator [21].

As mentioned in the Bechterew's experiment, unilateral vestibular lesions cause a proportional disequilibrium in the vestibular tonus, resulting in a sensation of movement (vertigo) and a spontaneous nystagmus, the slow phase of which beats to the side with less tonic activity, while the fast phase beats to the side opposite to the lesion.

Some vestibular disorders may lead to a dynamic disequilibrium during the head's rotation; in some circumstances, larger r-VORs result from head movements in the same direction.

Detection of Vestibular Deficits

Vestibular deficits are more easily detected employing stimuli with high accelerations, high velocities, and high frequencies. This is a consequence of the fact that the excitatory stimuli are more effective than the inhibitory ones (Ewald's second law). In order to maintain a target image at the retinal foveae, the eyes must perform a movement in the reverse direction of the head rotation, with the same speed and the same amplitude. A speed of 200°/s or more, however, renders the smooth pursuit system inoperative and unable to process the image stabilization, which will depend entirely on the VOR gain.

Another characteristic of the high-speed stimulation is that it acts on the phasic cells located at the apex of the crista ampullaris, while lower speeds stimulate mainly the tonic cells [31].

Figure 17 shows schematically the location of the phase and tonic cells in the crista ampullaris. Figure 18 details the mechanisms involved, depicting the lateral semicircular canals, the type I cells, the VOR paths, and the position of the eyes in reaction to a high-speed stimulus.

It should be noted that the head's rotation to the right stimulates mainly the right lateral semicircular canal; the rotation to the left stimulates mainly the left lateral semicircular canal. In a normal individual, the eyes stay fixed on the target object. In cases of vestibular areflexia, the eyes stay fixed for a small amount of time and then return to the target object with a saccadic movement. At intense accelerations, the lateral semicircular canal's endolymphatic current in the direction away from the utricle is unable to compensate the deficit [31, 32].

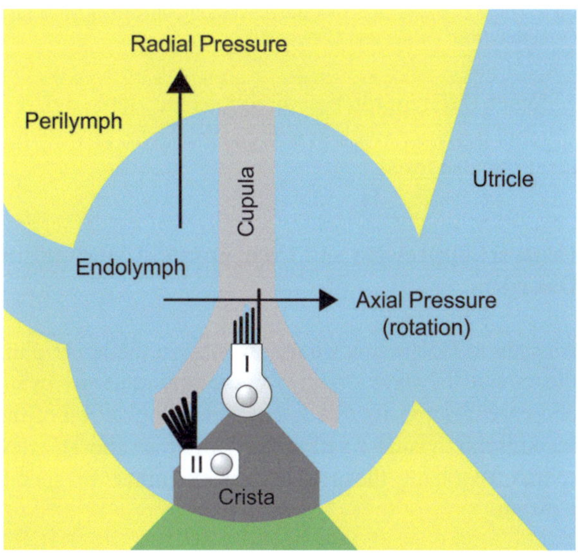

Fig. 17 A scheme of the position of the hair cells of the crista ampullaris. The kinocilium of the type I cells at the apex of the crista touches the cupula, but the stereocilia do not, while all of the cilia of the type II cell located at the base of the crista are immersed in the cupula. This configuration shows that these cells respond to different stimuli. (Adapted from Ulmer and Chays [27])

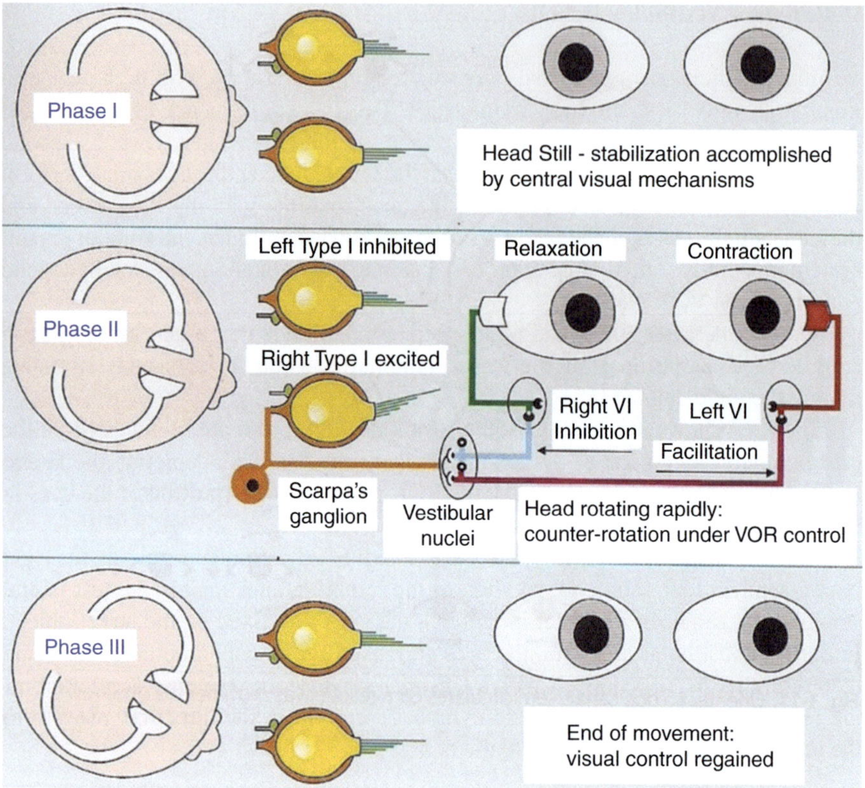

Fig. 18 The cupular movements stimulate the ipsilateral type I cells and inhibit the contralateral ones. Due to the high speed of the movement, only the ipsilateral cells actually stimulate the VOR. (Adapted from Ulmer and Chays [27])

When different rotation directions are employed, it is possible to study the anterior and posterior semicircular canals. These physiological data are the basis for the head impulse tests.

Central Suppression and Compensation Mechanisms in Vestibular Disorders

As seen in Bechterew's experiments, in the acute phase of a vestibular lesion, in the course of days or weeks, the spontaneous nystagmus may will gradually decrease in intensity due to compensating action of the central vestibular system. In addition, visual fixation can suppress the spontaneous nystagmus in bright rooms, requiring the use, by the examiner, of special techniques to avoid this fixation.

Anatomical Orientation of the Semicircular Canals and the Corresponding Eye Movements

The anatomical location of the semicircular canals makes it possible to predict the direction of the slow phase of the nystagmus. As a rule, the activation of a single canal, or the inhibition of the opposite canal of the same pair, induce a slow phase in a plane parallel to that of the canal. For instance, the stimulation of one of the posterior canals in a patient with benign paroxysmal positional vertigo (BPPV) will result in a nystagmus with a slow phase that will include rotatory and downbeat vertical directions.

When several canals are stimulated by the head movement, the resulting nystagmus may be determined by the sum of the vectors of each contributing canal. A complete unilateral lesion will emphasize the spontaneous activity of the normal side, producing a spontaneous nystagmus with a horizontal component (originating in the lateral canal) and a rotatory movement (originating from the anterior and posterior canals).

Eye Movements Resulting from the Otolithic Receptors

The hair cells of the utricle and saccule respond to inclinations of the head and promote a static ocular rotation. They also account for the compensatory slow phase of the *linear vestibulo-ocular reflex* (L-VOR).

Vascular Supply of the Inner Ear

The vascularization of the inner ear has important clinical implications.

The labyrinth is supplied by the labyrinthine artery, also called internal auditory artery, which usually originates from the anteroinferior cerebellar artery (AICA); occasionally, it may be a branch of either the basilar or the vertebral arteries (Fig. 19).

The internal auditory artery subdivides into the anterior vestibular artery and the common cochlear artery. The anterior vestibular artery supplies parts of the saccule, utricle, and semicircular ducts. The common cochlear artery, in turn, divides into the vestibulocochlear artery and the main cochlear artery. The vestibulocochlear artery supplies one half to two thirds of the basal coil of the cochlea, the greater part of the saccule, the body of the utricle, the posterior semicircular duct, and parts of the lateral and superior semicircular ducts. The main cochlear artery supplies the remaining parts of the cochlea.

Occasionally, the main cochlear artery may be missing; it is then replaced by the cochlear branch of the vestibulocochlear artery.

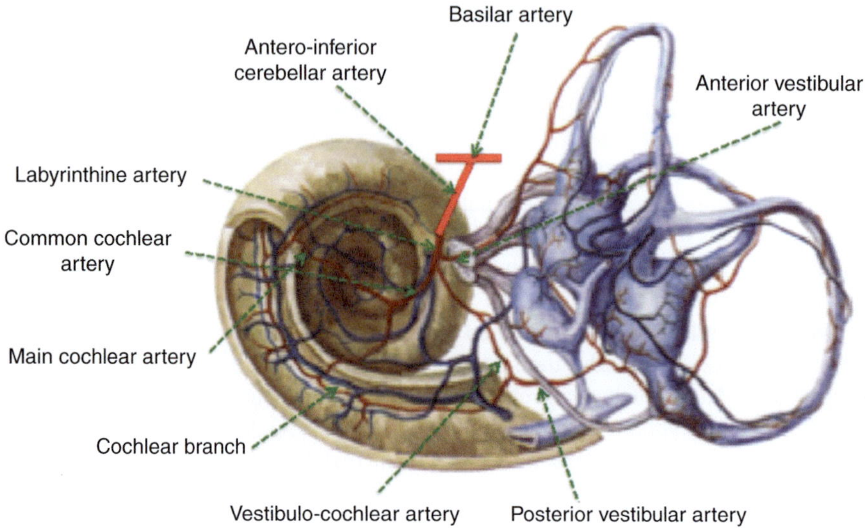

Fig. 19 Arterial supply of the inner ear. (Adapted from Hain, Ramaswamy and Hillman [33])

The labyrinthine venous drainage is via the vein of the cochlear aqueduct. The apical and basal spiral modiolar veins drain appropriate parts of the cochlea. There may be additional drainage routes of the cochlea formed by connections with vessels in the surrounding bone and with veins of the internal auditory meatus (the internal auditory veins). The venous drainage of the semicircular ducts and vestibule is provided by the anterior and posterior vestibular veins, which, in turn, drain into the vein of the cochlear aqueduct.

The following clinical considerations are directly related to the vascular supply of the inner ear:

1. The labyrinthine artery is a terminal artery; its occlusion and the occlusion of AICA cause total deafness and total loss of vestibular function on the affected side.
2. The anterior vestibular artery has no collateral arteries that can alternately supply its corresponding areas; its obstruction can result in a vertiginous episode. Occasionally, this obstruction liberates utricular otoliths that reach the posterior semicircular canal; in these cases, episodes of postural vertigo will occur after the compensation of the sudden vertigo (Lindsay-Hemenway syndrome).
3. The posterior vestibular artery has many intraosseous collaterals that may compensate its eventual obstructions.
4. A circulation deficit including the common cochlear and the posterior vestibular arteries may determine high-frequency hearing losses.

Central Projections of the Vestibular Organs

The central projections of the semicircular canals are mainly directed to the rostral portion of the vestibular nuclei – medial and superior vestibular nuclei. The projections of the otolithic organs are mainly directed to the caudal portion – lateral and inferior nuclei (Fig. 20).

For this reason, patients with infarction of the dorsolateral portion of the medulla oblongata (Wallenberg's syndrome) show a predominance of otolithic signs: body inclination and vertical diplopia resulting from the skew.

The vestibulospinal projections follow the lateral and spinal tracts, acting on the motor neurons of the anterior horn of the spinal cord, adjusting the muscular tone. Lesions of these pathways, when located below the vestibular nuclei, cause falls to one side of the body, but do not cause vertigo or vegetative symptoms.

The Eyes

Vision is an integral part of the body equilibrium, particularly in respect to the role of the eye movements.

These are performed by the six extraocular muscles of each eye (Fig. 21). Table 2 shows the muscles and their corresponding innervation.

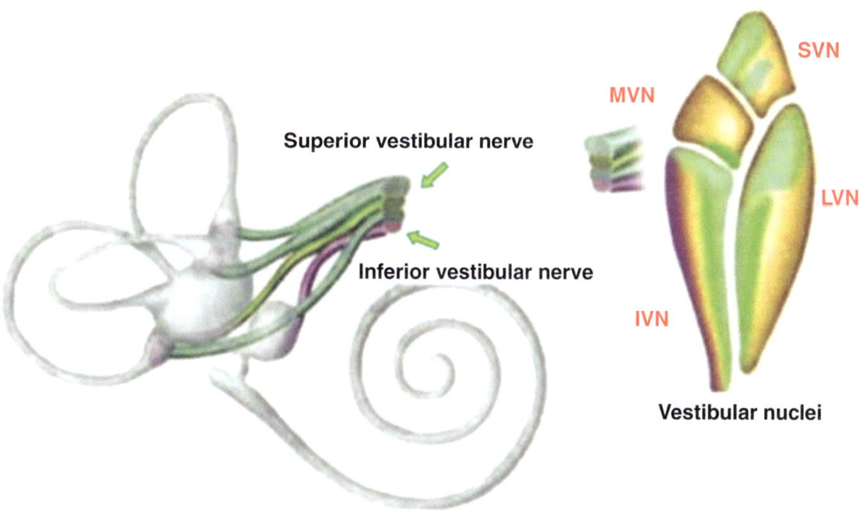

Fig. 20 Central projection of the vestibular organs

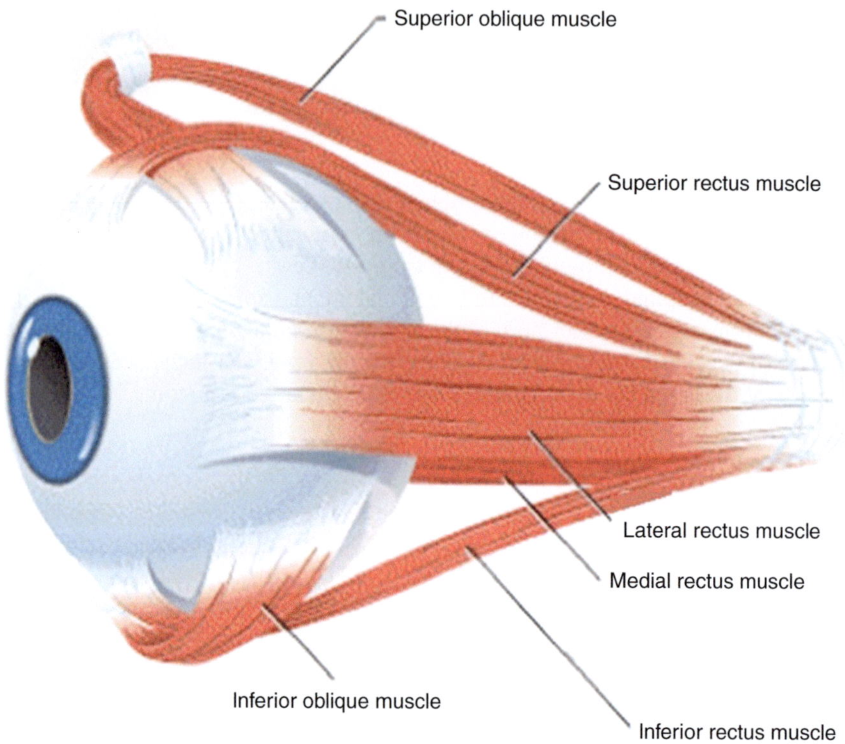

Fig. 21 The extraocular muscles

Table 2 Eye muscles and respective innervations

Muscle	Innervation
Superior rectus	Oculomotor nerve (III), superior branch
Inferior rectus	Oculomotor nerve (III), inferior branch
Lateral rectus	Abducens nerve (VI)
Medial rectus	Oculomotor nerve (III), inferior branch
Superior oblique	Trochlear nerve (IV)
Inferior oblique	Oculomotor nerve (III), inferior branch

Since only a small part of the eye – the fovea – provides sharp vision, the eye must move to follow a target, and these movements must be fast and precise. The III, IV, and VI cranial nerves are responsible for all of the eye movements, regardless of their speeds and latencies, but they need supranuclear information to generate these movements. As a rule, the eyes move symmetrically due to a *common pathway of conjugate eye movements* [32].

Each lateral semicircular canal connects to the lateral rectus muscle on the same side and to the contralateral medial rectus muscle. Each anterior semicircular canal connects to the ipsilateral inferior oblique muscle and to the contralateral superior

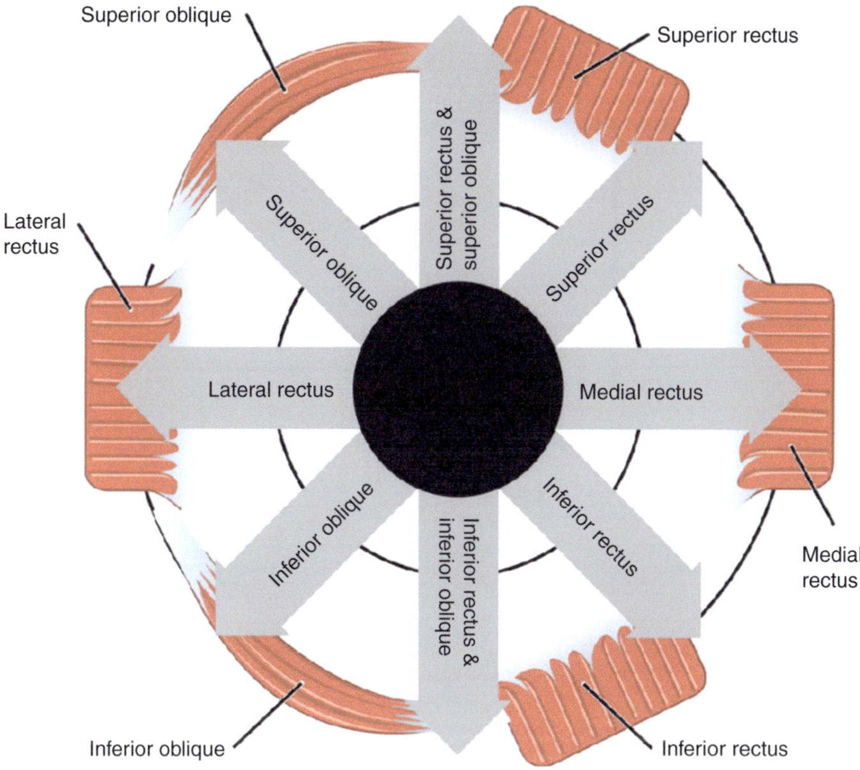

Fig. 22 The eye movements and the corresponding extraocular muscles. (Wikimedia Commons)

rectus muscle. And each posterior semicircular canal connects to the ipsilateral inferior rectus muscle and the contralateral superior oblique muscle. The muscles required for the different eye movements are shown schematically in Fig. 22. Figures 23, 24, and 25 show the pathways from the semicircular canals to the eye muscles. These schemes, however, do not include the connections to the cerebellum and the reticular formation.

It becomes evident that the commands for conjugate horizontal eye movements are directed from the vestibular nuclei to the nucleus of the abducens nerve (VI); the commands for vertical eye movements are directed to the nuclei of the oculomotor (III) and trochlear (IV) nerves. The main path for the stimuli is always the medial longitudinal fasciculus (Fig. 26).

Different systems are consigned to the functions of organizing and firing the different types of eye movements in order to stabilize the images. Two systems – vestibular and optokinetic – maintain the image at the retina; four others, saccades, smooth pursuit, vergence, and fixation, keep the image at the fovea.

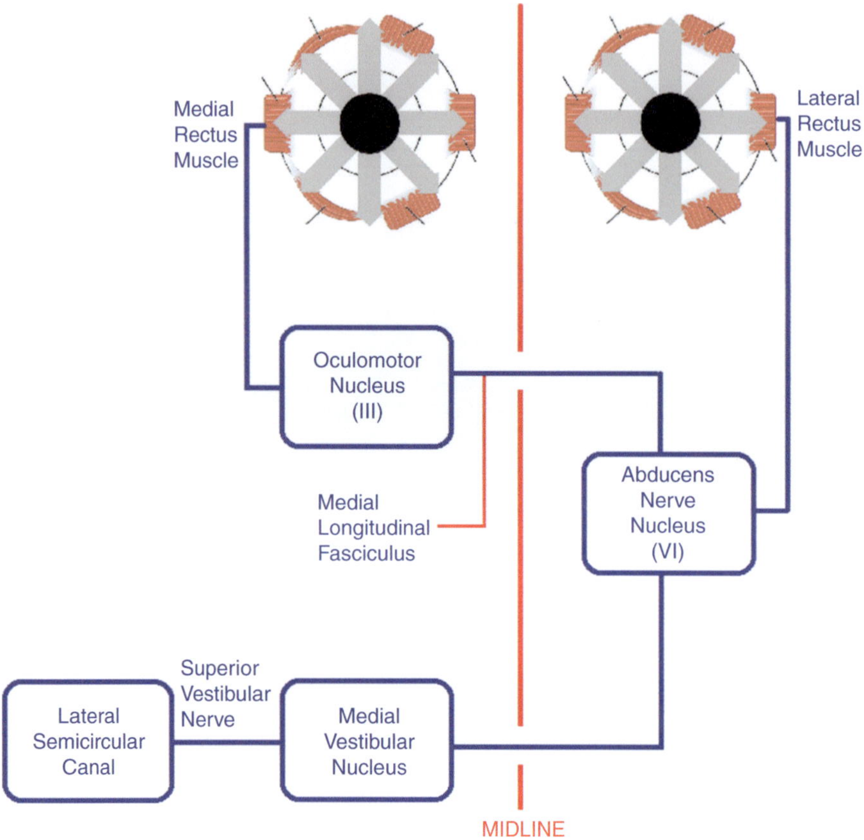

Fig. 23 The pathways that connect the lateral semicircular canals to the eye muscles

- *Vestibular system* – stabilizes the images during head movements, short latencies.
- *Optokinetic system* – dependent on visual stimuli, maintaining the images steady during continuous motions. It relies on the VOR at small speeds; for high speeds, it depends on subcortical pathways that are connected to the vestibular nuclei and cerebellum (Fig. 27).
- *Saccades* – place the image at the fovea. They are very fast movements. They may be voluntary, induced by vision, when looking at an object, and may be automatic, like the fast phase of the nystagmus or the rapid eye movements (REM) when we sleep. Their latencies, amplitudes, speeds, and durations are

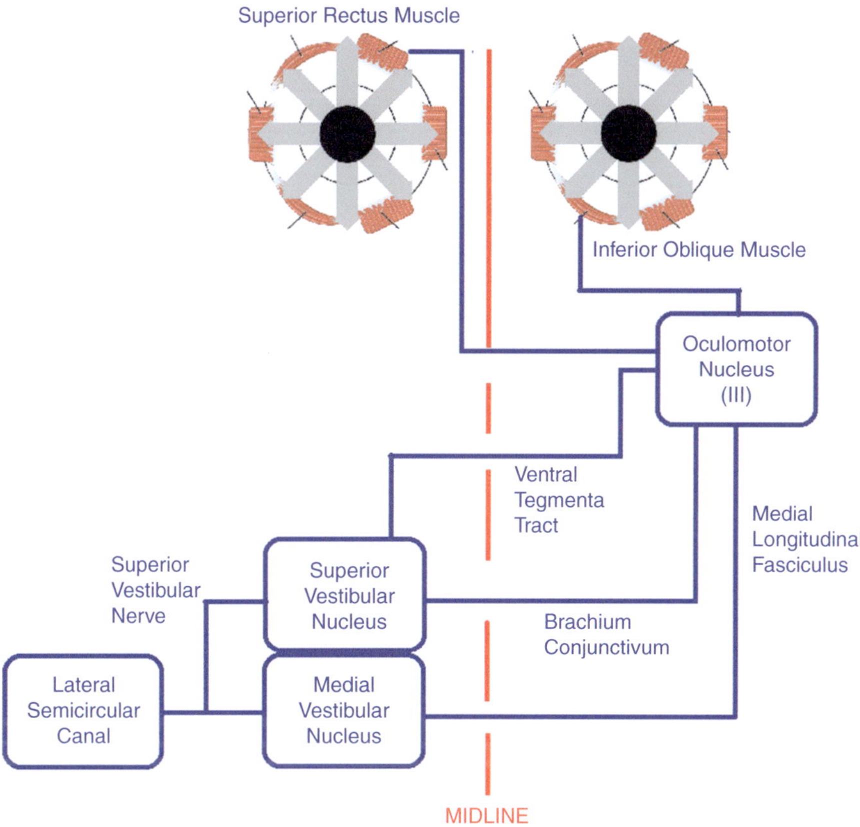

Fig. 24 The pathways that connect the anterior semicircular canals to the eye muscles

variable and are not voluntary. They are generated by a generator in the reticular formation and are liberated by the thalamus and frontal cortex (voluntary saccades) or the parietal cortex (visual saccades). The precision of the movements is controlled by the cerebellum; cerebellar disorders will affect these eye movements (Fig. 28).

- *Smooth pursuit* – maintains in the fovea the image of a moving object. The fovea informs the speed and direction of the movement of the object to an area of the frontal cortex named *frontal pursuit area* and to the temporal and parietal cortical areas. The information is processed by the brainstem, with a participation of the vestibular nuclei and then use the common conjugate pathways (Fig. 29).

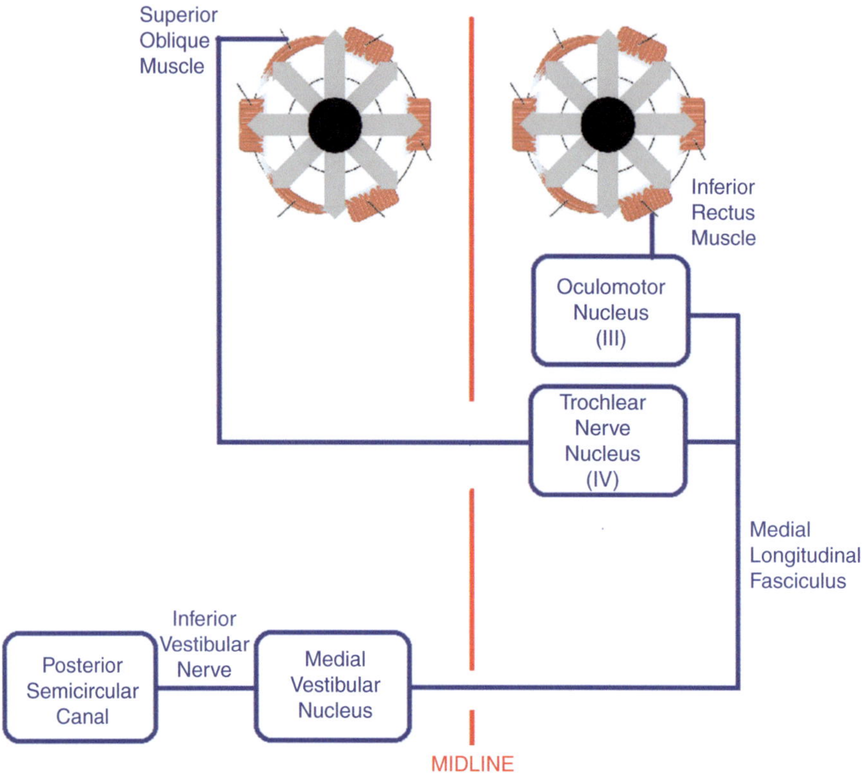

Fig. 25 The pathways that connect the posterior semicircular canals to the eye muscles

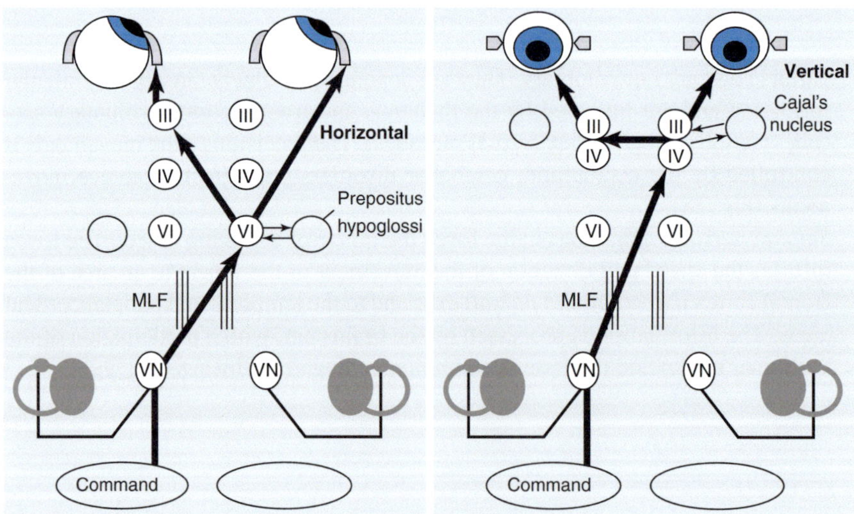

Fig. 26 Pathways for conjugate eye movements. (Adapted from Conraux [34])

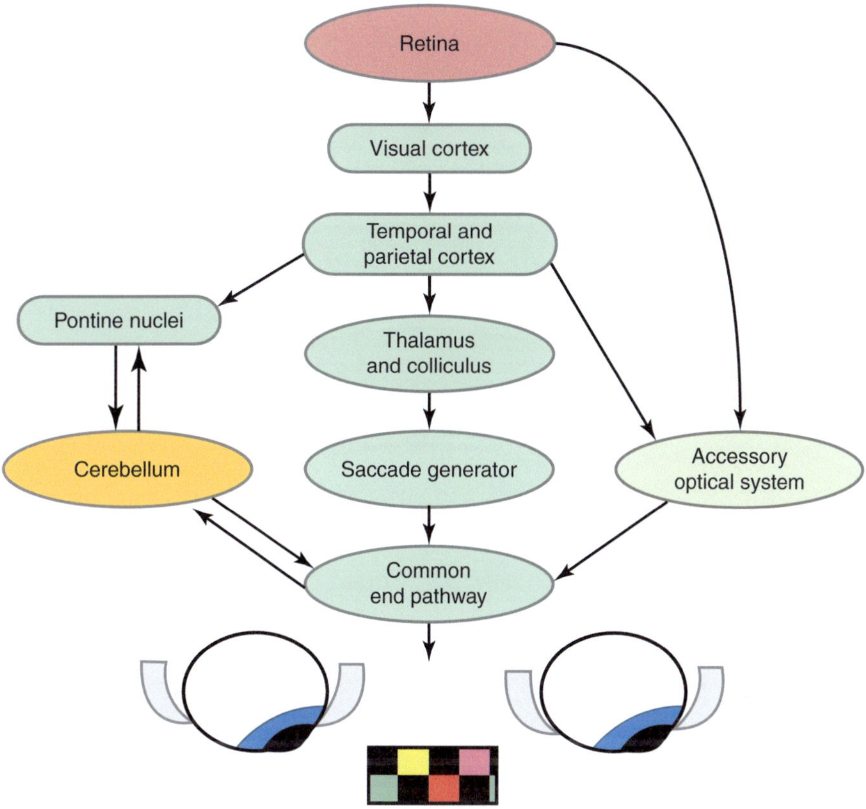

Fig. 27 The optokinetic system. (Adapted from Conraux [34])

- *Vergence* – moves the eyes in opposite directions to avoid image discrepancies in each fovea.
- *Fixation* – maintains the eyes in the acquired position following each of the mentioned mechanisms.

The Cerebellum

The cerebellum is extensively connected to the balance system and has many connections to the vestibular nuclei. It is not needed for the performance of body movements but is essential to the precision of these movements.

Three lobes can be distinguished within the cerebellum: the anterior lobe, the posterior lobe, and the flocculonodular lobe. The midline portion is the cerebellar vermis. The dorsal portion of the vermis acts in the precision of the eye movements.

The medial zone of the anterior and posterior lobes constitutes the spinocerebellum that acts mainly to add precision to the body and limb movements. The lateral

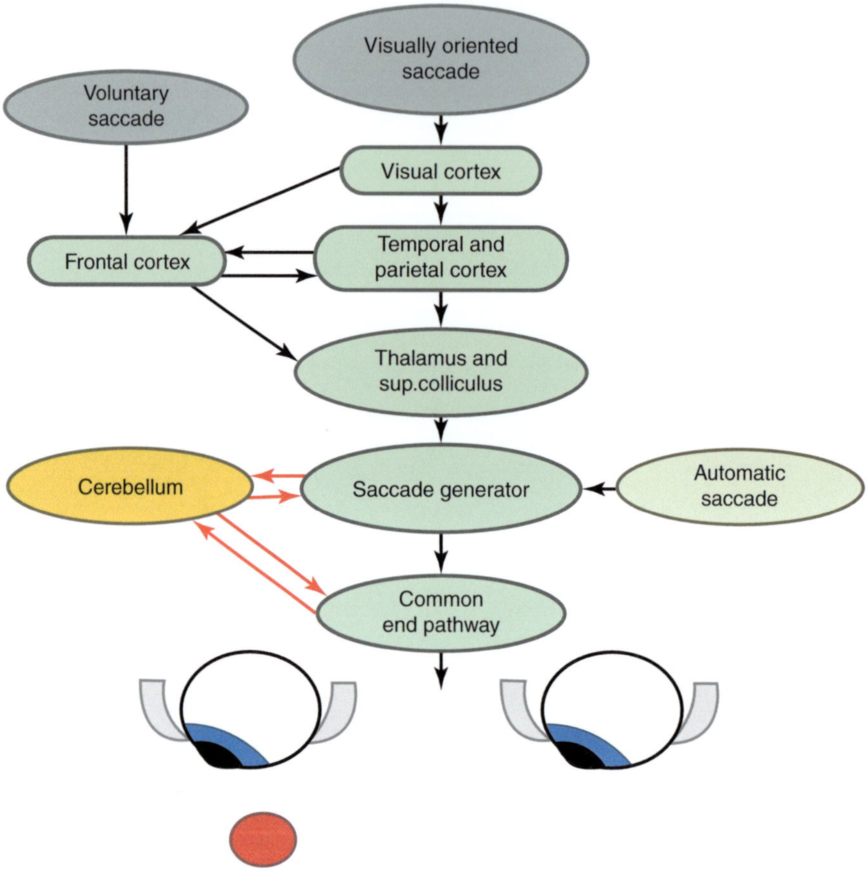

Fig. 28 Ocular saccades. (Adapted from Conraux [34])

zone, which is the largest part, constitutes the cerebrocerebellum, also known as neocerebellum. It is thought to be involved in planning movements before they are performed and in evaluating sensory information for action.

The most important part of the cerebellum, in terms of equilibrium, is the flocculonodular lobe, which is also called vestibulocerebellum. It is the oldest part, in evolutionary terms (archicerebellum), and participates mainly in balance and spatial orientation; its primary connections are with the vestibular nuclei, although it also receives visual and other sensory inputs. Damage to this region causes disturbances of balance and gait.

Sensorial Convergence

The perception of balance, like many other body systems, is not based on a single type of input. It employs several mechanisms, and each system is made more perfect with cross-informations and feedbacks in order to achieve more precision.

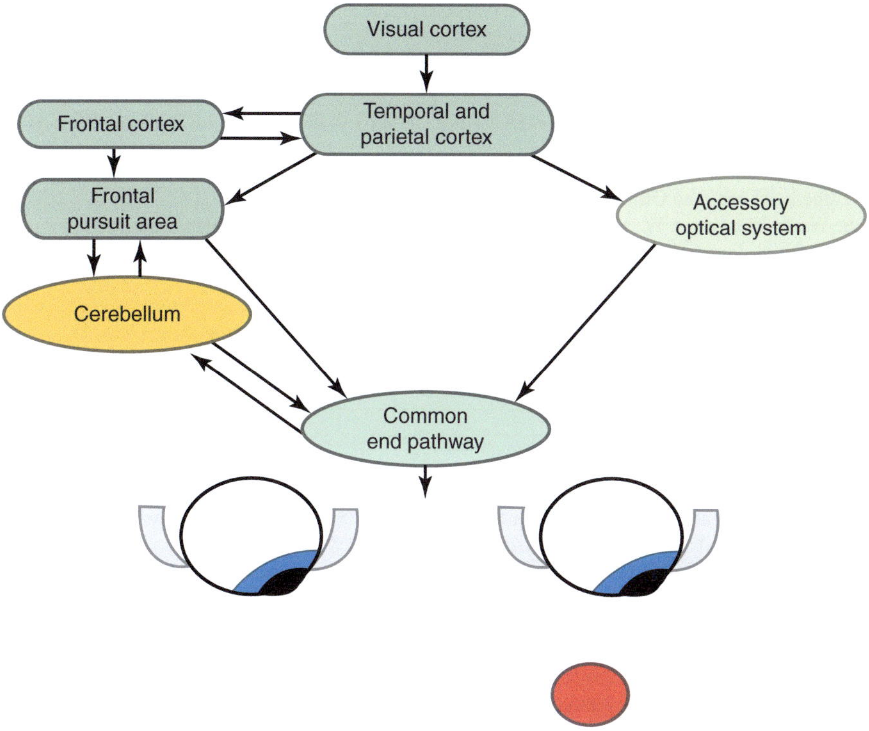

Fig. 29 The smooth pursuit pathways. (Adapted from Conraux [32])

The vestibular nuclei are the centers for these informations, receiving inputs from the vestibular end organs, from the eyes, and from the proprioceptive receptors. All of this information must be consistent and harmonious. Let us consider what happens when we walk: the vestibular system gathers the information about the resulting linear acceleration, the retina captures and records the displacement of the visual images, and the sensory and motor systems will do the same in order to accomplish our movement.

If the available information is not harmonious, disequilibrium or unsteadiness will result. One of the main tasks of the neurotologist is to diagnose the disorders that derive from the malfunction of all of these systems.

References

1. Hawkins JE, Schacht J. Sketches of otohistory. Part 8: the emergence of vestibular science. Audiol Neurotol. 2005;10:185–90.
2. Davis H. A sensory system in evolution. Quincy: Grass; 1977.
3. Schwander M, Kachar B, Müller U. Review series: the cell biology of hearing. J Cell Biol. 2010;190(1):9–20. https://doi.org/10.1083/jcb.201001138.
4. von Békésy G. DC resting potentials inside the cochlear partition. J Acoust Soc Am. 1952;24:72–6.

5. Smith CA, Davis H, Deatherage BH, Gessert CF. DC potentials of the membranous labyrinth. Am J Physiol. 1958;193:203–6.
6. Eldredge DH, Smith CA, Davis H, Gannon RP. The electrical polarization of the semicircular canals (Guinea pig). Ann Otol Rhinol Laryngol. 1961;70:1024–36.
7. Schuknecht H, Ishii T. Hearing loss caused by atrophy of the stria vascularis. Nihon Jibiinkoka Gakkai Kaiho. 1966;69:1825–33.
8. Kimura R, Perlman HB. Experimental obstruction of venous drainage and arterial supply of the inner ear. Ann Otol Rhinol Laryngol. 1957;66:537–46.
9. Wever EG, Bray CW. Auditory nerve impulses. Science. 1930;71:215–8.
10. Davis H, Fernandes C, McAuliffe DR. The excitatory process in the cochlea. Proc Nat Acad Sci USA. 1950;36:580–7.
11. Flourens M-J-P. Recherches expérimentales sur les proprietés et les fonctions du systeme nerveux dans les animaux vertebrés. Paris: Crevot. Quoted by Hawkins & Schacht; 1824.
12. Ewald JR. Physiologische Untersuchungen über das Endorgan des Nervus Octavus. 1892, Wiesbaden, JF Bergmann. Quoted by Mangabeira-Albernaz PL, Ganança M. Vertigem. 1976, 2 ed, São Paulo, Moderna.
13. Kingma H. What physics do I have to know to become a neuro-otologist? 3rd Bárány Teaching Course. 10th ed: Uppsala; 2013.
14. Curthoys IS. The new vestibular stimuli: sound and vibration – anatomical, physiological and clinical evidence. Exp Brain Res. https://doi.org/10.1007/s00221-017-4874y.
15. Schuknecht HF. Cupulolithiasis. Arch Otolaryngol. 1969;90:765–78.
16. Brandt T, Steddin S. Current view of the mechanism of benign paroxysmal positioning vertigo: cupulolithiasis or canalolithiasis? J Vestib Res. 1993;3:373–82.
17. Mangabeira-Albernaz PL. A Evolução de um Sistema Sensorial Thesis, Escola Paulista de Medicina, 1989.
18. Vidal PP, Cullen K, Curthoys IS, Du Lac S, Holstein G, Idoux E, Lysakowski A, Peusner K, Sans A, Smith P. The vestibular system. In: Paxinos G, editor. The rat nervous system. 4th ed. Elsevier; 2015. https://doi.org/10.1016/B978-0-12-374245-2.00028-0.
19. Lysakowski A, McCrea RA, Tomlinson RD. Anatomy of vestibular end organs and neural pathways. In: Cummings CW, editor. Otolaryngology – head and neck surgery. Saint Louis: Mosby; 1996.
20. Marelli E. Anatomy and physiology pf the vestibular system. In: Carmona S, Libonati GA, editors. Neurotology. 1a ed. Buenos Aires: Akadia; 2014. p. 1–16.
21. Cohen B, editor. Vestibular and oculomotor physiology. New York: Academy of Sciences; 1981.
22. Leigh J, Zee D. The neurology of eye movements. 4th ed. Oxford: Oxford University Press; 2006.
23. Zee DS. Anatomy and physiology of the VOR. Syllabus of the vestibular testing master class. Baltimore: Johns Hopkins University; 2017.
24. Zuma e Maia FC, et al. Elementos práticos em otoneurologia. 2nd ed. Rio de Janeiro: Revinter; 2011. p. 17–9.
25. MacDougall H, Curthoys IS. Plasticity during vestibular compensation: the role of saccades. Front Neurol. 2012;3:21. https://doi.org/10.3389/fneur.2012.00021.
26. Termsarasab P, Thammongkolchai T, Rucker JC, Frucht SJ. The diagnostic value of saccades in movement disorder patients: a practical guide and review. J Clin Mov Disord. 2015;2:14. https://doi.org/10.1186/s40734-015-0025-4.
27. Optican LM. The role of omnipause neurons. Prog Brain Res. 2008;171:115–21. https://doi.org/10.1016/S0079-6123(08)00615-8.
28. Lorente de Nó R. Trab Lab Invest Biol Univ Madrid. 1928; 24–63. Quoted by Mangabeira-Albernaz PL, Ganança M. Vertigem. 1976, 2 ed, São Paulo, Moderna.
29. McCabe BF. The quick component of nystagmus: a presentation of a theory of its origin and mechanism involving the dynamic rhythmic inhibition of the slow component, based upon a

comprehensive review of prior work and additional experimental evidence. Laryngoscope. 1965;75:1619–46.
30. Bechterew W. Ergebnisse der Durchschneidung des N. Acusticus, nebst Erörterung der Bedeutung der semicircular Canale für das Körpergleichgewicht. Pflügers Arch ges Physiol. 1883;30:312–47. Quoted by Mangabeira-Albernaz PL, Da Reflexia Vestibular com Relação a Estímulos Mínimos. 1966, Thesis, Escola Paulista de Medicina.
31. Ulmer E, Chays A. Curthoys and Halmagyi head impulse test: an analytical device. Ann Otolaryngol Chir Cervicofac. 2005;122:84–90.
32. Aw ST, Halmagyi GM, Haslwanter T, Curthoys IS, Yavor RA, Todd MJ. Three- dimensional vector analysis of the human vestibuloocular reflex in response to high acceleration head rotations. II. Responses in subjects with unilateral vestibular loss and selective semicircular canal occlusion. J Neurophysiol. 1996;76:4021–30.
33. Hain TC, Ramaswamy TS, Hillman MA. Anatomia e fisiologia do sistema vestibular normal. In: Herdman SJ, editor. Reabilitação vestibular. 2nd ed. São Paulo: Manole; 2002. p. 3–24.
34. Conraux C, Gentine A. Vertiges: exploration clinique et functionnelle de l'appareil vestibulaire. CD-ROM: Strasbourg; 1980.

The Role of Clinical History in Neurotology

History is the most important part of evaluation in neurotology. Taking a good history can be tedious, as complaints are often vague and frequently filled with anxiety-provoked symptoms. In medical clinics, we learned that the greater the number of information given by the patient, the greater our ability to make a diagnosis. In case of dizzy patient, in a certain point excessive information confuses the doctor's diagnoses. In reality, neither patients nor physicians have a clear understanding of what the terms "dizziness" and "vertigo" mean.

During the past 15 years, a growing body of scientific evidence has demonstrated that the traditional approach to bedside diagnosis of patients with vertigo and dizziness is inadequate. Former teaching is that history taking should first rely on categorizing symptoms by type (e.g., vertigo, presyncope, disequilibrium, nonspecific dizziness). These traditional categories direct subsequent diagnostic inquiry, with vertigo prompting a search for vestibular causes, presyncope a search for cardiovascular causes, unsteadiness a search for neurologic causes, and nonspecific dizziness a search for psychiatric or metabolic causes [1].

These symptoms have been replaced by an emphasis on categorizing *timing and triggers* for vestibular symptoms, which focuses the clinician's attention on four key syndromic patterns: (1) acute, spontaneous, prolonged vestibular symptoms; (2) episodic, positional vestibular symptoms; (3) episodic, spontaneous vestibular symptoms; and (4) chronic unsteadiness (with or without oscillopsia).

According to *International consensus definitions for common vestibular symptoms* [2], it's absolutely fundamental to establish if the symptoms that led the patient to consultation is really *vertigo*, which means it's a sensation of self-motion when no self-motion is not occurring or the sensation of distorted self-motion during an otherwise normal head movement. This "internal" vestibular sensation is distinguished from the "external" visual sense of motion referred to in this classification as either external vertigo or *oscillopsia*. Another symptom as *dizziness* is the sensation of disturbed or impaired spatial orientation without a false or distorted sense of motions, and *unsteadiness or imbalance* is the feeling of being unstable while seated, standing, or walking without a particular directional preference.

P. L. M. Albernaz et al., *The New Neurotology*,
https://doi.org/10.1007/978-3-030-11283-7_2

Some authors [3] assume that the key factors that allow a first approximation of diagnosis identification are based on the *time profile*, *symptom profile*, and *trigger profile* of the disease. Based on this identification, they proposed an interesting mnemonic "SO STONED" that comprises eight different dimensions that characterize the vertigo-related complaints of the patients and guide the clinician in his or her decision scheme. All these letters "SO STONED" have a specific meaning: Symptoms, Often (frequency), Since, Trigger, Otology, Neurology, Evolution, and Duration.

In the German Center for Vertigo and Balance Disorders [4], it was concluded that five different categories with the following key symptoms provide a reliable and practical diagnostic guide for the general neurotologist and others who manage dizzy patients:

1. Paroxysmal positional vertigo (benign paroxysmal positional vertigo/central positional vertigo and or nystagmus)
2. Spontaneous recurrent vertigo attacks (vestibular migraine or Menière's disease)
3. Sustained rotational vertigo (vestibular neuritis or central pseudo-neuritis)
4. Frequent spells of dizziness or imbalance (vestibular paroxysmia/superior canal dehiscence syndrome)
5. Postural imbalance without other neurological symptoms (persistent postural-perceptual dizziness/bilateral vestibulopathy)

Besides that, once a patient has been assigned to one of the five syndromic categories, further differentiation of the underlying disorders is based on the following:

1. Type of vertigo
2. Duration of attacks
3. Frequency of attacks
4. Triggers/modulating factors
5. Associated symptoms

In our personal experience [5] the *duration of the episodes* is of fundamental importance, serving as a guide on physical examination:

1. *Seconds*: which means that there is no vestibular lesion but it's just a mechanical dysfunction (e.g., benign paroxysmal positional vertigo (BPPV)).
2. *Minutes/hours*: there is an organic lesion that is reversed in a short time and behaves episodically (e.g., vestibular migraine/Menière's disease/transient ischemic attack of the vertebrobasilar territory/perilymphatic fistula/seizure/microvascular compression/brainstem paroxysmal central vertigo/panic attack/phobic postural vertigo/alcoholic positional nystagmus).
3. *Days*: onset of symptoms abruptly producing a vestibular lesion (e.g., vestibular neuritis/otitis media/strokes/demyelinating disease).
4. *Persistent*: it is an injury that is slowly progressive (e.g., acoustic neuroma/cholesteatoma and other slow-growing tumors/vestibular bilateral areflexia).

To obtain a good history is an art. It's up to you to decide what is the best way.

References

1. Newman-Toker DE. Symptoms and signs of neuro-otologic disorders. Continuum (Minneap Minn). 2012;18(5):1016–40.
2. Bisdorff A, Von Brevern M, Lempert T, et al. Classification of vestibular symptoms: toward an international classification of vestibular disorders. J Vestib Res. 2009;19(1–2):1–13.
3. Wuyts FL, Van Rompaey V, Maes LK. "SO STONED": common sense approach of the dizzy patient. Front Surg. 2016;3:32. https://doi.org/10.3389/fsurg.2016.00032.
4. Brandt T, Strupp M, Dieterich M. Five keys for diagnosing most vertigo, dizziness, and imbalance syndromes: an expert opinion. J Neurol. 2014;261:229–31. https://doi.org/10.1007/s00415-013-7190-x.
5. Marelli E. El vertigo. In: Carmona S, Libonati GA, editors. Neuro-otologia. 3a ed. Buenos Aires: Libreria Akadia; 2012. p. 37–41.

An Introduction to Vestibular Disorders

Disorders of the vestibular system are related to several different symptoms, including dizziness, unsteadiness, vertigo, and oscillopsia [1].

Dizziness is the sensation of disturbed or impaired spatial orientation without a false or distorted sense of motion.

Unsteadiness, or imbalance, is the feeling of being unstable while seated, standing, or walking, without a particular directional preference.

Vertigo is a sensation of self-motion when no self-motion is occurring or a sensation of distorted self-motion during an otherwise normal head movement.

Oscillopsia is a visual sensation that stationary objects are swaying back and forth.

The symptom of vertigo is always related to the vestibular system. All of the others may be vestibular or non-vestibular.

These symptoms may be physiological, like motion sickness, fear of heights, the debarquement syndrome (unsteadiness felt when leaving a boat after a period of time in the sea), and the Coriolis effect (a disequilibrium caused by intense accelerations, often described in supersonic airplane flights). All of these physiological symptoms may be aggravated by actual vestibular disorders.

Most of the clinical syndromes associated with vestibular disorders do not correspond to known pathological changes. But there are some relative clinical correlations, which will be analyzed below.

Structural Defects

Some inner ear congenital defects may be associated with vestibular symptoms. Patients with Mondini dysplasia usually present only hearing loss, but there are cases with episodes of disequilibrium or vertigo [2].

P. L. M. Albernaz et al., *The New Neurotology*,
https://doi.org/10.1007/978-3-030-11283-7_3

Dehiscence of the superior semicircular canal, although probably congenital, does not cause symptoms in patients with less than 30 years of age. Vertigo is not an uncommon symptom in these patients [3].

The perilymphatic hypertension syndrome [4] is related to an enlarged cochlear aqueduct or a defect in the modiolus; these situations result in a direct communication of the spinal fluid spaces to the inner ear. It causes varying degrees of mixed hearing loss and may cause perilymphatic fistulas that may result in repeated episodes of meningitis. They also account for gushers of spinal fluid through the oval window during attempts to perform stapedectomies. Episodes of vertigo may occur, but they are infrequent.

Vertigo spells, on the other hand, are very common in patients with enlarged vestibular aqueducts [5, 6].

The Perilymphatic Space

Perilymphatic fistulas may occur in the semicircular canals or in the cochlear windows. They can be congenital, as the oval window fistulas of the Mondini dysplasia and the perilymphatic hypertension syndrome or the dehiscence of the superior semicircular canal. But they can occur in patients of many different age groups.

Fistulas of the lateral semicircular canal are often caused by cholesteatomas and are frequently associated with episodes of vertigo.

Round and oval window fistulas can be caused by barotrauma and are frequently seen in SCUBA divers. They cause sudden deafness, often accompanied by vertigo. There are reports [7] that they may render the divers totally disoriented, with severe risk of drowning; they usually have to be brought back to the surface by their diver companions.

The so-called spontaneous fistulas may cause sudden deafness, in many cases accompanied by vertigo. But there are chronic fistulas with fluctuant hearing loss, tinnitus, and episodes of vertigo, mimicking Menière's disease; most probably the perilymph hypotension allows for an expansion of the endolymphatic space.

The Endolymphatic Space

Endolymphatic hydrops is a common cause of episodic vertigo. It results from excessive formation of endolymph or inadequate reabsorption. It is most frequently caused by Menière's disease but may also be caused by cochlear malformations (such as Mondini dysplasia), tertiary syphilis, and tumors involving the endolymphatic sac. It has also been reported in rare cases of Alport syndrome. It is interesting to note that the receptor cells, both cochlear and vestibular, are not particularly affected by the endolymphatic hypertension.

A milder form of endolymphatic hydrops is related to metabolic ear problems that cause changes in the chemical composition of endolymph, with an increase in the concentration of sodium and a reduction in the concentration of potassium. These two mechanisms for hydrops can exist simultaneously.

Tumors of the endolymphatic sac may mimic Menière's disease; they are usually a result of von Hippel-Lindau disease, a genetic disorder caused by a mutation in the von Hippel-Lindau tumor suppressor gene. Meningiomas that reach the endolymphatic sac area can also mimic Menière's disease.

Receptor Cells

Loss of vestibular hair cells has been reported in many different conditions. Most of the histological evidence is related to the semicircular canals; there are few histological studies of acquired disease of the saccule and utricle.

Most of the hereditary disorders affecting the statoacoustic system affect primarily the cochlear cells, but loss of vestibular receptor cells has been described in Usher syndrome, usually linked to cerebellar ataxia. Only the more severe cases of Usher syndrome present these symptoms, and these patients also have gait disorders.

Viral diseases may cause losses, both in prenatal situations and throughout life.

Maternal rubella used to be a very common cause of congenital deafness, before vaccination became available. It usually does not affect the vestibular hair cells.

The epidemic parotiditis virus causes unilateral profound hearing losses in some children. Some rare bilateral cases have also been reported. The vestibular cells are not involved, but a few of these patients develop a late endolymphatic hydrops that occurs many years after the onset of the hearing loss.

Sudden loss of vestibular function was well described by Nylén in 1924 [8], with the name of *vestibular neuritis*. The patient has a violent episode of vertigo that may last for several weeks. A nystagmus can be observed, beating to the opposite side of the vestibular areflexia, and in the Romberg test the patient falls to the side of the lesion. A sudden sensorineural hearing loss may also be present. This is a unique episode; the patient, after the vestibular compensation, will not have other episodes of vertigo. This disorder is usually caused by a virus infection of the inner ear, but it may also be of vascular origin.

A variation of the vestibular neuritis, the *Lindsay-Hemenway syndrome* [9], is caused by an obstruction of the anterior vestibular artery; after the compensation of the vestibular areflexia, the patient begins to have episodes of positional vertigo.

Vascular disorders may result in loss of hair cells in the cupulae of the semicircular canals or ganglion cells. They may account for cases of episodic vertigo, related to hyporeflexia of some of the vestibular responses. This disorder was described by Dix and Hallpike in 1952 [10]. Their findings were described in relation to the stimulation of the lateral semicircular canals, since no adequate evaluation of the vertical canals was then available. It is possible that similar disorders can affect the anterior and posterior canals, their cristae, and their ganglion cells.

It has been experimentally demonstrated that acoustic and physical trauma can cause loss of hair cells, both cochlear and vestibular [11, 12].

Many elderly patients present *presbyastasis* – age-related disequilibrium. Loss of vestibular hair cells is one of the possible causes of presbyastasis, but most of the time there are multiple factors involved.

Cupulae and Semicircular Ducts

Several circumstances may cause detachment of otoliths from the otolithic membrane, and this may cause a deposit of inorganic material in the cupula and semicircular canal (cupulolithiasis [13]) or in one of the ducts (ductolithiasis – also referred as canalolithiasis [14]), the consequence of which is a disorder called *benign paroxysmal positional vertigo – BPPV.* It is now known that sometimes more than one canal or one duct may be involved.

BPPV has been known for many years, having been originally described by Adler in 1887. Bárány, in 1921, described the symptoms in detail, and Dix and Hallpike, in 1952, gave it the present name and created maneuvers to improve its diagnosis [15]. But the mechanical origin of the disease has only been established after Schuknecht's pathology observations in 1969 [13].

Maculae and Otolithic Membranes

For many years the study of the saccular and utricular function involved the use of very expensive research systems designed to register responses to linear acceleration.

The clinical evaluation of the saccular and utricular function is rather recent, with the development of the *vestibular evoked myogenic potentials – VEMP.* These electric responses were at first described by Bickford et al. in 1964 [16], and in 1971 Townsend and Cody [17] demonstrated that these responses were mediated by activation of the vestibular apparatus. Other studies led to the conclusion that the cervical responses (cVEMP) involved the stimulation of the saccule and the ocular responses (oVEMP) dealt with the stimulation of the utricle.

These potentials have been demonstrated to be clinically significant in the diagnosis of Menière's disease, as the endolymphatic hydrops involves the saccule and utricle, as well as the cochlea and the semicircular canals. It is also very important in the diagnosis of the dehiscence of the superior semicircular canals; since it is a functional examination, it gives information that is more significant than that of the computerized tomography scans, since very thin bone covering the canal may be mistakenly interpreted as a dehiscence. There are also mentions of a contribution of these tests to the diagnosis of unilateral vestibular disorders and vestibular schwannomas.

It is interesting to note that the temporal bones of many patients that had been submitted to stapedectomies showed atrophies of the saccule, with loss of hair cells in the maculae, probably due to ruptures of the saccular membrane. Apparently these patients did not show any significant vestibular symptoms.

It is now known that otoliths may get detached from the otolithic membrane and remain loose in the endolymphatic space. Cupulolithiasis and ductolithiasis have been mentioned in this chapter. Electron microscopy scans have demonstrated that normal otoliths are quite different from those found in persons with vestibular disorders. Age is one of the factors that affect the uniformity of the otoliths. There is no question that BPPV is more common in persons above 40 years of age, but is sometimes seen in younger persons. BPPV that results from head trauma or stapedectomy may be observed in many different age groups.

The Vestibular Nerves

Compression of the vestibular nerves may cause episodes of vertigo.

Vestibular schwannomas rarely cause vertigo, because vestibular compensation usually occurs simultaneously with the slow growth of the tumor. But there are rare cases that mimic Menière's disease, causing vertigo, tinnitus, and hearing loss. The same occurs with meningiomas of the cerebellopontine angle.

Vascular loops around the nerves may also cause vertigo.

The Central Vestibular Disorders

Conventionally peripheral vestibular disorders are those that involve the inner ear and the vestibular nerve. Central disorders involve the vestibular nuclei and the vestibular pathways, all the way to the cerebral cortex. It is important to understand that the classification of neurotological disorders into peripheral and central is important for the clinical evaluation of vestibular diseases, but there are mixed entities and also peripheral disorders that may evolve to central disorders.

Central vestibular disorders may be caused by hemorrhagic or ischemic insults to the cerebellum, the vestibular nuclei, and their connections with the brainstem. They may also be caused but structural problems, brain tumors, infection, trauma, and degenerative diseases, particularly multiple sclerosis.

One of the significant structural problems is the Arnold-Chiari malformation that frequently causes vertigo. Normal pressure hydrocephalus is often associated with unsteadiness and gait disturbance, but it may eventually cause episodes of vertigo.

The neurotologist must be able to establish a differential diagnosis between a peripheral and a central vestibular disorder. This subject will be extensively dealt with in Chap. 8.

References

1. Bisdorff A, Von Brevern M, Lempert T, et al. Classification of vestibular symptoms: toward an international classification of vestibular disorders. J Vestib Res. 2009;19(1–2):1–13.
2. Mangabeira-Albernaz PL, Fukuda Y, Chammas F, Ganança MM. The Mondini dysplasia – a clinical study. ORL J Otorhinolaryngol Relat Spec (Basel). 1981;43:131–52.
3. Minor LB, Solomon D, Zinreich J, Zee DS. Sound and/or pressure-induced vertigo due to bone dehiscence of the superior semicircular canal. Arch Otolaryngol. 1998;124:249–58.
4. Mangabeira-Albernaz PL, Hidal LBT, Iorio MCM. The Perilymphatic hypertension syndrome. Acta Otolaryngol. 1992;112:306–10.
5. Hill JH, Freint AJ, Mafee MF. Enlargement of the vestibular aqueduct. Am J Otolaryngol. 1984;5(6):411–4.
6. Yang CJ, Lavender V, Meinzen-Derr JK, Cohen AP, Youssif M, Castiglione M, Manickam V, Bachmann KR, Greinwald JH. Vestibular pathology in children with enlarged vestibular aqueduct. Laryngoscope. 2016;126(10):2344–50. https://doi.org/10.1002/lary.25890.
7. Caldas NCR, Mangabeira-Albernaz PL. Fístula perilinfática. In: Mangabeira-Albernaz PL, Ganança MM, House WF, editors. Surdez neuro-sensorial. São Paulo: Moderna; 1978. p. 135–51.
8. Nylén CO. Some cases of ocular nystagmus due to certain positions of the head. Acta Otolaryngol. 1924;6:106–19.
9. Lindsay JR, Hemenway WG. Postural vertigo due to unilateral sudden partial loss of vestibular function. Ann Otol Rhinol Laryngol. 1956;65(3):692–706.
10. Dix MR, Hallpike CS. The pathology, symptomatology and diagnosis of certain common disorders of the vestibular system. Proc R Soc Med. 1952;45:441–54.
11. Britton BH. Vestibular responses to pressure variations: a review. Otolaryngol Head Neck Surg. 1986;95:516. https://doi.org/10.1177/019459988609500417.
12. Mangabeira-Albernaz PL, Covell WP, Eldredge DH. Changes in the vestibular labyrinth with intense sound. Laryngoscope. 1959;69:1478–93.
13. Schuknecht HF. Cupulolithiasis. Arch Otolaryngol. 1969;90:765–78.
14. Brandt T, Steddin S. Current view of the mechanism of benign paroxysmal positioning vertigo: cupulolithiasis or canalolithiasis? J Vestib Res. 1993;3:373–82.
15. Susuki M. Positional Vertigo – past and present. In: Suzuki M, editor. Basic and clinical approach to BPPV based on model experimental results: Society for Promotion of International Oto-Rhino-Laryngology (SPIO). Tokyo: Japan; 2012. p. 10–4.
16. Bickford RG, Jacobson JL, Cody DT. Nature of average evoked potentials to sound and other stimuli in man. Ann NY Acad Sci. 1964;112:204–23.
17. Townsend GL, Cody DT. The averaged inion response evoked by acoustic stimulation: its relation to the saccule. Ann Otol Rhinol Laryngol. 1971;80(1):121–31.

The Bedside Tests: Practical Key Strategies to the Diagnosis of Vestibular and Oculomotor Disorders

The recent developments in neurotology brought new possibilities for the examination of patients in emergency clinics or in hospitals. These new tests are usually referred as *bedside tests*.

In order to derive adequate information from these tests, it is necessary to follow certain basic strategies that are required to obtain adequate interpretation of these tests. These strategies are the understanding of the eye movements, an essential knowledge of the anatomy and neurophysiology of the vestibular and oculomotor systems, and a detailed patient's history. These strategies will be discussed prior to the details of the bedside tests.

The First Practical Key Strategy: Understanding the Six Eye Movements

The movements of the eyes are carried out by the six pairs of extraocular muscles; they are capable of moving the globes in the six cardinal movements.

The six different eye movements have special characteristics and involve different parts of the brain. They may be divided in two categories: the actions that hold the images of a target steady on the retina and those that direct the object of interest precisely to the fovea (Fig. 1).

The former category includes:

1. A *fixation system* that holds the image of a stationary object on the fovea when the head is immobile
2. The vestibular system, by means of the *vestibulo-ocular reflex* (VOR), which holds the image of a target steady on the retina during brief head movements
3. The *optokinetic system*, which holds the image of a target steady on the retina during sustained head movements

P. L. M. Albernaz et al., *The New Neurotology*,
https://doi.org/10.1007/978-3-030-11283-7_4

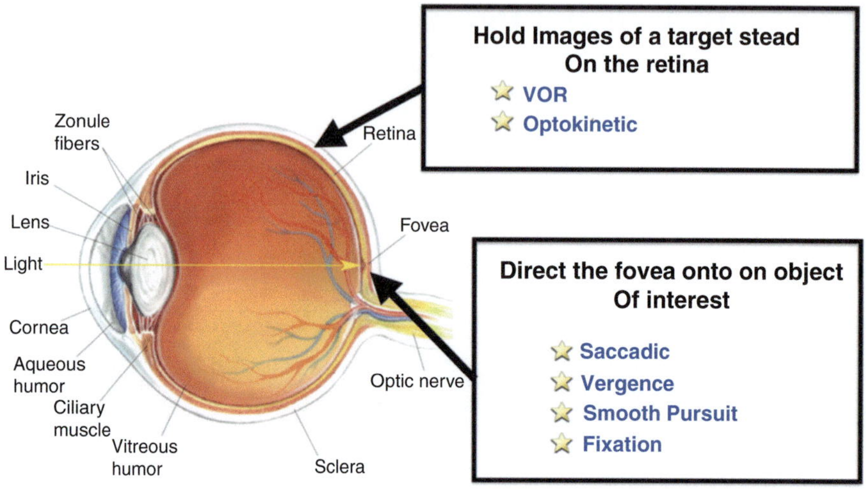

Fig. 1 The characteristics of the six eye movements

The latter category that comprises the systems that direct the object of interest to the fovea includes:

1. The *saccadic system* that brings the image of an object of interest rapidly onto the fovea
2. The *smooth pursuit system* that holds the image of a small, moving target on the fovea
3. The *vergence system*, which moves the eyes in an opposite direction (i.e., convergence and divergence), so that images of a single object are held simultaneously on each of the two foveae [1]

With the exception of voluntary saccades and vergence/divergence saccades, all other types of eye movements are reflexive movements.

The Second Practical Key Strategy: The Essential Knowledge of Anatomy and Physiology of the Vestibulo-Ocular Reflex (VOR) and the Brainstem Centers for Triggering and Controlling Eye Movements

As shown in detail in Chap. 1, VOR stabilizes retinal image during head motion by counterrotating the eyes at the same speed as the head but in the opposite direction. Information about the motion passes from the vestibular sensors in the inner ear to the VOR circuitry in the brainstem, which computes an appropriate eye velocity command. Thus, the function of the VOR is to generate the best eye orientation that compensates for the changes in position and orientation of the head. It contributes, therefore, to optimize visual acuity during head motion, enhances balance control, and allows detection of self-motion and orientation relative to gravity.

When the head moves, *both vestibular and visual information are available*, but they have different latencies and velocities to accomplish the task. The vestibular labyrinths act as very sensitive sensors of head acceleration and tilt; vestibular information takes only about 7–15 ms to travel from the vestibular sensors, through the brainstem, to the ocular motor neurons. With this short latency, the eyes can easily compensate for the rapid oscillation of the head. Visual information takes about 100 ms to travel from the visual cortex, through a series of brain structures, to the ocular motor neurons in charge of moving the eyes. This delay is much too long for the eyes to keep up with an oscillating object, or other similar conditions.

In fact, several systems contribute to motion and tilt perception: semicircular canals, maculae, eyes, and proprioceptive receptors. Both visual and somatosensory systems can only process relatively slow body movements and can be modeled with a cutoff frequency of about 0.2 Hz. The otolith organs detect low-frequency linear accelerations up to 1 Hz, whereas the semicircular canals detect angular velocities between 0.1 and 10 Hz [2].

Only a few brainstem centers, which have clearly allocated functions, are important for triggering and controlling the eye movements. This circumstance enables the physician to localize the specific area in the brainstem that causes the disturbance, the *midbrain*, *pons or medulla*, or *cerebellum* (in particular the *flocculus*), rendering their pathological anatomy easy to understand (Fig. 2).

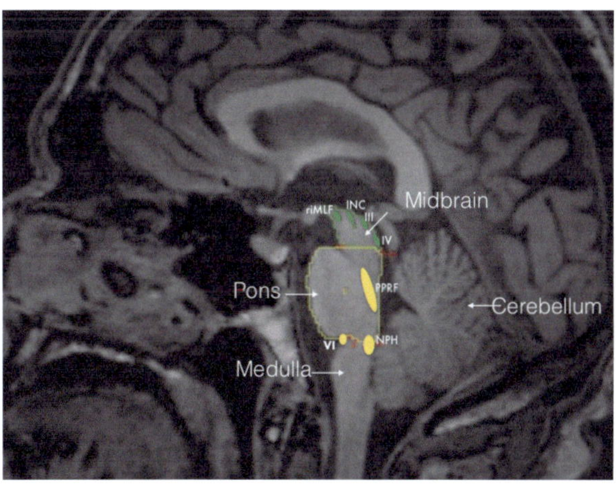

Fig. 2 Important specific areas in the brainstem (midbrain, pons, or medulla) and cerebellum (in particular the flocculus) for triggering and controlling eye movements that enable the physician to localize the disturbance. VI abducens nucleus, NPH nucleus prepositus hypoglossi, PPRF paramedian pontine reticular formation, IV trochlear nucleus, III oculomotor nucleus, INC interstitial nucleus of Cajal, riMLF rostral interstitial nucleus of the medial longitudinal fasciculus

The following simple clinical rules apply:

- *Horizontal eye movements* are generated and controlled in the pontine region – *paramedian pontine reticular formation* (*PPRF*) – and the neural integrators are the *nucleus prepositus hypoglossi* and the *medial vestibular nucleus* (*NPH-MVN*), respectively.
- *Vertical and torsional eye movements* are generated and controlled in the midbrain – *rostral interstitial nucleus of the medial longitudinal fasciculus* (*riMLF*) and *interstitial nucleus of Cajal* (*INC*), respectively.

The *cerebellum* has a central role in the control of the eye movements, both by immediate "online" control and long-term adaptive mechanisms that optimize ocular motor performance to meet the needs of the visual system [3].

Distinct regions within the cerebellum are associated with specific aspects of the control of eye movements [4]:

1. The flocculus and paraflocculus, (cerebellar tonsil), for high-frequency (brief) vestibular responses, *sustained pursuit eye movements*, *gaze holding*, and *VOR cancelation*
2. The nodulus and ventral uvula, for low-frequency (sustained) vestibular responses, modulating *velocity-storage mechanism* within the vestibular nuclei, and *tilt suppression* of post-rotatory VOR and head-shaking nystagmus [5]
3. The dorsal vermis (lobules VI and VII) and the underlying caudal fastigial nuclei, for *saccade amplitude* and *pursuit initiation*

The neural circuitry that controls vestibular eye movements is intertwined with a larger network within the brainstem and cerebellum that also controls other types of conjugate eye movements (Fig. 3).

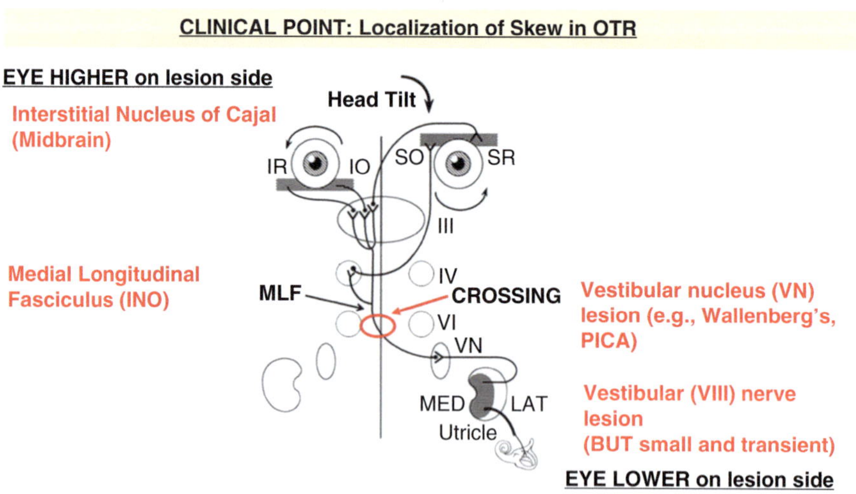

Fig. 3 The neural circuits that control the eye movements

The Third Practical Key Strategy: A Detailed Patient History

Clinical history is of utmost importance in neurotology, beginning with the precise understanding of the patient's symptoms. Newman-Token et al. [6] proposed a simplified approach to neurotological diagnosis named TiTrATE:

TiTrATE = Timing, **Tr**iggers, **A**nd **T**arget **E**xamination

Timing and triggers are the most important elements of the clinical history. Timing refers to the onset, duration, and evolution of the dizziness or vertigo. Triggers refer to actions, movements, or situations that provoke the onset of dizziness or vertigo. The targeted examination – examination suggested by the timing and triggers – will be discussed in the next topic.

Using *timing*, patients can be classified into the three main vestibular syndromes, as defined by the Bárány Society: *episodic vestibular syndrome* (patients with repeated episodes of dizziness or vertigo), *acute vestibular syndrome* (almost always a single vertiginous attack), and *chronic vestibular syndrome* (vertigo that lasts for long periods of time.

Using *triggers*, each of these syndromes may be spontaneous (not related to trigger factors) or consequent to head or body movements, ototoxicity, cranial trauma, etc.

Table 1 presents a classification of the most frequent vestibular disorders, based on timing and triggering. The serious disorders are represented in red.

Table 1 Timing and Triggering of the most frequent Neurotological Disorders

Clinical history		Disorders
Episodic symptoms	Spontaneous	Vestibular migraine Menière's disease Hypoglycemia Panic syndrome Transient ischemic attack Cardiac arrhythmia
Episodic symptoms	Positional	Orthostatic hypotension BPPV Central PPV
Acute or continuous symptoms	Spontaneous	Vestibular neuritis Herpes zoster oticus Viral or bacterial encephalitis Cerebral vascular accident
Acute or continuous symptoms	Post event	Drug intoxication Postoperative Cranial traumatism Wernicke's encephalopathy

The Fourth Practical Key Strategy: Systematic Clinical Bedside Examination

The visual and vestibular systems *are overlapped and use the same output: the neural circuitry that controls the eye movements* [7] (Fig. 3). This circumstance leads to some strategies when performing a clinical bedside examination. It is important to study the eyes alone, the vestibular system alone, and the eyes and vestibular system together.

Static Observation of the Two Systems

Head Tilt

There are two situations in which the head will appear tilted: (1) patients with a *trochlear nerve palsy* that usually tilt their head in the direction of the lower eye and (2) patients with an *ocular tilt reaction (OTR)* that appears when there is an imbalance in the otolith-ocular and otolith-spinal pathways [8]. In cases of *peripheral vestibular damage* or lesions within the *vestibular nuclei* (in the medulla or caudal pons), there will be a *head tilt toward the affected side.* For lesions within the rostral pons and midbrain (commonly in the medial longitudinal fasciculus), there is usually a *head tilt away from the affected side* [9].

Subjective Visual Vertical (SVV)

A tilt of the subjective visual vertical (SSV) is a sensitive sign of a disturbance in the otolith-ocular pathway [10] and often occurs together with the OTR. The SVV can be measured at the bedside using the bucket method [11] or other devices.

Spontaneous Nystagmus

Spontaneous jerk nystagmus is the hallmark of a tone imbalance between the inputs from the semicircular canals of the two labyrinths. When nystagmus is peripheral in origin, it characteristically increases or only becomes apparent when fixation is eliminated. In cases of central origin (e.g.,Wallenberg's syndrome), the eyes are often deviated toward the side of the lesion under closed lids so that when the eyes open, there is a corrective saccade back to straight-ahead fixation.

Examination of the Eye Movements with the Head Still (Without the Participation of the Vestibular System)

Ocular Alignment: The Cover Test

The examination of the alignment of the eyes can provide important information about otolith-ocular pathways. *Cover testing* is used in the same way as when evaluating any patient with diplopia or ocular misalignment.

The patient is asked to fix his gaze on a small visual target, e.g., the tip of a pen. The examiner looks for movements of the eye that has just been uncovered. When there is a vertical misalignment, the usual differential diagnosis is between trochlear nerve palsy and a skew deviation. In the fourth nerve palsy, the affected left eye is excyclorotated and deviates upward when covered, i.e., when the non-affected eye is viewing. In skew deviation, the higher eye is incyclorated (Fig. 4).

In summary, in skew deviation, there is no or little torsional disparity. In superior oblique palsy, there is a torsional disparity with the lines pointing to the side of the paretic eye.

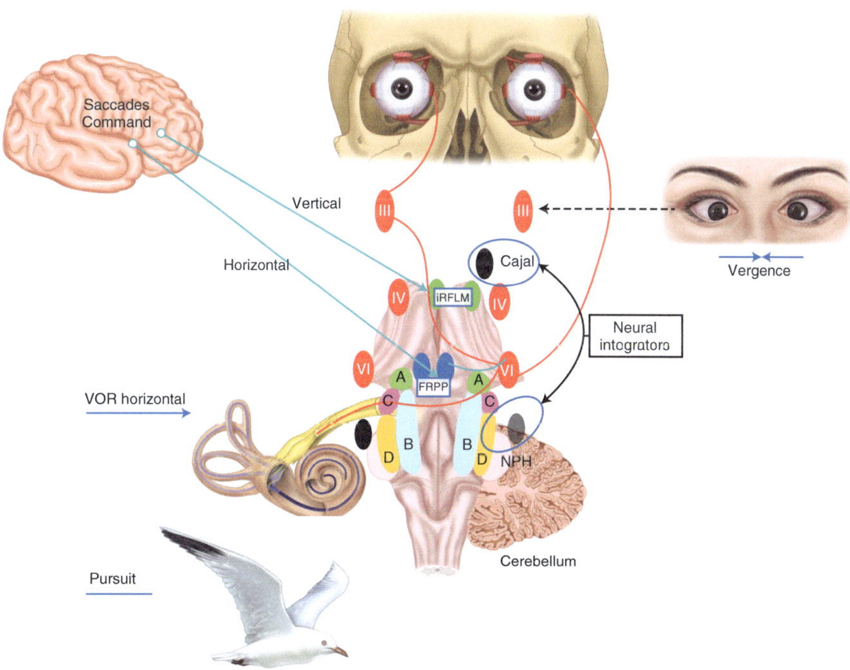

Fig. 4 Localization of skew in ocular tilt reaction (OTR). (Adapted from Leigh and Zee [16])

Spontaneous Nystagmus Pattern with and Without Fixation (Frenzel Lenses to Remove Fixation) and Gaze-Evoked Nystagmus

The effect of removing fixation on nystagmus can be appreciated using Frenzel goggles, or during occlusive ophthalmoscopy, when one eye is covered and the fundus of the other eye observed for the appearance of, or increase in amplitude of, any spontaneous drift [12].

For examination of the gaze-evoked nystagmus, the patient is asked to fix his gaze on a small target 20° to the left and the right from the central position, during 20 s.

When a horizontal nystagmus only appears in one direction of eccentric gaze, the cause may be a mild unilateral peripheral vestibular lesion. Spontaneous nystagmus may also occur in patients with lateral canal BPPV, with the head upright. This is likely due to the natural inclination of lateral semicircular canals in relation to the horizontal plane. The nystagmus typically stops after forward flexion of the head in the sitting position [13].

The pathologic gaze-evoked nystagmus due to brainstem or cerebellar lesions can also be accompanied by signs of vestibular imbalance. The combination may manifest as low-frequency, large-amplitude nystagmus on looking toward the lesioned side and high-frequency, small-amplitude nystagmus on looking away from the lesion.

Characteristics of Peripheral Lesions

1. Peripheral vestibular nystagmus increases or only appears with the removal of fixation.
2. Increases in intensity when looking in the direction of quick phase (Alexander's law).
3. Mixed horizontal-torsional nystagmus is characteristic of complete unilateral loss of function.
4. The peripheral nystagmus obeys Ewald's first law: the eye rotates in a plane parallel to the stimulated canal, independently of the position of the eye in the orbit.

Characteristics of Central Lesions

1. Fixation suppression of nystagmus is usually impaired in patients with unilateral brainstem or cerebellar lesion.
2. Pure vertical or pure torsional nystagmus which remains as such on eccentric gaze is always central.
3. Central nystagmus is often considerably modulated with vergence.
4. Central nystagmus has smaller amplitude when the eyes move in the direction of the quick phase.

Saccades

Saccades are best examined at the bedside by having a patient look alternately at two targets held apart horizontally or vertically, such as the examiner's finger and nose. The velocity, accuracy, trajectory, and ability to conjugate should be noted [1, 12].

For horizontal saccades:

1. A discrete lesion of the PPRF causes a conjugate horizontal saccadic palsy to the same side.
2. A lesion of the medial longitudinal fasciculus causes ipsilateral adduction palsy, the cardinal manifestation of internuclear ophthalmoplegia.
3. A lesion of NPH-MVN (leaky integrator) causes horizontal gazed-evoked nystagmus.

For vertical saccades:

1. A lesion of riMLF causes slowing of downward saccades.
2. A lesion of INC (leaky integrator) causes torsional nystagmus.

Saccade abnormalities can also be detected, within the hierarchy of saccades, by assessing (in order):

1. *Quick phases*: an optokinetic nystagmus is elicited by using an optokinetic drum; the loss of quick phases is usually due to a *lesion of premotor burst neurons* in the brainstem.
2. *Voluntary saccades to command*: the patient is asked to make rapid saccades between two stationary targets; the loss of voluntary saccades, with preservation of quick phases, is characteristic of acquired oculomotor apraxia.
3. *Predictive, anticipatory saccades*: the examiner holds both hands up and asks the patient to make a saccade when one of the examiner's fingers moves; with predictable timing, first a finger on one hand is moved and then a finger on the other. The cycle is repeated several times, occasionally not moving one finger to determine if the patient makes a predictable saccade. Defects of predictable saccades control are common in *Parkinson's disease*.
4. *Anti-saccades*: Hold both hands up and move a finger on one hand suddenly. Ask the patient to look away from the moving finger (i.e., look to the finger that does not move). Errors on anti-saccades task are common in *lesion of the prefrontal cortex*.
5. *Hypermetric saccades*: These can be easily seen and relate to lesions of the nucleus fastigius.
6. *Hypometric saccades*: These low-amplitude saccades are seen in patients with lesions in the cerebellar vermis.

Smooth Pursuit

In this strategy, the patient is asked to track a small target with the head still.

1. Catch-up saccades are seen when the gain is low.
2. Backup saccades are observed when the gain is high.

Vergence

The patient is asked to fixate on a small target as it is brought toward the nose. The vergence system is the first system to be affected by fatigue, alcohol, and other drugs, and defective vergence is a common cause of strabismus and diplopia [1].

Optokinetic Nystagmus

Optokinetic nystagmus (OKN) is induced reflexively by motion of a larger visual scene, which causes an illusionary sensation of self-rotation in the opposite direction.

The OKN test may be performed to see whether the patient has a lesion in the pons or midbrain or just has normal eyes' saccade movements in the horizontal and vertical plans.

Stimulation of the Vestibular System (Without Participation of the Vision)

These tests must be performed with the patient wearing Frenzel lenses.

Positional Test

Positional testing is an essential part of the vestibular examination in all patients with the complaint of dizziness. The positional maneuvers are best performed with the patient wearing Frenzel lenses to remove fixation (see chapter on BPPV).

The two maneuvers that should be performed are:

1. The Dix-Hallpike maneuver, to detect canalolithiasis of a posterior semicircular canal. The patient is moved from the sitting to the head-hanging position with the head rotated about 45° right or left relative to the trunk.
2. The supine-roll maneuver to detect a canalolithiasis or cupulolithiasis of the lateral semicircular canals.

Vibration-Induced Nystagmus

Low-frequency vibration (60 Hz or 100 Hz), applied to the mastoid tip or vertex, may induce nystagmus in patients with unilateral loss of vestibular function and occasionally in other conditions, such as superior canal dehiscence [8]. In the case of a unilateral loss of function, the slow phase of the nystagmus usually beats toward the side of the paretic ear. When vibration elicits a vertical nystagmus, a central lesion should be suspected. A vibration-induced torsional or vertical nystagmus may also occur with a superior canal dehiscence [14].

Head-Shaking Nystagmus (HSN) and Head-Shaking Tilt Suppression (HSTS)

The head-shaking nystagmus (HSN) test is considered a useful clinical tool for detecting asymmetries between the vestibular labyrinths and provides some insight into the integrity of the velocity storage system [15]. Shaking the head with an oscillation about 2 Hz for approximately 20 s in the horizontal plane may cause a horizontal nystagmus where the fast phase beats toward the unaffected labyrinth [16]. This finding suggests a peripheral vestibular hypofunction; the duration of the nystagmus will be as long as 6 s in the post-acute stage [16]. The presence of a vertical nystagmus after a horizontal head shaking typically suggests pathology affecting the central vestibular pathways [17]; downbeating nystagmus has been reported as very common, after horizontal head shaking, in patients with vestibular migraine [18].

For the HSTS test, the patient is instructed to tilt his head forward until the chin rests on the upper thorax, immediately after the passive horizontal head shaking. They remain in this position for 60 s [5]. The authors suggest that tilting of the head forward after first applying horizontal head-shaking (HSTS test) is much less effective at suppressing the induced nystagmus in patients with a central cause for their vestibular-like symptoms.

Hyperventilation-Induced Nystagmus

Hyperventilation is performed in a sitting position through quick and deep respiratory cycles for 70 s: this duration is usually sufficient to cause the metabolic and neurophysiological effects of the hyperventilation [19].

Hyperventilation often induces nystagmus in patients with compression of the vestibular nerve by a tumor (e.g., vestibular schwannoma) or small blood vessel loops (microvascular compression) or with demyelinating diseases affecting the central pathways (e.g., multiple sclerosis) [8].

Valsalva-Induced Nystagmus

The Valsalva maneuver can induce nystagmus either by increasing intracranial pressure (straining against closed glottis as in lifting a heavy weight) or by increasing pressure in the middle ear (blowing out against pinched nostrils). The nystagmus may be induced in patients with cranio-cervical junction anomalies, such as Arnold-Chiari malformation, with perilymphatic fistulas, or superior canal dehiscence. Jugular venous compression may also increase the intracranial pressure and induce a nystagmus similar to that of the Valsalva maneuver [8].

Tullio's Phenomenon

Tullio's phenomenon (noise-induced nystagmus and oscillopsia) often occurs in patients who have Valsalva-induced nystagmus and is commonly associated with superior canal dehiscence [7] and perilymphatic fistulas.

Stimulation of the Vestibular System (with Participation of the Vision)

Dynamic Visual Acuity

Dynamic visual acuity is assessed by asking the patient to read while his head is oscillated horizontally, vertically, or in the roll plane (from ear to shoulder) at a relatively high frequency of about 2 Hz [8]. Normal individuals may lose one or two lines of acuity with head rotation, whereas patients with vestibular abnormalities often lose more than two.

With unilateral vestibular hypofunction, DVA is symmetric during pitch (vertical) and roll (torsion) but not yaw (horizontal) rotation; DVA is degraded more during yaw rotations toward the paretic than toward the healthy ear [20].

Visually Enhanced Vestibular Ocular Reflex (VVOR)

The VVOR test requires a low-frequency stimulation.

The subject is asked to stare at a fixed dot on the wall at a distance of 1.5 m. His head is slowly moved at about 0.5 Hz and with an amplitude of 10° in the horizontal plane. The patient is asked to maintain the fixation on the dot during the whole test.

Patients with unilateral vestibular hypofunction exhibit catch-up saccades beating to the healthy side following the head rotation to the affected side. Patients with bilateral vestibular hypofunction exhibit catch-up saccades beating to the *opposite* side of the head movement, for both sides. Patients with cerebellar lesion exhibit catch-up saccades to the *same* side of head movement for both sides.

Vestibulo-Ocular Reflex Suppression (VORS)

For the VORS the patient looks at a finger of his extended arm, while he turns smoothly at the waist, from side to side with the arm, trunk, and head en bloc. Patients with unilateral vestibular hypofunction exhibit catch-up saccades to the healthy side when the head is moved to this side, while patients with bilateral vestibular hypofunction do not show catch-up saccades during head movement to either side. Failure of VORS in the absence of spontaneous nystagmus indicates a supratentorial lesion [21].

Head Impulse Test

Instruct the patient to maintain fixation on the examiner's nose, and then rotate the patient's head slowly to each side, then briskly back to midline, or briskly from midline to each side. This is a high-frequency stimulation.

Normally, the VOR is able to match the velocity of head rotation, and the gaze fixation never leaves the nose. With a vestibulopathy on the side to which the head is quickly rotated, the impaired VOR causes the eyes to lag behind during the rapid head movement, fixation is lost, and a corrective saccade back to the target occurs. The catch-up saccade indicates peripheral vestibular hypofunction on the side toward which the head was rotated [22].

Examination of the Vestibulospinal Reflex

A simple test for the vestibulospinal reflex is the Romberg test performed on a rubber foam pad. The foam minimizes the proprioceptive input from the feet. The patient stands with his feet together, hands by the sides, and eyes closed. The test is very sensitive to identify patients with unilateral or bilateral vestibular loss, who tend to fall to one of the sides. In the absence of a vestibular deficit, the Romberg test on foam is also positive in patients with midline cerebellar disorders, who tend to fall forward or backward [23].

The HINTS Protocol

Kattah et al. [24] and Newman-Toker et al. [25] proposed a simple protocol to be used, in emergency clinics, to identify the central vestibular syndromes. This protocol has been used in many different clinics, with good results [26–28].

HINTS = **H**ead **I**mpulse + **N**ystagmus + **T**est of **S**kew

The combination of these tests that have been described in this chapter is particularly useful in the differential diagnosis of acute spontaneous disorders, including vestibular neuritis, bacterial labyrinthitis, herpes zoster oticus, cerebral vascular accidents (either ischemic or hemorrhagic), brainstem encephalitis, etc., in emergency clinics. Audiological tests must be added to the HINTS protocol to increase its sensitivity.

In cases of cerebral vascular accidents, the HINTS protocol gives the following results:

1. Head impulse normal
2. Direction-changing nystagmus or fast-phase alternating nystagmus
3. Refixation on test of skew (cover test)

Abnormal results with the head impulse test usually indicate peripheral disorders. Vertical deviation on the test of skew is always central and usually precedes the findings in magnetic resonance images for 24 h or more.

References

1. Wong AMF. Eye movement disorders. New York: Oxford University Press; 2008.
2. Kingma H, Van der Berg R. Anatomy, physiology and physic of the peripheral vestibular system. Handb Clin Neurol. 2016;137:1–16. (3rd series), Neuro-Otology. https://doi.org/10.1016/B978-0-444-63437-5.00001-7.
3. Kheradmand A, Colpak ZD. Eye movements in vestibular disorders. Handb Clin Neurol. 2016;137. (3rd series) Neuro-Otology. J.M. Furman and T. Lempert, Eds.
4. Kheradmand A, Zee DS. Cerebellum and ocular motor control. Front Neurol. 2011;2:53. https://doi.org/10.3389/fneur.2011.00053. eCollection 2011.
5. Zuma e Maia FC, Cal RV, D'Albora R, Carmona S, Schubert MC. Head shaking tilt suppression: a clinical testy to discern central from peripheral cause of vertigo. J Neurol. 2017;264:1264. https://doi.org/10.1007/s00415-017-8524-x.
6. Newman-Toker DE, Edlow JA. TiTrATE: a novel approach to diagnosing acute dizziness and vertigo. Neurol Clin. 2015;33(3):577–99. https://doi.org/10.1016/j.ncl.2015.04.011.
7. Strupp M, et al. Central ocular motor disorders, including gaze palsy and nystagmus. J Neurol. 2014;261(Suppl 2):542. https://doi.org/10.1007/s00415-014-7385-9.
8. Kheradmand A, Zee DS. The bedside examination of the vestibular reflex (RVO): an update. Paris: Elsevier Masson SAS; 2012.
9. Brandt T, Dieterich M. Skew deviation with ocular torsion: a vestibular brainstem sign of topographic diagnostic value. Ann Neurol. 1993;33(5):528–34.
10. Dieterich M, Brandt T. Ocular torsion and tilt of subjective visual vertical are sensitive brainstem signs. Ann Neurol. 1993;33:292–9.
11. Zwergal A, Rettinger N, Frenzel C, Dieterich M, Brandt T, Strupp M. A bucket of static vestibular function. Neurology. 2009;72:1689–92.
12. Leigh RJ, Zee DS. The neurology of eye movements. 5th ed. New York: Oxford University Press; 2015.
13. De Stefano A, Kulamarva G, Citraro L, Neri G, Croce A. Spontaneous nystagmus in benign paroxysmal positional vertigo. Am J Otolaryngol. 2011;32:185–9.
14. White JA, Hughes GB, Ruggieri PN. Vibration-induced nystagmus as an office procedure for the diagnosis of superior semicircular canal dehiscence. Otol Neurotol. 2007;28:911–6.

15. Katsarkas A, Smith H, Galiana H. Head-shaking nystagmus (HSN): the theoretical explanation and the experimental proof. Acta Otolaryngol. 2000;120(2):177–81.
16. Lee YJ, Shin EJ, Park MS, Kim JM, Na BR, Kim CH, Park HJ. Comprehensive analysis of head-shaking nystagmus in patients with vestibular neuritis. Audiol Neurootol. 2012;17:228–34. https://doi.org/10.1159/000336958.
17. Kim YE, Kim JS, Yang HJ, Yun JY, Kim HJ, Ehm G, Kim JM, Jeon BS. Perverted head-shaking and positional downbeat nystagmus in essential tremor. Cerebellum. 2016;15(2):152–8. https://doi.org/10.1007/s12311-015-0683-7.
18. Kim CH, Shin JE, Song CI, Yoo MH, Park HJ. Vertical components of head-shaking nystagmus in vestibular neuritis, Meniere's disease and migrainous vertigo. Clin Otolaryngol. 2014;39(5):261–5.
19. Califano L, Mellilo MG, Vassalo A, Mazzone S. Hyperventilation-induced nystagmus in a large series of vestibular patients. Acta Otorhinolaryngol Ital. 2011;31(1):17–26.
20. Schubert M, Migliaccio AA, Ng TWC, Shaikh A, Zee DS. The Under-Compensatory Roll aVOR does not Affect Dynamic Visual Acuity. J Assoc Res Otolaryngol. 2012;13:517–25.
21. Halmagyi GM, Gresty MA. Clinical signs of visual-vestibular interaction. J Neurol Neurosurg Psychiatry. 1979;42:934–9.
22. Halmagyi GM, Curthoys IS. A clinical sign of canal paresis. Arch Neurol. 1988;45:737–9.
23. Straumann D. Bedside examination. Handb Clin Neurol. 2016;137:91–101. (3rd series) Neuro-Otology. J.M. Furman, T. Lempert, eds. https://doi.org/10.1016/B978-0-444-63437-5.00007-8.
24. Kattah JC, Talkad AV, Wang DZ, Hsieh YH, Newman-Toker DE. HINTS to diagnose stroke in the acute vestibular syndrome: three-step bedside oculomotor examination more sensitive than early MRI diffusion-weighted imaging. Stroke. 2009;40(11):3504–10. https://doi.org/10.1161/STROKEAHA.109.551234.
25. Newman-Toker DE, Kerber KA, Hsieh YH, Pula JH, Omron R, Saber Tehrani AS, Mantokoudis G, Hanley DF, Zee DS, Kattah JC. HINTS outperforms ABCD2 to screen for stroke in acute continuous vertigo and dizziness. Acad Emerg Med. 2013 Oct;20(10):986–96. https://doi.org/10.1111/acem.12223.
26. Carmona S, Martínez C, Zalazar G, Moro M, Batuecas-Caletrio A, Luis L, Gordon C. The diagnostic accuracy of truncal Ataxia and HINTS as cardinal signs for acute vestibular syndrome. Front Neurol. 2016;7:125. https://doi.org/10.3389/fneur.2016.00125. eCollection 2016.
27. Jaynstein D. HINTS for differentiating peripheral from central causes of vertigo. JAAPA. 2016;29(10):56–7. https://doi.org/10.1097/01.JAA.0000496966.42862.e1.
28. Batuecas-Caletrío A, Yáñez-González R, Sánchez-Blanco C, González-Sánchez E, Benito J, Gómez JC, Santa Cruz-Ruiz S. Vértigo periférico frente a vértigo central. Aplicación del protocolo HINTS. Rev Neurol. 2014;59(8):349–53.

Clinical Evaluation of the Vestibular System: The Vestibular Laboratory Tests

The functional examination of the vestibular system is complex, since these evaluations depend entirely on motor responses, particularly eye movements and postural changes.

The basis for most vestibular tests is induced head movements. These movements, as a rule, stimulate the vestibular organs on both sides, and this makes it more difficult to diagnose unilateral disorders. The development of new tests, however, has made it possible to examine the right and left vestibular organs separately.

There are many tests of vestibular function that can be performed by means of special equipment, in a laboratory specifically dedicated to clinical investigations in patients with disorders of the vestibular system. The reasons for performing these tests can be listed as follows [1]:

1. To confirm the preliminary diagnosis derived from the clinical history, the physical examination, and the bedside tests
2. To identify oculomotor abnormalities by means of more sensitive analysis of eye movements
3. To determine if additional diagnostic tests, such as imaging studies, or clinical laboratory tests, will be needed

One must take into consideration that vestibular tests are functional. They may inform the site of the lesion, but they cannot, as a rule, establish the type of disease that causes it. The results of the vestibular tests, therefore, must be analyzed together with the clinical history, physical examination, and, eventually, laboratory tests, imaging, and other tests, to establish a diagnosis.

On the other hand, vestibular tests are the only available tests for the brainstem reticular formation [2].

P. L. M. Albernaz et al., *The New Neurotology*,
https://doi.org/10.1007/978-3-030-11283-7_5

Electronystagmography and Videonystagmography

The majority of the vestibular laboratory tests involve the recording of the eye movements induced by vestibular stimulation.

According to Henriksson [3], there were many early attempts to record the eye movements, carried out by Berlin in 1891, Buys in 1909, Ohm in 1914, Struyken in 1918, and Dohlman in 1925. They employed optical, mechanical, and photographical methods, with the objective of improving their studies of the nystagmus.

Emil du Bois-Reymond, the developer of experimental electrophysiology, reported, in 1849, that the amplitude of the corneo-retinal potentials varied with different eye movements. This is the basis of electronystagmography (ENG) , which, however, only began to be employed in the 1950s [4, 5].

ENG has been the method of choice for recording eye movements for many years. It records horizontal movements and, changing the position of the electrodes, vertical movements. It does not, however, record rotatory movements. A variation devised by Pansini and Padovan [6], named vectornystagmography, allowed for a recording of rotatory movements as oblique and has been used in an attempt to record responses from the vertical semicircular canals [7].

More recently videonystagmography (VNG), introduced in 1995 [8], became the favored method to record eye movements. VNG has many advantages, as shown in Table 1 [9].

The Vestibular Tests

The words electronystagmography and videonystagmography are often employed to enclose all of the tests that require records of the eye movements. But they do not constitute a single test. They involve several procedures that will be described one by one.

Table 1 Differences between ENG and VNG

Electronystagmography (ENG)	Videonystagmography (VNG)
Uses electrodes to record corneo-retinal potential	Records eye movements directly with infrared cameras
Recording sensitivity = 2	Recording sensitivity = 0.1
Artifacts (blinking, electromagnetic disturbances, and EEG activity)	Not affected by any extrinsic factors
Detailed oculomotor tests are not possible	All oculomotor tests can be studied in detail
Cannot record rotatory eye movements	Rotatory eye movements can be recorded
It is not possible to review or replay tests	Videos can be reviewed and played in slow motion
Each eye can be recorded separately, but this requires more channels or more time	Each eye can be recorded separately
Cannot be used in blind patients	It is not affected by any eye condition, except congenital blindness

Spontaneous Nystagmus

Nystagmus is an involuntary eye movement that is part of the vestibulo-ocular reflex (VOR). It is characterized by a slow phase, which is a smooth pursuit movement in one direction, and a fast phase – a saccadic movement – in the opposite direction.

The patient is asked to look forward at a stationary object. Patients with normal vestibular organs do not show nystagmus on direct observation, but it may be present in recordings. The presence of spontaneous nystagmus is caused by an asymmetry in peripheral or central vestibular pathways.

Spontaneous nystagmus is usually horizontal, or horizontal with a torsional component. But it can be vertical, with a torsional component, in focal lesions involving the anterior or posterior semicircular canals. In peripheral disorders the fast phase beats in the direction of the normal ear.

Pure vertical nystagmus is almost always central, except for small intensity upbeating nystagmus that may be seen in normal elderly patients. Both downbeating and upbeating nystagmus with fixation denote a central lesion in the cerebellum or the medulla. There are many possible causes including congenital malformations, tumors, or ischemic events.

The intensity of spontaneous nystagmus is related to the severity of symptoms. Low-intensity spontaneous nystagmus may be recorded in normal individuals, with slow component velocities not exceeding 4°/s for VNG and 6°/s for ENG [1, 10, 11].

In patients with acute peripheral disorders, the nystagmus is accompanied by vertigo. The amplitude of the nystagmus decreases with eye fixation (eyes open or lights on). The absence of the fixation effect indicates that the nystagmus is of central origin. In patients with central spontaneous nystagmus, there is little or no vertigo.

Patients with central vestibular disorders occasionally present *alternating nystagmus*, the eyes beating in one direction and then changing to the opposite direction. *Dissociated nystagmus* – different eye movements in each eye – is also seen in central disorders.

Some patients present *congenital ocular nystagmus*. These eye movements almost never present a slow and a fast phase, they are usually pendular movements.

Both spontaneous nystagmus and congenital optical nystagmus interfere with the vestibular tests and have to be taken into consideration when studying labyrinthine function.

Gaze Nystagmus

The patient is asked to look at an object placed 20° to 30° away from the central vision, to the left, to the right, up and down. Further eye deviation should be avoided, because most patients have some nystagmus at extreme eye positions.

In patients with spontaneous nystagmus caused by peripheral disorders, the amplitude of the gaze nystagmus increases when the patient moves the eyes in the direction of the fast phase.

In patients with central vestibular disorders the following conditions may be found:

1. Patients without spontaneous nystagmus and gaze nystagmus
2. Patients with unilateral gaze nystagmus
3. Patients with bilateral horizontal gaze nystagmus
4. Patients with multiple nystagmuses – horizontal to the left for the left gaze, to the right for the right gaze, up-beating for the up gaze, and down-beating for the down gaze

Conditions 1 and 2 may occur in peripheral patients, but the fixation effect is not present in central cases. Conditions 3 and 4 are always central [11].

Smooth Pursuit

The patient is instructed to follow a computer-generated visual target that moves slowly in the horizontal plane. The patient is also instructed not to move his or her head while following the target. Some neurotologists also employ vertical movements.

The stimulus is usually sinusoidal. In normal persons the recordings follow the sinusoidal pattern of the stimulus (type I eye tracking), with eventually a few intervening saccades (type II eye tracking). Type III eye tracking shows the superposition of a spontaneous nystagmus on the sinusoid tracing. Type IV is an anarchic trace found in central disorders [11].

Saccade Tests

These tests evaluate rapid eye movements [12, 13]. The patient is instructed to follow a computer-generated visual target that jumps back and forth with randomized amplitude, randomized direction, and sometimes randomized timing. The patient is also instructed not to move his or her head.

The parameters for this test include velocity, accuracy, and latencies that are recorded for saccades in different directions. Latency is of approximately 200 ms, and the eye movements match the targets, with occasional overshoots or undershoots, that are normal.

Slow Saccades

Slow saccades, affecting both eyes, either in one or in both directions, are seen in patients with degenerative diseases of the central nervous system or may be caused by some medications [14]. In very severe cases, the patient may be unable to make fast eye movements.

Dysmetric Saccades

These are characterized by consistent overshoots or undershoots, either in one or both directions. They are usually caused by cerebellar lesions. An unusual type of saccadic dysmetria is lateropulsion, in which there are overshoots in one direction and undershoots in the opposite direction; this is usually caused by an infarct of the posterior inferior cerebellar artery. In rare cases it can result from an infarct of the contralateral superior cerebellar artery [1].

Internuclear Ophthalmoplegia

This is characterized by the slowing of the adducting saccades, either in one of the eyes or in both eyes (bilateral). The abducting eye usually has nystagmus immediately after the saccade. Internuclear ophthalmoplegia denotes a central lesion in the medial longitudinal fasciculus on the side of slow adduction. It is often seen in patients with demyelinating diseases, but it can also occur with infarcts or brainstem tumors [15].

Optokinetic Test

This is a recording of the eye movements that are recorded as the patient views a series of images moving either to the right or to the left. These images may be supplied by a computer or by a simple drum. There is no stimulation of the peripheral vestibular organs, but the vestibular system plays an important role in the production of the optokinetic nystagmus that presents well-defined slow and fast phases.

The optokinetic responses arise from retinal stimulation. The pathways studied by the optokinetic test are basically the same of the smooth pursuit test.

In normal patients the optokinetic responses for each direction are symmetrical. The presence of spontaneous nystagmus, either in peripheral or central cases, renders the optokinetic nystagmus asymmetrical; asymmetry in the absence of spontaneous nystagmus is always central, usually characterizing cerebral hemisphere damage.

The optokinetic response may also be dysrhythmic or absent in central cases.

Dynamic Positional Tests

These are tests that are employed to identify patients with benign paroxysmal positional vertigo (BPPV), which is the most common cause of dizziness. There are at present several diagnostic tests for different conditions. This topic is extensively discussed in Chap. 10.

Rotatory Chairs

Rotatory tests stimulate the vestibular system by means of the head movements induced by the chair. The head movements, or the chair movements, are compared with the slow-phase velocity of the nystagmus that results from the stimulation.

There are several types of tests that can be performed with rotatory chairs. The most important are the high-frequency rotation (original or modified Bárány's tests) and the slow harmonic sinusoidal testing that alternate clockwise and anticlockwise movements. There are several types of chairs that can be used, with different degrees of sophistication.

Bárány used the rotatory chair to study the vertical canals that he could not investigate with the caloric tests. Bárány's chair was a modification of earlier chairs that were used in hospitals for patients with mental disorders. The rotatory vestibular tests proposed by Bárány are presently restricted to the investigation of patients with suspicion of bilateral loss of vestibular function; they may be employed, however, in special cases of patients with neurological disorders and for training military pilots, conditioning them to use their instruments rather than trust their visual perceptions [16].

The classical tests with the Bárány chair are shown in Table 2. They can be performed either with an old Bárány chair or with a modern computerized chair.

Computerized chairs allow for a choice of different frequencies and different periods of time, but there are no standardized procedures.

The slow sinusoidal tests can be performed with constant amplitude movements, in computerized chairs, or with decreasing amplitudes; these latter can also be performed with chairs that have torsion bars or springs. These tests are commonly called *torsion swing tests*. They have been created by Mach [17], but its clinical use began with Hennebert in 1956 [18]. The long period of lapsed time derived from the circumstance that per-rotatory nystagmus must be recorded for these tests, which are usually conducted in the dark.

The anatomical structures involved in rotatory tests are the same that are stimulated in the caloric tests, with the difference that both right and left lateral canals are

Table 2 Vestibular tests with the Bárány chair

	Tests 1 and 2	Tests 3 and 4	Tests 5 and 6
	Head tilted 30° downward	Head 60° tilted backward	Head tilted 90° over right shoulder
Chair turns	10 turns in 20 s	10 turns in 20 s	5 turns in 10 s
Canal(s) stimulated by clockwise motion	Left lateral	Right anterior and posterior canals	Right posterior canal
Resulting post-rotational nystagmus	Left horizontal	Anticlockwise rotatory nystagmus	Downbeating vertical nystagmus
Canal(s) stimulated by anticlockwise motion	Right lateral	Left anterior and posterior canals	Left posterior canal
Resulting post-rotational nystagmus	Right horizontal	Clockwise rotatory nystagmus	Upbeating vertical nystagmus

stimulated simultaneously. In spite of the extensive previous clinical experience, the indications for the rotatory tests are nowadays relatively limited. They are used mainly in the following situations:

1. Cases of bilateral canal paresis
2. Cases with inconclusive results in other tests
3. Tests for special populations: pediatric or handicapped
4. Control of ototoxicity, particularly in patients undergoing chemotherapy
5. Evaluation of vestibular compensation

The results take in consideration asymmetry of the gain in the clockwise and anticlockwise movements. The more sophisticated equipments allow for measuring latency and phase.

Caloric Tests

Caloric tests induce nystagmus mainly by creating convection currents in the endolymph. Only the lateral canals can be stimulated, since the vertical canals are anatomically distant from the external acoustic meatus. The structures involved are the lateral semicircular canal, the superior vestibular nerve, and the central structures.

The caloric tests have been the most important tests of peripheral vestibular function for many years, for they were the only tests that allowed for the separate study of each ear. But it must be taken into consideration that they are not a physiological test; the vestibular organs are sensors of accelerations, not of temperature changes. And the results of these tests are quite variable, so they are useless for following a patient's vestibular disorder. A study of caloric tests performed in the morning, in the afternoon, and in the evening in a group of patients demonstrated that the results were not consistent [19].

It has also been established [20] that the caloric tests stimulate the vestibular organs at frequencies below 0.1 hertz, much lower than most of the system's activity (Fig. 1).

Furthermore, the examination is often uncomfortable, occasionally causing nausea and vomiting. Therefore, after the advent of the head impulse tests, there is a tendency to abandon the caloric tests. They are still employed by many neurotologists, and for this reason an analysis of its contributions must be included in this chapter.

According to Gernandt [21], Charles Brown-Séquard, in 1860, verified that a thermal stimulation of the vestibular system induced a sensation of vertigo, and Josef Breuer, in 1889, observed that this stimulation produced nystagmus. The clinical use of the caloric test began with Bárány in 1906 [22]. A major contribution to perfect it was presented by Fitzgerald and Hallpike in 1942 [23].

The test is administered with the patient in supine position, with the head elevated 30°, thus placing the lateral semicircular canals in the plane of gravity. According to the classical Hallpike test, each ear is irrigated twice, once with water

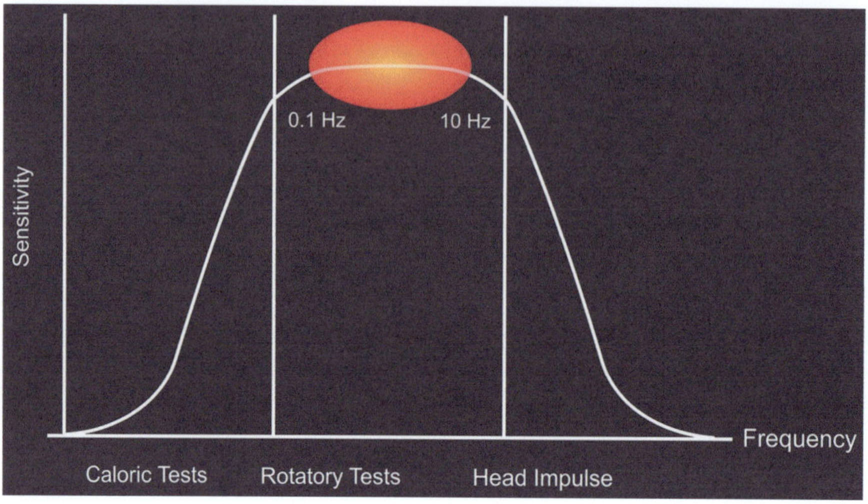

Fig. 1 The frequency spectrum of the vestibular system and the area stimulated by different tests. (Adapted from Kingma [20])

at 30° C and once with water at 44° C. An air stimulus can be used instead of water, at temperatures of 42° C and 20° C.

In normal patients the thermal stimulation with warm stimulus produces a nystagmus beating to the stimulated side; the cold stimulus produces a nystagmus to the opposite side. The speed of the slow phase of the post-caloric nystagmus is measured, and the responses are approximately the same for these patients.

Patients with abnormal vestibular responses may show *hyporeflexia*, when one of the ears presents smaller responses, both for the warm and the cold stimulation, or *directional preponderance*, when the nystagmus in one direction is larger than that of the opposite direction, regardless of the temperature of the stimulus. Directional preponderance is attributed to a latent spontaneous nystagmus.

In patients with *areflexia*, either unilateral or bilateral, a stronger stimulus is used: water at 18° C or air at 10° C. Patients with bilateral areflexia that do not respond to these colder stimuli may have bilateral loss of vestibular function, but this diagnosis requires the presence of marked disequilibrium, no responses in high-frequency rotatory stimulation and no responses in the video head impulse test [24].

Hyperreflexia, or unusually intense responses, is common in patients with metabolic inner ear disorders, deriving from changes in the density of endolymph. It may be central in some cases, but in these patients, there are other indications of central disorders.

The findings in caloric tests that are indicative of central lesions are the following [25]:

1. Absence of the fixation effect in the post-caloric responses.
2. Absence of the fast component of the nystagmus – this characterizes a bulbopontine lesion involving the reticular formation.

3. Perverted nystagmus – the post-caloric nystagmus is vertical or oblique, rather than horizontal; this results from a partial destruction of the vestibular nuclei.
4. Inverted nystagmus – rarer than the perverted nystagmus but also resulting from a partial lesion of the vestibular nuclei.
5. Cochleovestibular dissociation – this is a rare condition in which a patient with total disequilibrium and many neurological symptoms presents normal hearing and complete absence of vestibular responses; it is caused by a complete destruction of the vestibular nuclei. The condition is rare because it rapidly leads to the patient's death.

The Video Head Impulse Test: vHIT

The head impulse test (HIT) was described in 1988 by Halmagyi and Curthoys [26], initially as a simple bedside test of the VOR function. It consists of observing the patient's eyes as the head is rotated using small-amplitude, high-velocity, and high-acceleration movements. These movements stimulate the phasic receptor cells in the crista of one of the lateral semicircular canals, the contralateral one being inhibited by the quick movement, of the order of 200°/s. Aw et al. [27] verified that with the patient's head in different positions, it was possible to investigate each of the six semicircular canals. It was then demonstrated that the reliability and sensitivity of the test were improved when the eye movements were recorded [28]. The video head impulse test (vHIT) is easier to interpret, particularly in relation to the vertical canals.

A special chapter will deal extensively to vHIT, which is now the most important part of the vestibular laboratory tests.

Vestibular-Evoked Myogenic Potentials: VEMPs

VEMPs are short-latency electromyographic potentials that are evoked in response to loud acoustic sounds. It is now known that the VEMPs originate in the vestibular system, since they disappear after the section of the vestibular nerves but is still present in patients with profound hearing loss [29, 30].

The electrodes are most frequently placed on the neck, over the sternocleidomastoid muscles, cervical VEMP or cVEMP, and the extraocular eye muscles, ocular VEMP or oVEMP. The cVEMP responses originate from the sacculus, the oVEMP ones from the utricle. It should be noted that before the advent of the vestibular myogenic potentials, the utricle and the saccule could only be studied by complex linear acceleration systems available only in a few research centers.

The sound stimuli for the VEMPs are usually clicks or tone bursts, delivered by air conduction or bone conduction. Bone-conducted stimuli are particularly useful in patients with mechanical hearing loss, but it must be noted that they stimulate both sides.

The cVEMP recordings require a contraction of the sternocleidomastoid muscle. Certain head positions (head turned away from the ear being tested or elevated) generate better responses. For the oVEMPs the patient is asked to raise the head approximately 30°.

Figures 2 and 3 show the central pathways for these potentials.

The following parameters are employed for the interpretation of the responses [1]:

Latencies The latencies of P_1 or N_1 are affected by the type of stimulus (click or tone burst and stimulus frequency) but are not influenced by the stimulus intensity. Abnormal latencies have been reported in some otologic diseases, but most of the time, they are seen in patients with central vestibular disorders, particularly in multiple sclerosis. As a rule, the latencies are not as clinically useful as other parameters

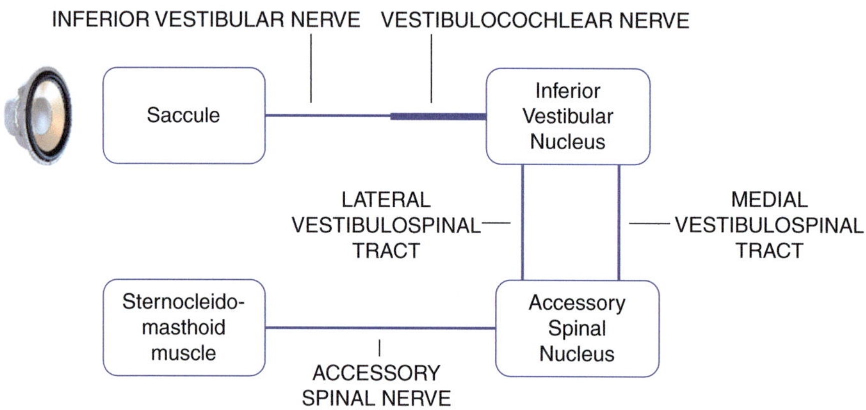

Fig. 2 Pathways of the cVEMP

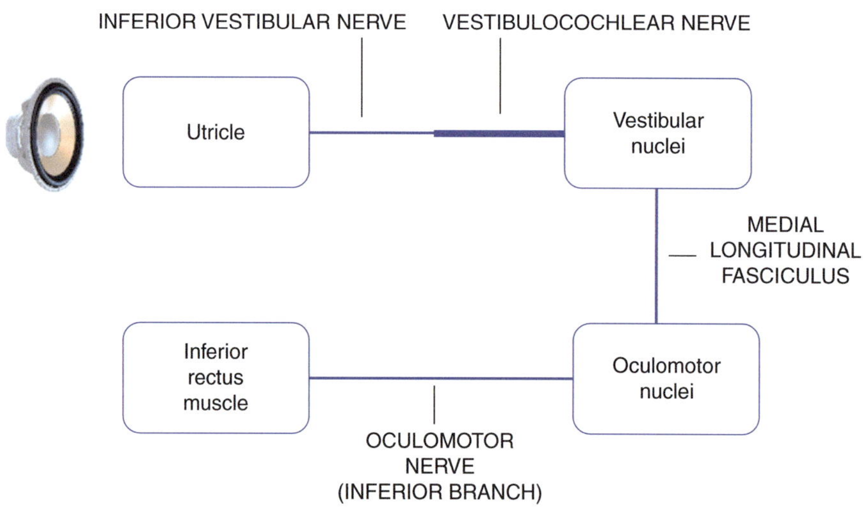

Fig. 3 Pathways of the oVEMP

Amplitudes These are usually defined as the difference between the averaged levels of P_1 and N_1. They may vary from a few μv to 300 μv, or more, for the cVEMPs; oVEMP's amplitudes are usually smaller. The oVEMP's responses are affected by the gaze direction, the stronger response being obtained at the 30° upward gaze.

Asymmetry This is usually defined as the difference between the amplitude of each side divided by their sum. Values of 35–40% are considered clinically significant. In patients with vestibular neuritis or vestibular schwannoma, VEMPs can identify the involved branch of the vestibular nerve. About half of the patients with Menière's disease have abnormal VEMP asymmetries.

Thresholds This is the minimal sound intensity that produces a response. In cases of suspected superior canal dehiscence, the thresholds are more useful than the amplitude or asymmetry. Low thresholds (less than 80 dB HL) are considered abnormal and are found in all patients that complain of symptoms resulting from loud sounds, particularly the Tullio phenomenon.

Comments

During many years the clinical evaluation of the vestibular system relied on the studies of the spontaneous, gaze, and optokinetic nystagmus, rotatory tests, and caloric tests.

The advent of the video head impulse test and the VEMP tests brought the possibility of evaluating of all of the vestibular sensory organs – the receptors of the six semicircular canals and of both utricles and saccules; furthermore, the studies of the saccadic eye movements brought new neurophysiological information on the vestibular oculomotor reflexes.

These new neurophysiological data suggest that in the near future, the clinical evaluation of the vestibular organs will depend essentially on the study of the nystagmus, saccades, vHIT, and VEMPs, leaving rotatory and caloric tests to a smaller number of special cases.

References

1. Barin K. Interpretação dos Testes de Função Vestibular – Tendências Futuras. In: Zuma e Maia FC, Mangabeira-Albernaz PL, Carmona S, editors. Otoneurologia atual. Rio de Janeiro: Revinter; 2014. p. 199–231.
2. Cohen B, Henn V. Unit activity in the pontine reticular formation associated with eye movements. Brain Res. 1972;46:403–10.
3. Henriksson NG. Speed of the slow component and duration in caloric nystagmus. Acta Otolaryngol Suppl. 1956;125:1–29.
4. Henriksson NG. An electrical method for registration and analysis of the movements of the eyes in nystagmus. Acta Otolaryngol. 1955;45(1):25–41.

5. Aschan G, Bergstedt M, Stahle J. Nystagmography: recording of nystagmus in clinical neuro-otological examinations. Acta Otolaryngol Suppl. 1956;129:1–103.
6. Pansini M, Padovan I. Three derivations in electronystagmography. Acta Otolaryngol. 1969;67:303–9.
7. Mangabeira-Albernaz PL, Ganança MM, Caovilla HH, et al. Atlas de Vecto-Electronistagmografia. São Paulo: Aché; 1984.
8. Vitte E, Sémont A, Freyss G, Soudant J. Videonystagmoscopy: its use in the clinical vestibular laboratory. Acta Otolaryngol Suppl. 1995;520(Pt 2):423–6.
9. Pietkiewicz P, Pepas R, Sulkowski WJ, Zielinska-Blizniewska H, Olszewski J. Electronystagmography versus videonystagmography in diagnosis of vertigo. Int J Occup Med Environ Health. 2012;25(1):59–65. https://doi.org/10.2478/s13382-012-0002-1.
10. Zuma e Maia FC, Carmona S, Costa SS. Avaliação clínica do paciente vertiginoso. In: Zuma e Maia FC, Mangabeira-Albernaz PL, Carmona S, editors. Otoneurologia atual. Rio de Janeiro: Revinter; 2014. p. 25–51.
11. Albertino S, Albertino RS. Videonistagmografia. In: Zuma e Maia FC, Mangabeira-Albernaz PL, Carmona S, editors. Otoneurologia atual. Rio de Janeiro: Revinter; 2014. p. 147–65.
12. Wong AMF. Eye movement disorders. New York: Oxford University Press; 2008.
13. Yacovino DA. Neurociência dos Movimentos Oculares no Envelhecimento e nas Doenças Neurológicas. In: Zuma e Maia FC, Mangabeira-Albernaz PL, Carmona S, editors. Otoneurologia atual. Rio de Janeiro: Revinter; 2014. p. 53–68.
14. Leigh RJ, Zee DS. The neurology of eye movements. New York: Oxford University Press; 2006.
15. Zee DS. Internuclear ophthalmoplegia: pathophysiology and diagnosis. Baillière's Clin Neurol. 1992;1(2):455–70.
16. Mangabeira-Albenaz PL. Cadeira rotatória. In: Zuma e Maia FC, Mangabeira-Albernaz PL, Carmona S, editors. Otoneurologia atual. Rio de Janeiro: Revinter; 2014. p. 167–74.
17. Hawkins JE, Schacht J. Sketches of otohistory – Part 8/; the emergence of vestibular science. Audiol Neurootol. 2005;10:185–90.
18. Hennebert PE. Les réactions vestibulaires aux épreuves rotatoires sinusoidales. Acta Otolaryngol. 1956;46:221–6.
19. Tello A. Habituación vestibular ante los estímulos calóricos repetidos. Rev Otorrinolaringol (Chile). 1961;21:15–25.
20. Kingma H, van de Berg R. Anatomy, physiology, and physics of the peripheral vestibular system. Handb Clin Neurol. 2016;137:1–16. https://doi.org/10.1016/B978-0-444-63437-5.00001-7.
21. Gernandt BE. Vestibular mechanisms. In: Handbook of physiology, section I, neurophysiology, vol. 1. Washington, DC: American Physiological Society; 1959. p. 549–80.
22. Bárány R. Some new methods for functional testing of the vestibular apparatus and the cerebellum. Nobel lecture. Nobelprizeorg 3 Dec 2012. Retrieved from http://www.nobelprize.org/nobel_prizes/medicine/laureates/1914/barany-lecture.html.
23. Fitzgerald G, Hallpike CS. Studies in human vestibular function. I. Observations on directional preponderance ("Nystagmusbereitchaft") of caloric nystagmus resulting from cerebral lesions. Brain. 1942;65:115–37.
24. Mangabeira-Albernaz PL, Cusin FS. The video head impulse test in a case of suspected bilateral loss of vestibular function. Int Arch Otorhinolaryngol. 2015;20:84–6. https://doi.org/10.1055/s-0034-1395999.
25. Mangabeira-Albernaz PL, Ganança MM. Vertigem. 2nd ed. São Paulo: Moderna; 1976.
26. Halmagyi GM, Curthoys IS. A clinical sign of canal paresis. Arch Neurol. 1988;45:737–9.
27. Aw ST, Halmagyi GM, Black RA, Curthoys IS, Yavor RA, Todd MJ. Head impulses reveal loss of individual semicircular canal function. J Vestib Res. 1999;9:173–80.

28. Macdougall HG, McGarvie LA, Halmagyi GM, Curthoys IS, Weber KP. The video Head Impulse Test (vHIT) detects vertical semicircular canal dysfunction. PLoS One. 2013;8(4):e61488. https://doi.org/10.1371/journal.pone.0061488.
29. Welgampola MS, Colebatch JG. Characteristics and clinical applications of vestibular- evoked myogenic potentials. Neurology. 2005;64(10):1682–8.
30. Cal R, Zuma e Maia FC, Araújo MS, Brusco TR. Potenciais Evocados Miogênicos Vestibulares (VEMP). In: Zuma e Maia FC, Mangabeira-Albernaz PL, Carmona S, editors. Otoneurologia atual. Rio de Janeiro: Revinter; 2014. p. 105–19.

The Video Head Impulse Test (vHIT)

In 1988, Halmagyi and Curthoys [1] described a bedside-type examination that was useful to identify uni- or bilateral loss of vestibular function. For this test the examiner executes a quick impulse on the patient's head, with high acceleration, high velocity, and short amplitude. Meanwhile, the patient is asked to maintain his eyes focused on a fixed target that may be the examiner's nose or some mark on the wall of the examination room.

They stated that in a high percentage of cases, the short and quick head movements induce saccadic eye movements and demonstrated that these saccades resulted from the stimulation of phasic receptor cells in the crista of one of the lateral semicircular canals, the contralateral one being inhibited by the quick movement of the order of 200°/s. These physiological principles have been confirmed by other investigators [2].

Aw et al. [3], in 1999, and Halmagyi et al. [4], in 2001, verified that with the patient's head in different positions, it was possible to investigate each of the six semicircular canals.

When the vestibular function is normal, in spite of the high acceleration, the patient is able to maintain his eyes on the target, due to the rotational vestibulo-ocular reflex (r-VOR) – the high-speed connections that link the vestibular organs to the oculomotor muscles. Patients with unilateral vestibular hypofunction will be unable to maintain his eyes on the target, and the examiner will see corrective saccades that represent the patient's attempt to keep the target in his foveae. The presence of this saccadic movement indicates that there is a low r-VOR gain on this side.

Since its original description, this test, known as a head impulse test (HIT), has been used in all the world as an excellent bedside test to diagnose the losses of vestibular function.

HIT has the following important characteristics:

1. It can be done quite quickly and has good specificity when performed by an experienced examiner.

P. L. M. Albernaz et al., *The New Neurotology*,
https://doi.org/10.1007/978-3-030-11283-7_6

2. It tests each of the six semicircular canals, due to the physiological principle that the excitatory vestibular responses are more intense than the inhibitory ones, so that, even with asymmetry in the levels of vestibular stimulation in high speeds, the excitatory response modulates the r-VOR.
3. It may test the vertical semicircular canals, but these tests are more difficult to interpret.

In spite of these characteristics and its worldwide use, HIT has some disadvantages:

1. It requires an experienced examiner, able to identify the presence of corrective saccades; this degree of experience is uncommon in emergency departments' physicians.
2. The sensitivity of the test is approximately 50%.
3. It is difficult to test the vertical semicircular canals.
4. It is a qualitative test; the r-VORs gain cannot be measured.
5. The results cannot be recorded.

In view of these disadvantages, in the last 20 years, there were many attempts to develop a video system that would allow a recording of the results and a mensuration of the r-VOR gains for each of the six semicircular canals. Magnusson et al. [5] in 2002, demonstrated that the reliability and sensitivity of the test were definitely improved by using video-oculography. Several studies [6–15] confirmed and validated the use of the vHIT in neurotological diagnosis.

Commercially available systems, capable to record head and eye movements and calculate r-VOR gain by means of mathematical algorithms, have existed only in the last 6 years.

In order to understand the operation of the video-oculography systems, it is necessary to review the mechanisms involved in the vestibulo-ocular reflex and the saccadic eye movements.

Vestibulo-Ocular Reflex (VOR)

The main function of the vestibulo-ocular reflex (VOR) is to stabilize the image in the retina during rapid head movements. In order to achieve this action, it emits signals to the oculomotor system that give rise to eye movements of the same speed of the head movements but in opposite direction. In other words, VOR produces eye movements that compensate for the head movements.

VOR's reflex arc involves three or four neurons – vestibular ganglion, vestibular nuclei, and oculomotor nuclei – and has special features that enable it to produce very rapid movements that occur, for instance, when we walk, run, or practice sports.

VOR's latency is of approximately 8 ms. This short latency allows for the permanence of the image in the fovea even when the head movements are very rapid. Its frequency varies from 0.5 to 5.0 Hz, and its maximal angular velocity varies from 30 to 150°/s. Ideally this speed should be above 100°/s; for lower speeds other eye movements, like smooth pursuit and optokinetic nystagmus, will help in maintaining the image in the retina.

The output of the vestibular sense organs is transmitted by the fibers of the vestibular nerves to the vestibular nuclei, located at the bulbopontine transition of the floor of the forth ventricle. From the vestibular nuclei, the nerve fibers join the medial longitudinal fasciculus, reaching the nuclei of the oculomotor nerves: oculomotor (cranial nerve III), trochlear (CN IV), and abducens (CN VI). The pathways from each semicircular canal to the corresponding eye muscles can be found in chapter 1.

In order to provide adequate precision to the eye movements, so that they reproduce the head movements in the opposite direction, each semicircular canal stimulates only one specific pair of ocular muscles, so that the eyes move approximately in the same plan of the canal. The cerebellum and the reticular formation are involved in maintaining the precision of the movements.

It must be noted that when one of the semicircular canals yields an excitatory stimulus, the contralateral synergic canal will yield an inhibitory stimulus; the excitatory stimuli will induce a contraction of the corresponding eye muscles, while the inhibitory stimulus will provide a relaxation of the antagonist muscles. VOR, therefore, is a combination of excitatory and inhibitory stimuli, always with a preponderance of the excitatory stimuli over the inhibitory ones, according to Ewald's second law.

Corrective Saccades

A person with an intact vestibular system is capable of maintaining his eyes fixed on a target even when he rotates his head, as a consequence of his normal VOR. On the other hand, a patient with a unilateral vestibular hypofunction will be unable to maintain his eyes on the target when he rotates his head to the malfunctioning side. His eyes will move with the head, and the target's image will leave the fovea until, at the end of the head movement, the eyes will make a voluntary corrective saccade to bring the target back to his visual field.

This corrective saccade is perceived by the examiner when he performs the clinical HIT and is called an *overt saccade*. The presence of an overt saccade is an indirect indication of hypofunction of the semicircular canal ipsilateral to the side of the head rotation.

When the corrective saccade occurs during the head's rotation, it cannot be seen by the examiner. This is called a *covert saccade* and contributes to false-negative results in the clinical HIT tests. Covert saccades are not visible to the human eyes; they can only be observed in video-oculography records.

Saccades are very rapid eye movements, the function of which is to bring the visual stimuli to the foveae. Their latencies are approximately 100 ms, their angular velocity may reach 600°/s, and they are very brief (30 to 100 ms). They are very precise and end abruptly.

Saccades have a central stimulation pathway and their firing stimuli are visual. Visual stimuli are electromagnetic, different from the mechanical vestibular stimuli. For this reason, the saccade's latency is ten times greater than that of the VOR. The mechanisms involved in the production of saccades, as well as the nuclei and pathways, are explained in chapter 1.

Equipment

There are several commercially available video-oculography instruments that can be used to perform the vHIT test. This chapter discusses general principles that do not apply exclusively to any of the existing systems.

Most of the instruments have lightweight glasses, weighing approximately 60 g, a high-speed infrared television camera (250 frames/s), an accelerometer, a gyroscope, and a mirror. The system records the eye movements (both nystagmus and saccades) and provides graphics at the end of the examination. There is also a sensor with nine axes that measures the head movements, so that they can be compared to the eye movements. Two laser dots are projected alternately to calibrate the system.

The glasses are firmly fixed on the patient's head by an elastic band, so that they cannot be displaced during the examination.

There is also a commercially available system that employs a high-precision television camera, situated at a fixed distance from the patient, not making use of glasses.

Examination

The patient is seated at a distance of at least 1.5 m from a target fixed at a wall. Smaller distances may generate vergence movements, impacting on the calculations of the VOR gain. The amount of light in the room must be adjusted to avoid the presence of reflections over the patient's pupil at any point of the head's excursions.

The glasses must be firmly fixed to the patient's head, since any displacement during the examination will cause a *phase-shift* artifact.

A precise calibration is absolutely essential, requiring from the examiner a previous knowledge of the instrument's software.

After the careful placement of the glasses, the instrument's camera will automatically detect the patient's pupil, and its area will be projected in the computer's screen. From this moment on, all eye movements will be recorded. Eye makeup may render the pupil's detection more difficult and may introduce artifacts. Oriental patients, who usually have narrow eyelid clefts, require very careful positioning of the glasses in order to identify the pupil.

The examiner stands behind the patient, placing his hands on the patient's head without touching the glasses.

The head impulses are performed in three different conditions:

1. *To examine the lateral semicircular canals*: The patient's head is rotated quickly to one of the sides. It is convenient to choose left or right rotation at random, so that the patient cannot expect the movement. The amplitude of the movement is approximately 15° to 20°, with a speed of 120 to 150°/s and an acceleration of approximately $3000°/s^2$.
2. *To examine the left anterior and the right posterior semicircular canals (LARP)*: The examiner places his dominant hand on the top of the patient's head and the other hand under his chin. The patient's head is positioned 45° to the right and is quickly moved up and down at random.
3. *To examine the right anterior and the left posterior semicircular canals (RALP)*: The examiner places his dominant hand on the top of the patient's head and the other hand under his chin. The patient's head is positioned 45° to the left and is quickly moved up and down at random.

For each part of the examination, the patient has to maintain his eyes on the target all the time.

For the vertical canals, the amplitude of the movements shall be approximately 15° to 20°, with a speed of 100 to 200°/s and the same high acceleration of about $3000°/s^2$.

vHIT Parameters

Gain

Gain is the ratio between the eye speed and the head speed. In patients with normal vestibular function, VOR gains vary from 0.8 to 1.0. It is important to know that if the speed of the impulses is less than 120°/s, other oculomotor systems will get involved and the measure of the VOR gain will be compromised.

Corrective Saccades

When the VOR gain is smaller than 0.8, the quick head rotation will make the patient's eye loose the fixed target, and that gives origin to a corrective saccade, in the opposite direction of the head's rotation, to bring the target back to the fovea.

When corrective saccades are seen in the examination graphics, they must be analyzed for their *consistency*, that is, whether they are present in most of the impulses.

They are two types of corrective saccades. The *overt* or *catch-up* saccades occur immediately after the head's rotation, with a latency of 100 ms or less after the end of the impulse. A trained observer can easily identify them in the HIT.

The *covert* saccades appear during the head impulse and cannot be identified in the HIT tests; they are, however, identified with the vHIT.

The direction of the saccades must coincide with the slow phase of the VOR. Inverted saccades are suggestive of central vestibular disorders; they may happen, however, when the patient loses his attention during the examination and stops looking at the target.

Clinical Applications

vHIT is presently an essential part of the laboratory vestibular examination for patients with a suspected acute or chronic vestibular disorder. A reduced VOR gain and/or the presence of corrective saccades leads to the diagnosis of a vestibular hypofunction. The test provides a quantitative evaluation of the six semicircular canals and information concerning the VOR.

There are many differences between the vHIT and the caloric tests that for many years have been the only test capable of examining the ears separately. These differences are shown in Table 1.

The main indications to vHIT are the following:

Table 1 Characteristics of the vHIT and the Caloric Tests

vHIT	Caloric tests
Investigates all three semicircular canals	Investigate only the lateral canals
Performed rapidly	Require 20 minutes or more to be performed
Well tolerated	Uncomfortable
Tests the vestibular organs in high frequency (optimal working range)	Test the vestibular organs in low frequency (below working range)
Little influenced by medications	Influenced by many types of medications
No influence from external and middle ear anatomy	Very influenced by external and middle ear anatomy
Repeated tests control the patient's evolution	Repeated tests show too many variations
May be applied to all patients	May not be performed, or not tolerated, by many patients
May be used in acute vestibular disorders and as a bedside test	Usually performed after the disease's acute phase
Small and portable equipment	Large equipment, usually not portable

1. It helps in the differentiation of peripheral and central vestibular disorders, alone or as a part of the HINTS protocol (the HINTS protocol is detailed in chapter 4.
2. It allows a mensuration and follow-up of the vestibular function in patients that will be submitted to treatments potentially ototoxic, like intratympanic gentamicin or some chemotherapeutic medications.
3. Pre- and postoperative monitoring for patients submitted to cochlear implant surgery, to prevent bilateral loss of vestibular function.

For Menière's disease, vHIT results are not consistent. This is probably due to the clinical variableness of the disease in relation to the severity and duration of the symptoms and association with other pathologies, such as vestibular migraine and benign paroxysmal positional vertigo (BPPV). The caloric tests show a larger number of alterations in Menière's disease than the vHIT, but it has been recently demonstrated that the changes in the caloric tests may derive from a reduction of convective fluid movement due to the endolymphatic hydrops and does not represent an actual change in vestibular function [16, 17].

In patients with vestibular migraine, abnormal vHIT responses are found in 9% to 12% of the cases [18, 19]. In patients with BPPV, it would be expected to obtain normal vHIT responses, since it is, from a pathophysiologic point of view, a mechanical disorder. In one study that included 14 patients with BPPV, vHIT was normal in 12 (85%) [20].

vHIT Artifacts

Artifacts are errors that appear in some graphic representations of a test result, due to different factors; they must be recognized so that they will not affect the interpretation and the clinical decisions. Errors in the vHIT results may happen for the following reasons [21]:

1. *Artifacts related to the equipment*: When the glasses are not properly fixed to the head by the elastic band, a small inertial displacement may occur during the impulses. This will cause a false increase in the VOR's gain or may cause a VOR phase change.
2. *Artifacts related to the examiner*: The examiner without experience in the clinical HIT may find some difficulties in moving the patient's head at speed greater than 150°/s, particularly for the impulses related to the vertical canals (RALP and LARP). This may render a false normal result. The inadequate head position, with wrong angles, for the vertical canal tests will result in abnormally low VOR gains.
3. *Artifacts related to the patient*: Excessive makeup, or ophthalmological situations that result in a difficult identification of the pupil, may cause many different artifacts, in particular the loss of the pupillary track.

The SHIMP Test

This test called *suppression head impulse paradigm,* or SHIMP, is a derivative of the vHIT test, described in 2016 [22].

The patient is instructed to focus on a target that moves with his head. When the vestibular function is normal, the slow phase of the VOR directs his eyes in the opposite direction during the head impulse, and this requires an *anti-saccade* in the direction of the target and in the opposite direction of the VOR.

In patients with unilateral or bilateral vestibular hypofunction, due to reduced or absent VOR, the eyes will not be directed in the opposite direction to the head impulse, and therefore only small amplitude anti-saccades will occur or will be totally absent.

The SHIMP test assures the examiner of the VOR gains seen in the vHIT. The other important contribution of this test is that the presence of the anti-saccade is a significant indication of residual vestibular function.

Conclusion

The vHIT is a valuable method to evaluate patients with acute and chronic vestibular disorders. It requires, however, an understanding of the neurophysiology of the vestibular system, as well as an adequate experience with the instruments employed in order to avoid artifacts.

It is quite useful to evaluate vertiginous patients in emergency departments, being an important part of the HINTS protocol.

References

1. Halmagyi GM, Curthoys IS. A clinical sign of canal paresis. Arch Neurol. 1988;45:737–9.
2. Wuyts F. Principle of the head impulse (thrust) test or Halmagyi head thrust test. B-ENT. 2008;4:23–5.
3. Aw ST, Halmagyi GM, Black RA, Curthoys IS, Yavor RA, Todd MJ. Head impulses reveal loss of individual semicircular canal function. J Vestib Res. 1999;9:173–80.
4. Halmagyi GM, Aw ST, Cremer PD, Curthoys IS, Todd MJ. Impulsive testing of individual semicircular canal function. Ann N Y Acad Sci. 2001;942:192–200.
5. Magnuson M, Karlberg K, Halmagyi M, et al. The video-impulse test enhances the possibility of detecting vestibular lesions. J Vest Res. 2002;11:241–4.
6. Halmagyi GM, Black RA, Thurtell MJ, Curthoys IS. The human horizontal vestibulo-ocular reflex in response to active and passive head impulses after unilateral vestibular differentiation. Ann N Y Acad Sci. 2003;1004:325–36.
7. Black RA, Halmagyi GM, Thurtell MJ, Todd MJ, Curthoys IS. The active head-impulse test in unilateral peripheral vestibulopathy. Arch Neurol. 2005;62:290–3.
8. Ulmer E, Chays A. Curthoys and Halmagyi head impulse test: an analytical device. Ann Otolaryngol Chir Cervicofac. 2005;122:84–90.

9. Weber KP, Aw ST, Todd MJ, McGarvie LA, Curthoys IS, Halmagyi GM. Head impulse test in unilateral vestibular loss: vestibulo-ocular reflex and catch-up saccades. Neurology. 2008;70:454–63.
10. Weber KP, Aw ST, Todd MJ, McGarvie LA, Curthoys IS, Halmagyi GM. Horizontal head impulse test detects gentamicin vestibulotoxicity. Neurology. 2009;72:1417–24.
11. Weber KP, MacDougall HG, Halmagyi GM, Curthoys IS. Impulsive testing of semicircular-canal function using video-oculography. Ann N Y Acad Sci. 2009;1164:486–91.
12. Kaźmierczak H, Pawlak-Osin'ska K, Kaźmierczak W. The value of the Halmagyi-Curthoys test in neurological diagnostic procedures. Otolaryngol Pol. 2009;63:364–7.
13. MacDougall HG, Weber KP, McGarvie LA, Halmagyi GM, Curthoys IS. The video head impulse test: diagnostic accuracy in peripheral vestibulopathy. Neurology. 2009;73:1134–41.
14. Olszewski J, Pietkiewicz P, Milonski J, Bielinska M. The use of VHIT (videonystagmography head impulse test) in the diagnostics of semicircular canal injuries. Otolaryngol Pol. 2010;64:32–5.
15. Curthoys IS. The interpretation of clinical tests of peripheral vestibular function. Laryngoscope. 2012;122:1342–52.
16. Welgampola MS, Akdal G, Halmagyi GM. Neuro-otology – some recent clinical advances. J Neurol. 2017;264:188–203. https://doi.org/10.1007/s00415-016-8266-1.
17. Choi JE, Kim Y-K, Young SC, Lee K, Park HW, Yoon SH, Kim H-J, Chung W-H. Morphological correlation between caloric tests and vestibular hydrops in Ménière's disease using intravenous Gd enhanced inner ear MRI. PLoS One. 2017;12(11):e0188301. https://doi.org/10.1371/journal.pone.0188301.
18. Blödow A, Heinze M, Bloching MB, von Brevern M, Radtke A, Lempert T. Caloric stimulation and video-head impulse testing in Ménière's disease and vestibular migraine. Acta Otolaryngol. 2014;134(12):1239–44. https://doi.org/10.3109/00016489.2014.939300.
19. Yuan Q, Zhang Y, Liu DL, Zhang XL, Zhang QF. Vestibular function tests for vestibular migraine: clinical implication of video head impulse and caloric tests. Lin Chung Er Bi Yan Hou Tou Jing Wai Ke Za Zhi. 2017;31(13):984–7. https://doi.org/10.13201/j.issn.1001-1781.2017.13.003.
20. Mangabeira Albernaz PL, Zuma e Maia FC. The video head impulse test. Acta Otolaryngol. 2014;134:1245–50. https://doi.org/10.3109/00016489.2014.942439.
21. Mantokoudis G, Saber Tehrani AS, Kattah JC, Eibenberger K, Guede CI, Zee DS, et al. Quantifying the vestibulo-ocular reflex with video-oculography: nature and frequency of artifacts. Audiol Neurootol. 2015;20(1):39–50. https://doi.org/10.1159/000362780.
22. MacDougall HG, McGarvie LA, Halmagyi GM, Rogers SJ, Manzari L, Burgess AM, Curthoys IS, Weber KP. A new saccadic indicator of peripheral vestibular function based on the video head impulse test. Neurology. 2016;87(4):410–8. https://doi.org/10.1212/WNL.0000000000002827.

The Role of Audiology in Neurotology

The word *audiology* was coined by Hallowell Davis to distinguish this discipline from *otology*. Both otology and audiology deal with the ear, but in a totally different manner.

Surprisingly, audiology was not born in the area of medicine. For many years it stayed in the realm of telephone engineers and experimental psychologists, and most of its basic principles were established in the Bell Telephone Laboratories. In order to build telephones, there was a practical need to know how the ear worked and which frequencies were necessary for the word messages to be understood. And at that time physicians did not have this information. The tuning fork tests that they employed were of no help for those needs.

Initially the audiological studies followed the "black box" principles of experimental psychology, employing different stimuli and observing the corresponding responses. How the "black box" worked was of no concern.

Audiology came to medicine at the time of the fenestration operation. This was a procedure pioneered by Gunnar Holmgren, in Sweden, and Maurice Sourdille, in France, and perfected by Julius Lempert in the United States. It consisted of making a new "window" for the sound to get into the inner ear, and it was indicated for patients that had their oval windows blocked by otosclerotic bone. Lempert, however, never used audiological tests; he just asked his patients whether they were hearing better. But Theodore Walsh, in Saint Louis, and George Shambaugh Jr., in Chicago, began to test their patients [1, 2]. Walsh was close to the Central Institute for the Deaf and asked Hallowell Davis to establish a protocol to test his patients. Shambaugh had the help of the new Experimental Psychology group in Northwestern University. Both of them contributed to establish the indications and limits of the procedure and to improve the results. Gradually all otologists began to employ audiological tests that became mandatory in otology, and its contributions became increasingly important.

Medicine added neurophysiology to audiology, abandoning the "black box" principles. This led to important developments, such as supraliminary tests, immittance tests, otoacoustic emissions, and electrical responses. These different tests will be considered separately.

P. L. M. Albernaz et al., *The New Neurotology*,
https://doi.org/10.1007/978-3-030-11283-7_7

The inner ear is a unit that uses its ciliated cells to respond both to sound and accelerations. In spite of possessing different types of cells to exert different functions, they share the same fluids, the same arteries, the same veins, and the same type of complex innervation. Many of the disorders of the inner ear, therefore, involve both auditory and vestibular changes, which makes audiology an important area in neurotology.

Basic Audiological Tests

Classical audiology deals with four basic dimensions: thresholds, discrimination, recruitment of loudness, and adaptation.

Thresholds

The word *threshold* that designates a piece of wood or stone placed beneath a door is used in audiology to represent the line that must be reached to elicit a response, or, in other words, the minimal amount of energy that results in a response. Thresholds are usually obtained for tones and for human voice.

The thresholds for tones may use pure tones of different frequencies, or warble tones, which are frequency-modulated. Warble tones are useful when testing patients that complain of tinnitus, who sometimes have difficulty in responding to pure tones of frequencies similar to their tinnitus. The thresholds for the human voice usually employ two-syllable familiar words.

The early investigators already had a reliable unit for frequencies, the Hertz (Hz), equivalent to one cycle per second. But they had to create a unit for sound pressure, which is related to intensity. The human ear has a very large dynamic range in terms of sound intensities. The ratio of a sound capable of causing inner ear damage to a sound at threshold is approximately 1 trillion. For this reason, they decided to create a logarithmic unit, the Bel, named in honor of Alexander Graham Bell. The Bel proved to be too large for practical use, and the decibel (dB) became the widely used unit for sound pressure.

Logarithmic scales only express ratios, so the value of 20 microPascals (μPa) was established as a zero for physical reference. This decibel is named decibel sound pressure level (dB SPL).

The thresholds for pure tones in persons with normal hearing were first obtained by Sivian and White at the Bell Telephone Laboratories [3]. They found that the normal ear responded to frequencies of 16–16,000 Hz, but the thresholds for different frequencies were different. The ear was found to be more sensitive to frequencies of 1000–4000 Hz and less sensitive to lower and higher frequencies, the thresholds of which are higher, requiring more energy.

Some primitive electronic instruments to measure hearing have been built since 1903. The first modern-type audiometer, however, was created by Edmund P. Fowler, an otologist, and physicists Harvey Fletcher and Robert Wegel in 1922, employing frequencies at octave intervals. They also introduced the words *audiometry* and *audiogram*.

The audiometers do not use the physical sound pressure level as reference; the zero for each frequency is the respective threshold for normal ears. The decibel used in audiometers is referred as *decibel hearing level* (dB HL).

Air and Bone Conduction

The nineteenth-century otologists, using tuning forks, defined two types of hearing loss, *conduction hearing loss* and *perception hearing loss*, and devised different types of tests (Schwabach's, Rinne's, Weber's, Gellé's, and Bing's tests) to reach these diagnoses. Most of these tests originated in the 1880s. Their proposers had the notion that in bone conduction the sounds reached the inner ear directly, bypassing the external and middle ears.

This is not true. Bárány [4] and Békésy [5] demonstrated that the ossicles play an important part in bone conduction.

There are two basic mechanisms involved. One is the inertia of the ossicular chain. Particularly in low frequencies, the tuning fork makes the skull vibrate as a whole. This implies on a movement of the skull while the ossicles remain stationary, which results in inner ear stimulation in the same way that we normally hear, with the skull stationary and the ossicles moving. The other mechanism is compression. For higher frequencies the vibration of the skull creates alternately compressed and expanded portions. When the labyrinth is compressed, the larger amount of endolymph connected to the scala vestibuli (which includes the semicircular canals) creates a movement in the direction of the round window, resulting in a sound stimulation. Both inertial and compression mechanisms work together all the time, although the proportion of their actions will vary with the sound frequency. In a patient with a fixed stapes footplate, the inertial component disappears, but the compression component is increased by the inability of the endolymph to move the stapes.

One problem with bone conduction audiometric tests is that there is no radiating energy to be measured. For the early audiometers, the audiometric zeros for bone conduction were obtained by testing three or four normal hearing persons; afterward an *artificial mastoid* was developed in order to achieve this calibration.

But what is the energy level of the bone-conducted sound? It has been observed that most animals have a special system for reducing the intensity of the bone-conducted sounds, so that they do not interfere with the air-conducted ones. Without this rejection, the human voice would sound extremely loud, as well as the noises while chewing. One exception is the serpent, that has its body close to the soil and uses bone conduction to listen to soil-transmitted sounds.

Zwislocki [6] made a study of human bone conduction in free fields and concluded that the bone conduction thresholds are approximately 60 dB higher than those of the air conduction. This number matches the maximum amount of decibels observed in patients with air-bone gaps. It also explains why audiometers are capable of emitting sounds up to 120 dB in most frequencies, while the maximal stimuli for bone conduction do not exceed 75 dB. The frequency range of the bone conduction thresholds that can be obtained with precision is from 500 to 4000 Hz, while air conduction thresholds are obtained from 250 to 8000 Hz.

Types of Hearing Loss

Presently we prefer to use the expressions *mechanical hearing loss* and *sensorineural hearing loss*, rather than conductive and perception loss. For the mechanical losses, the bone conduction thresholds are lower than those of the air conduction losses and usually normal or close to normal. For sensorineural losses the air and bone thresholds are essentially the same.

Sometimes there is a combination of mechanical and sensorineural elements, configuring a *mixed hearing loss*, in which the bone conduction thresholds are lower than the air conduction ones but are not normal. We now know that mechanical and mixed hearing losses may originate in the inner ear.

Figures 1, 2, and 3 show typical audiograms with mechanical, sensorineural, and mixed hearing loss. Normal thresholds are up to 25 dB, and socially normal thresholds are up to 40 dB for frequencies 500, 1000, 1500, and 2000 Hz.

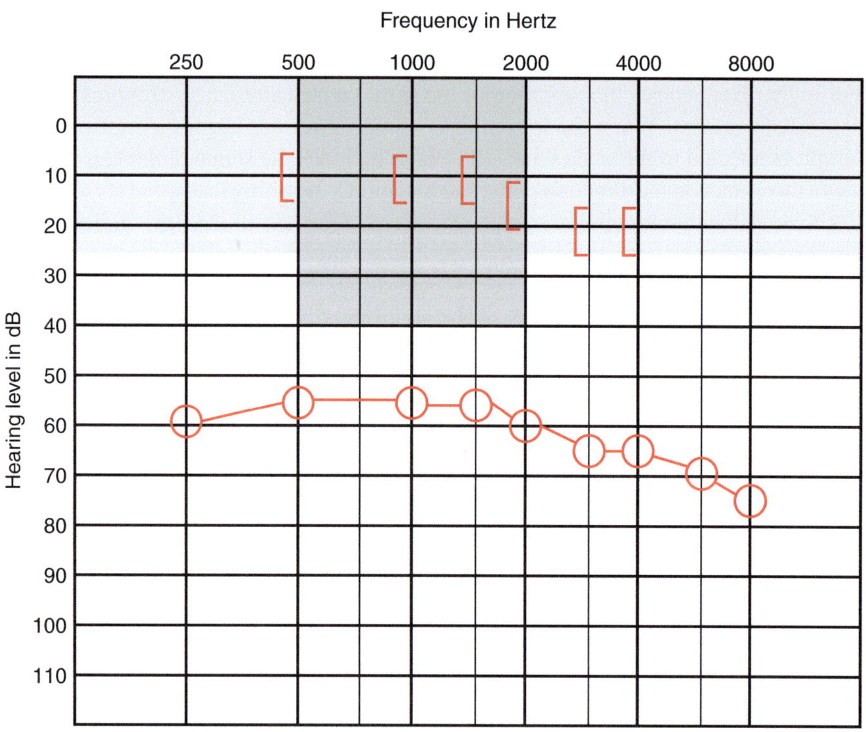

Fig. 1 Audiogram of a patient with a mechanical hearing loss. For the sake of clarity, only the thresholds of the left ear were represented. The symbol **O** represents the right ear air conduction thresholds. The symbol [represents the right ear air conduction thresholds

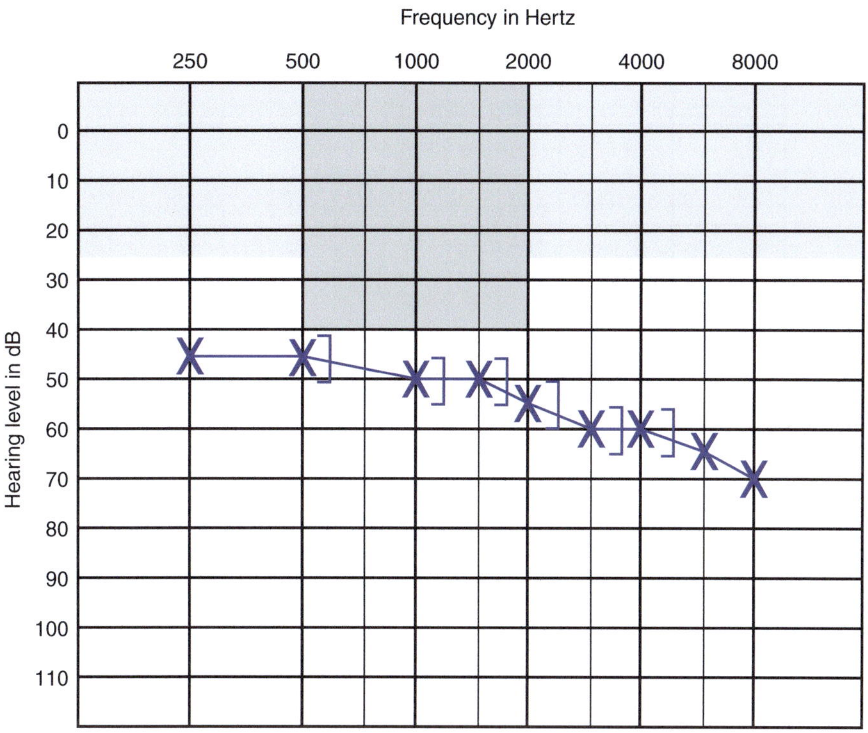

Fig. 2 Audiogram of a patient with a sensorineural hearing loss. For the sake of clarity, only the thresholds of the right ear were represented. The symbol **X** represents the left ear air conduction thresholds. The symbol **]** represents the left ear air conduction thresholds

Discrimination

Theoretically the word *discrimination* relates to the ability to distinguish different sounds. We can use it to measure distinction between different frequencies or between different intensities. Most of the time, however, we use the word in reference to *speech discrimination*, that is, the ability to understand words. The capacity of the human ear to analyze vocal sounds in fact includes the ability to distinguish different frequencies and intensities.

It has been demonstrated that the most difficult speech discrimination tests are those employing isolated monosyllables. Disyllables are a little easier, and sentences are used as the easiest tests. There are recorded words of phonetically balanced words and sentences lists that are presented to the patients so that they can repeat them. In situations of intense or profound losses, these tests can be performed as a *closed set* – the patient can see the sentences or word lists. These tests are often used for patients submitted to cochlear implants. For the *open set* tests that are more commonly used, the patient has no previous knowledge of the words in the list.

The open set tests with isolated monosyllables, or with isolated meaningless monosyllables, being the most difficult, are the most important for the audiological diagnosis.

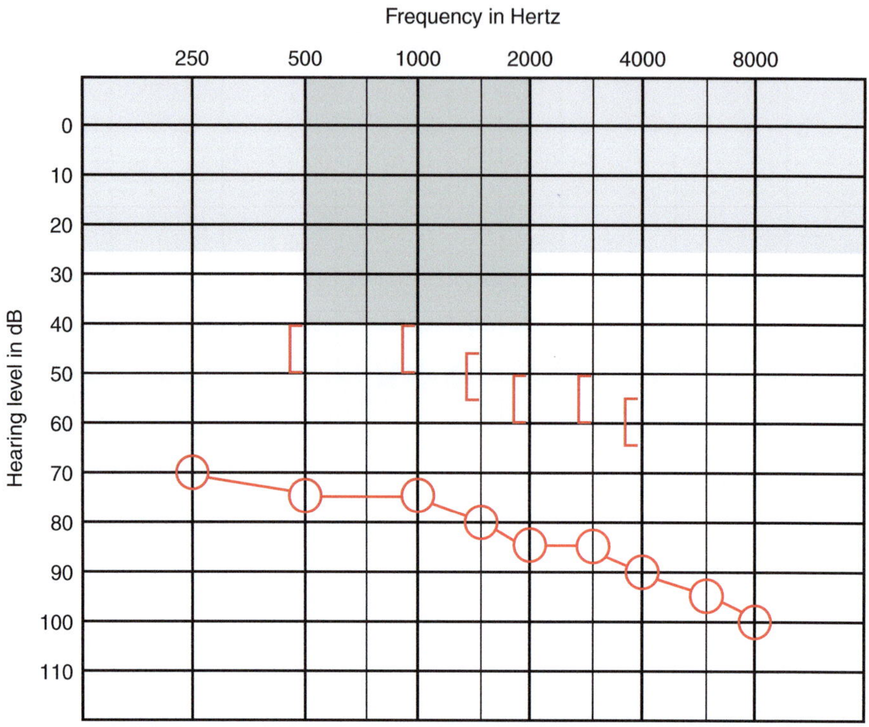

Fig. 3 Audiogram of a patient with a mixed hearing loss. For the sake of clarity, only the thresholds of the right ear were represented. The symbol **O** represents the right ear air conduction thresholds. The symbol **[** represents the right ear air conduction thresholds

Recruitment of Loudness

This is a phenomenon characterized by an abnormal growth of the sensation of loudness in relation to the physical increase in intensity. A patient with recruitment may not hear a low-intensity sound but will perceive a high-intensity sound as being very loud. This was described in 1928 by Fowler [7], and the name was suggested by Lorente de Nó, who felt that the high-intensity sound would "recruit" more nerve fibers to be transmitted to the higher centers.

Patients with Menière's disease usually have intense recruitment. Dix, Hallpike, and Hood [8], in 1948, suggested the use of recruitment tests to differentiate between Menière's disease and vestibular schwannomas. Actually, the phenomenon is usually absent in large tumors, but it may be present in small intrameatal tumors.

In patients with unilateral hearing loss, the recruitment may be measured by the loudness balance test described by Fowler. In patients with bilateral hearing loss, it may be identified by measuring the difference limen for intensity, that is, the smaller intensity difference that the patient is able to identify. The SISI test (short increment sensitivity index), proposed by Jerger [9], uses a fixed intensity difference that is identified only by patients with recruitment and has been extensively used for the measurement of recruitment before the advent of the immittance tests.

Adaptation

Neural adaptation, or sensory adaptation, is a change over time in the response of a sensory system to a stimulus.

There are two kinds of adaptation. Fast adaptation occurs immediately after the presentation of the stimulus; slow adaptation may take minutes, hours, or even days. These two types of adaptation depend on different physiological mechanisms.

The amount of adaptation in the normal human ear is very small, but it may become significant in patients with central auditory disorders. A simple clinical test for abnormal adaptation is the *tone decay test*, in which a pure tone is maintained for a period of 1 minute [10]. Normally the patient continues to hear the tone; in the presence of pathological adaptation, the audiologist has to increase the intensity of the tone one or more times so that it continues to be heard.

Immittance Tests

The middle ear is essentially an impedance transformer, so the concept of performing impedance tests became a significant area of research. Zwislocki made a major contribution by designing an acoustic impedance bridge [11]. This instrument, however, was later replaced by Terkildsen's electroacoustic bridge [12] that is simpler to use.

Since the bridge tests both impedance and admittance (the inverse of impedance), the word *immittance* was adopted in relation to these tests.

In addition to the measure of immittance, these tests include tympanometric curves that evaluate the air pressure in middle ear space and the thresholds of the tympanic reflexes. Metz, in 1952 [13], demonstrated that the thresholds of the reflex contractions of muscles of the middle ear were directly related to recruitment of loudness. At present the immittance tests are almost always the only tests performed to estimate recruitment. In normal patients the thresholds of the tympanic reflexes are 70–90 dB higher than the respective tonal thresholds. For the recruiting ears, the levels are lower.

Mechanical hearing losses interfere with the tympanic reflexes. They cannot be recorded when the air conduction thresholds are 40 dB or greater in the ear contralateral to the instrument's probe and 5 dB or greater in the side of the probe.

Since the stapedius muscle is innervated by a branch of the facial nerve, its contraction does not occur in the respective side in a patient with facial paralysis.

The early electroacoustic bridges could also be used to test adaptation, but the recently built ones that perform the tests automatically do not allow the use of longer stimulation times.

Otoacoustic Emissions

Otoacoustic emissions are sounds generated in the inner ear that are picked up by an especially calibrated microphone and recorded. They were first demonstrated by Kemp [14] in 1978, and it has been verified that these sounds result from the contractions of the external hair cells of the cochlea. These emissions may be spontaneous, but the significant audiological observations are those obtained with sound stimuli.

The primary purpose of otoacoustic emission tests is to determine cochlear status, specifically hair cell function. This information can be used to screen hearing (particularly in neonates, infants, or individuals with developmental disabilities) and differentiate between the sensory and neural components of sensorineural hearing loss. This information can even be obtained from comatose patients, because no behavioral response is required.

There are two basic types of otoacoustic emissions recorded with acoustic stimulation:

(a) Transient otoacoustic emissions: these are the emissions that result from acoustic stimuli of very short duration (clicks or tone bursts).
(b) Distortion product otoacoustic emissions: these are the emissions that result from two simultaneous tones of different frequencies.

It has been found that distortion product otoacoustic emissions provide more information for detecting mild hearing loss in high frequencies.

Transient otoacoustic emissions are the basis of a simple test for hearing defects in newborn babies, and many countries now have programs for the universal hearing screening of neonates. The probability of hearing defects in babies with normal external hair cells is very small, but there are rare disorders of the inner hair cells and higher centers in the auditory system – *auditory neuropathy* – for which the normal results of the screening tests will be misleading.

Electrical Response Audiometry

Hallowell Davis was the father of the electrical response audiometry [15, 16]. In addition to his many previous studies, he also pioneered the use of computers for averaging cortical auditory responses, and gradually other tests were developed. Davis always felt that these responses were not actually "evoked"; he merely called them "electrical responses." The word "evoked," however, is now frequently employed.

Table 1 Potentials evoked in the auditory system

Site of origin	Normal latencies
Cochlea (hair cells)	
Cochlear microphonics	0
Summating potential	0
Auditory nerve	
Eighth nerve action potential – wave I	2.0 ms
Brainstem	
Wave II – eighth nerve	3.0 ms
Wave III – cochlear nuclei	4.1 ms
Wave IV – lateral lemniscus	5.3 ms
Wave V – inferior colliculus	5.9 ms
Middle latencies	
N_0	8–10 ms
P_0	13 ms
N_a	22 ms
P_a	34 ms
N_b	44 ms
Vertex potential – auditory cortex	
P_1	50 ms (variable)
N_1	90 ms
P_2	180 ms
N_2	250 ms
P_{300}	300 ms

Table 1 shows the most frequently used evoked response auditory tests.

Electrocochleography

Electrocochleography (ECochG) was developed almost simultaneously by Yoshie in Japan [17], Sohmer and Feinmesser in Israel [18], and Aram in France [19]. The transtympanic electrode proposed by Aram [19] is the one that allows the best recording conditions, for being closer to the cochlea than the other types of electrodes, which allows for a tenfold increase in voltage.

The ECochG traces are a combination of cochlear microphonics (CM), summating potentials (SP), and action potentials (AP) of the acoustic nerve in the cochlea. Figure 4 shows the ECochG recordings for a normal ear, at different intensities.

ECochG was extensively used to obtain hearing thresholds in small children but has been almost totally replaced by the auditory brainstem response test, since it does not require a physician to insert the electrode nor an anesthesiologist.

ECochG is now employed for patients with Menière's disease, for monitorization of the auditory nerve during surgery on the brainstem or cerebellum, and for enhancement of wave I of the auditory brainstem response in patients with intense hearing loss. It may also be used to assist in the diagnosis of auditory neuropathy.

Fig. 4 A normal ECochG

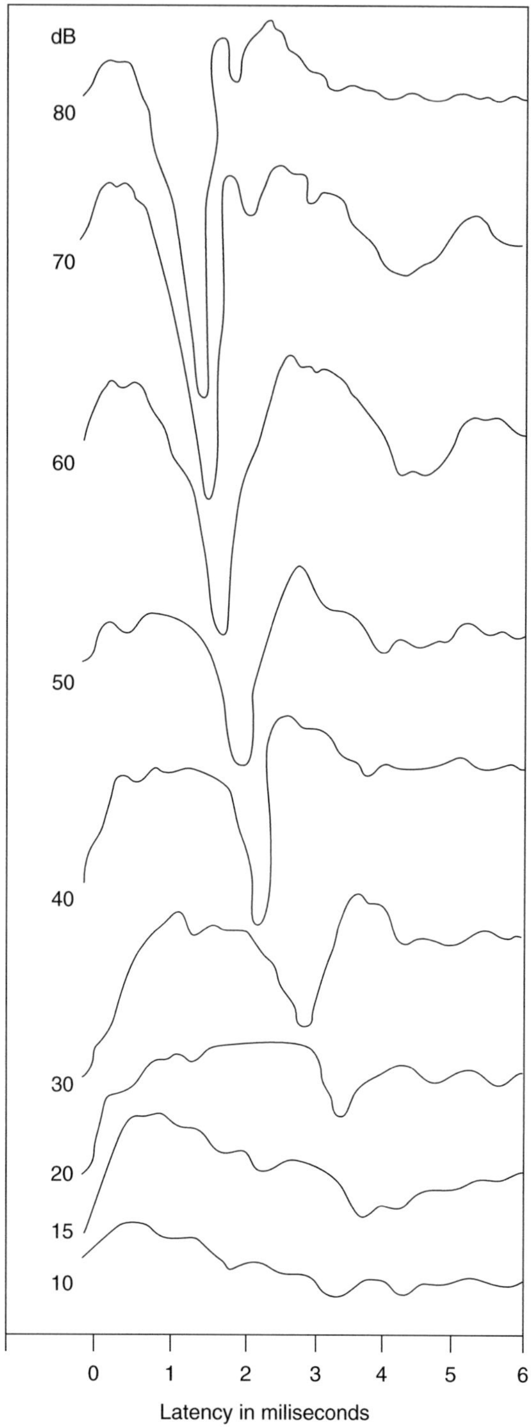

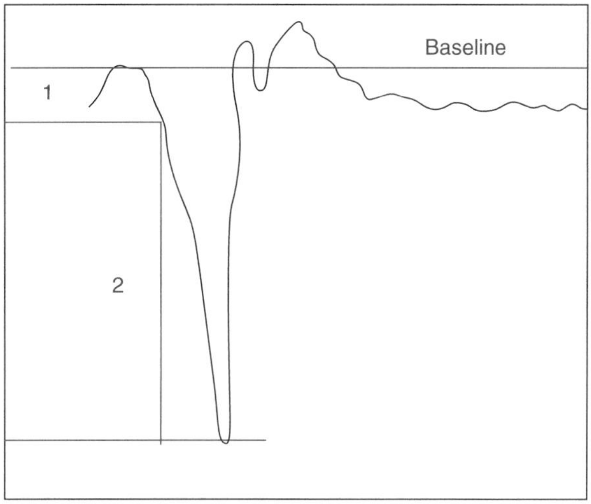

Fig. 5 Relation of the summating potentials (SM) and the action potentials (AP) in a normal ECochG. 1 = SP amplitude; 2 = AP amplitude

The electrocochleographic diagnosis of Menière's disease is based on a greater amplitude of the SP in relation to the AP. This is usually expressed as a ratio, since the amplitudes vary considerably in these tests. Recently it was found that the relation between the areas of these potentials is more sensitive than that of the amplitudes [20–22].

These abnormal relations are not seen in Menière's disease patients that have severe hearing losses. On the other hand, they are commonly found in the better ears of patients with apparently unilateral cases, indicating that these patients have bilateral asymmetrical disease [22, 23].

Figure 5 shows the normal relation between the SP and the AP.

Auditory Brainstem Responses (ABR)

ABR is also called *brainstem evoked response audiometry*, or *BERA*. The brainstem responses were first recorded in humans by Sohmer and Feinmesser [18] in 1967. Jewett and Williston [24], in 1971, gave a clear description of the human ABR and interpreted the waves as arriving from the brainstem. Jewett's name and nomenclature are usually employed to designate the ABR responses.

Figure 6 shows the normal ABR responses. Wave I is the response obtained in ECochG (an intracochlear acoustic nerve response). Wave II is an extracochlear acoustic nerve response. Wave III arises from the cochlear nucleus, wave IV from the lateral lemniscus, and wave V from the inferior colliculus. Waves VI and VII are mesencephalic and thalamic potentials. Wave V is the largest and most easily identified.

In 1974, Hecox and Galambos [25] showed that the ABR could be used for threshold estimation in adults and infants, and this test became the routine investigation for obtaining hearing thresholds in small children. In 1975, Starr and Achor [26] reported on the results of the ABR tests in pathological disorders of the brainstem.

Fig. 6 A normal ABR recording

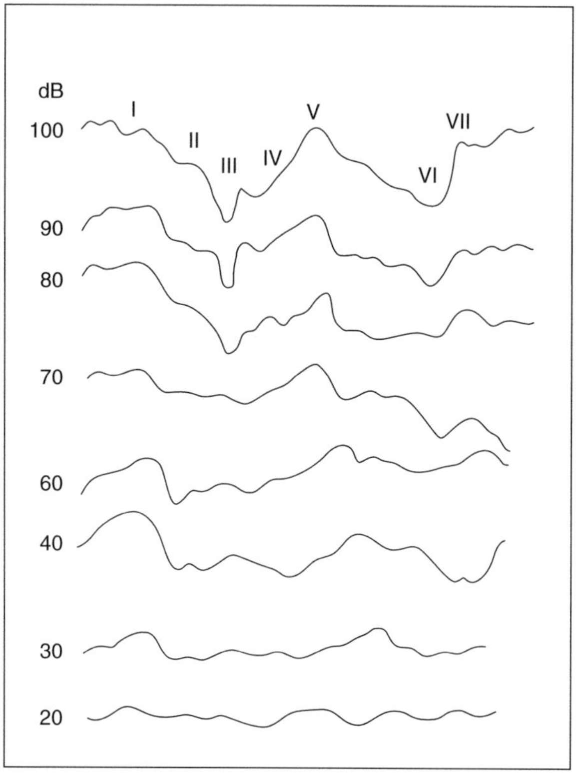

In 1977, Selters and Brackmann [27] published their findings on prolonged interpeak latencies in patients with vestibular schwannomas. Don et al. [28], in 2005, introduced the *stacked ABR* that increases the sensitivity of the test for the detection of small tumors. The stacked ABR is the sum of the synchronous neural activity generated from five frequency regions across the cochlea in response to click stimulation and high-pass pink noise masking. The development of this technique was based on the eighth cranial nerve compound action potential work done by Teas, Eldredge, and Davis [29] in 1962.

Another modification of the ABR was the *auditory steady-state response (ASSR)*, an auditory evoked potential, elicited with modulated tones that can be used to predict hearing sensitivity in patients of all ages. The responses to its very short sound stimuli create a statistically valid estimated audiogram [30].

Middle Latency Responses (MLR)

The middle latency responses were described by Goldstein and Rodman in 1967 [31]. The first wave is N_a (negative), followed by P_a (positive), N_b, P_b, and, in some recordings, N_c and P_c. The most important and most constant wave is P_a, which

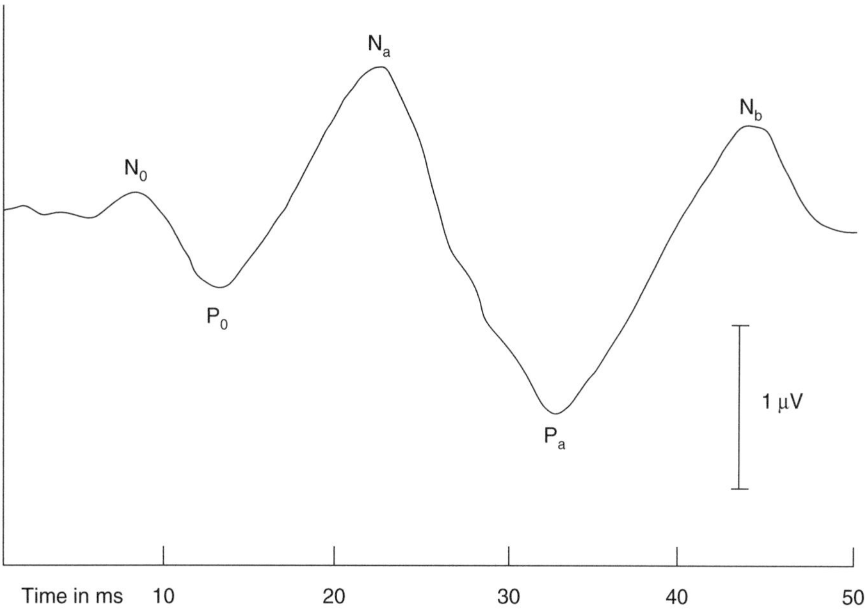

Fig. 7 The middle latencies auditory evoked responses. (Adapted from Brackmann et al. [22])

occurs between 10 and 80 ms after the acoustic stimulus. This response has multiple generators: thalamus-cortical pathways, inferior colliculus, and reticular formation. Figure 7 shows a recording of the middle latency waves.

These responses may be useful in the evaluation of children with language disorders and also in distinguishing lesions from functional alterations in the central nervous system.

Cortical Electrical Response Audiometry

This was the first electrical response test to be employed [32, 33], and it was found to be very reliable for obtaining auditory thresholds. It requires, however, cooperative patients, since these responses are sensitive to the use of anesthesia or sedation. Figure 8 shows the most important cortical evoked responses, usually referred to as the vertex potentials.

P_{300}

This electrical response that occurs approximately 300 ms after the stimulus is an event-related response. Even though it is commonly studied with acoustic stimuli, it may be excited by other types of stimuli.

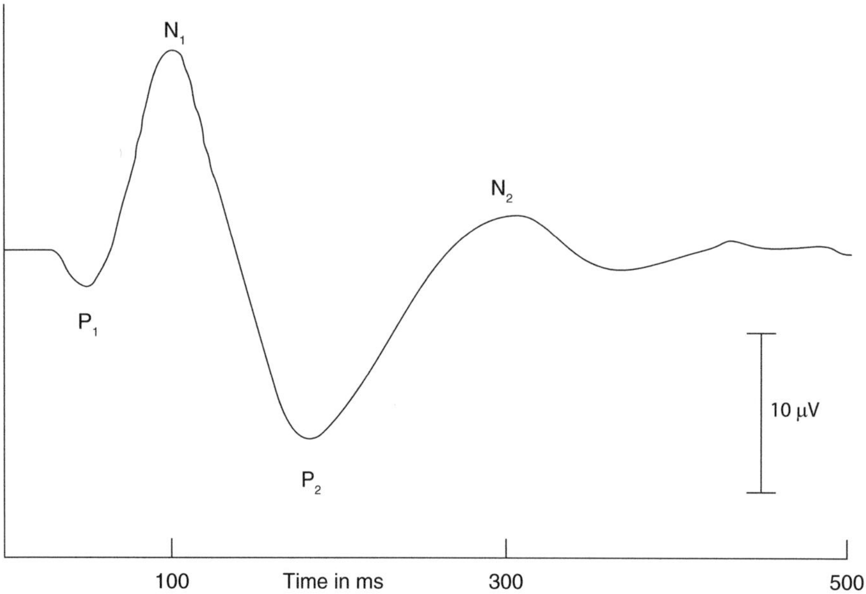

Fig. 8 Cortical auditory evoked responses. (Adapted from Brackmann et al. [22])

P_{300} depends on the patient's attention. Two stimuli of different frequencies are employed, and the patient has to make a signal every time he hears the "different" stimulus. The latencies change with age: they are longer in children and in elderly persons, reaching the lowest peak at age 18.

It has been used in children or elderly patients with central auditory processing disorders and to diagnose cognition disturbances in elderly patients. It is also employed to establish a differential diagnosis between organic and psychological brain disorders.

Evoked Responses to Electrical Stimulation

Both ABR and MLR can be elicited by electrical stimuli, and this has been very significant for the patients that need cochlear implants.

These tests are now being performed in the operating rooms to check whether the cochlear implant electrodes are adequately positioned and are working in a satisfactory manner.

These tests are also very useful to make the necessary adjustments to the cochlear implants in children. They allow the audiologists to estimate the adequate levels for each of the electrodes, something that is very easy to establish in post-lingual adults but used to be very difficult in pre-lingual children when these tests were not available.

Neurotological Aspects of Audiological Diagnosis

Normal Hearing

Patients with intense disequilibrium, neurological symptoms, and normal hearing have a rare condition named *cochleovestibular dissociation.* It is a consequence of a brain tumor that destroys the vestibular nuclei. It is rare because it rapidly leads to the death of the patient.

Middle Ear Mechanical Hearing Loss

Mechanical middle ear hearing loss is mostly related to otosclerosis and otitis media.

Otosclerosis is occasionally related to vertigo, most often in elderly women with unilateral disease [34]. Vertigo is also common after stapes surgery and may be persistent in cases in which the prosthesis employed is too long. Cases of benign paroxysmal positional vertigo (BPPV) have also been observed following stapedectomies.

Acute otitis media is a very common disorder. Most of the time it is cured without sequelae but occasionally evolves to chronic otitis media. But there are patients in whom the bacteria access the inner ear and the mechanical hearing loss will turn into a profound hearing loss, often accompanied by vertigo.

Patients with cholesteatoma often have fistulas in the lateral semicircular canal and may have sudden severe vertiginous attacks after which they will usually develop a profound hearing loss. In rare cases cholesteatomas may cause meningitis or a brain abscess.

Inner Ear Mechanical Loss

According to Hallowell Davis [35], "any inefficiency in the physical process of sound conduction, up to and including the bending of the cilia of the receptor cells, is functionally a mechanical loss."

This would include presbycusis that he considered as caused by the increased rigidity of the ear membranes with age. He felt that other types of hearing loss in elderly persons would be caused by additional vascular, metabolic, or autoimmune diseases and would not be actually age-dependent.

Tonndorf [36], in an experimental study with models, was able to demonstrate that the early hearing losses in Menière's disease were of purely mechanical origin.

Sudden Sensorineural Hearing Loss

Patients with sensorineural hearing losses may have sudden or progressive losses.

Sudden hearing losses are usually unilateral and may have different causes. Approximately 10% of them in adult patients are caused by vestibular schwannomas; it is important to submit these patients to magnetic resonance scans to discard this etiology.

The majority of the cases are due to mechanical, viral, vascular, or autoimmune disorders. They may be accompanied by sudden vertigo.

Mechanical sudden hearing losses are a result of a perilymphatic fistula. Vascular involvement of labyrinthine vessels has to be discarded in patients prone to vascular problems. Severe autoimmune diseases may account for bilateral sudden losses, fortunately rare.

Children with epidemic parotiditis may present viral unilateral profound hearing loss. A few of these cases evolve to delayed endolymphatic hydrops after a span of many years.

Progressive Sensorineural Hearing Loss

Most patients with sensorineural hearing loss have progressive losses. Usually the progression is slow, but there are some cases of rapidly progressive losses.

The etiological diagnosis of sensorineural hearing loss may involve all kinds of audiology tests, but some orientation may be obtained by the analysis of the pure tone audiograms and speech discrimination tests.

For most sensorineural losses, the discrimination scores are somewhat reduced, but severe discrimination losses are infrequent, except in tertiary syphilis and autoimmune diseases.

The audiograms of patients with sensorineural hearing loss may show flat curves, or elevated thresholds for low frequencies, or elevated thresholds for high frequencies, or elevated thresholds for both low and high frequencies, usually named inverted U shape.

Flat curves (Fig. 9) are usually seen in patients with atrophic degeneration of the stria vascularis, which is a genetic disorder [37]. Experimentally this type of hearing loss has been associated with reduction or absence of the endocochlear potential [38].

Elevated thresholds for low frequencies (Fig. 10) are usually seen in early cases of Menière's disease. They are usually associated with the presence of recruitment, which may be estimated by immittance tests. If there is a marked discrimination loss, it is important to rule out syphilis, autoimmune vasculitis of the inner ear, or general autoimmune diseases.

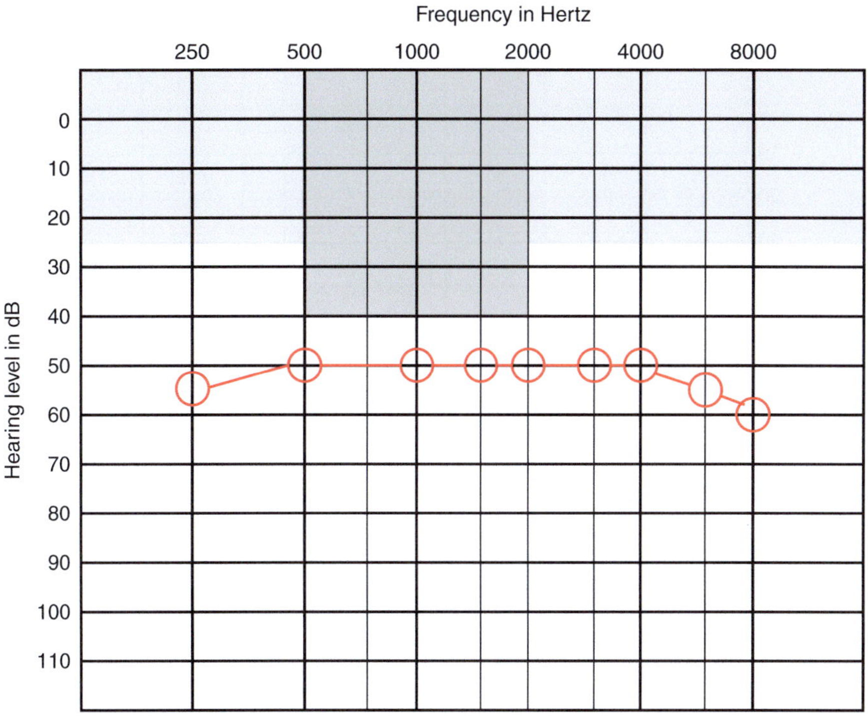

Fig. 9 Audiogram of a patient with a flat hearing loss, suggestive of genetical atrophy of the stria vascularis. For the sake of clarity, only the thresholds of the right ear were represented. The symbol **O** represents the right ear air conduction thresholds

Elevated thresholds for high frequencies (Fig. 11) are very common audiometric curves, often related to vascular problems. But they may also be related to physical trauma. Acoustic trauma usually affects the frequency of 4000 Hz more intensely than other frequencies (Fig. 12). Discrimination losses may occur, particularly when the descending curve reaches the frequency of 1500 Hz.

Patients with less than 30% discrimination for sentences will be candidates for a cochlear implant. In patients with autoimmune diseases, the discrimination sometimes improves with medical treatment.

A particular kind of high-frequency loss is the ski slope curve (Fig. 13). In most cases this is of perinatal origin, resulting from lack of oxygenation during the delivery; but it may also result from physical trauma. Cochlear implants with simultaneous sound stimulation may be indicated for these patients.

Inverted U-shape curves (Fig. 14) are usually seen in metabolic hearing loss. These hearing losses are usually mild and may often be improved or reverted with treatment [39].

Figure 15 shows an audiogram with no responses. The symbol ↓ is employed to represent the absence of response, and it is placed at the point of maximal energy

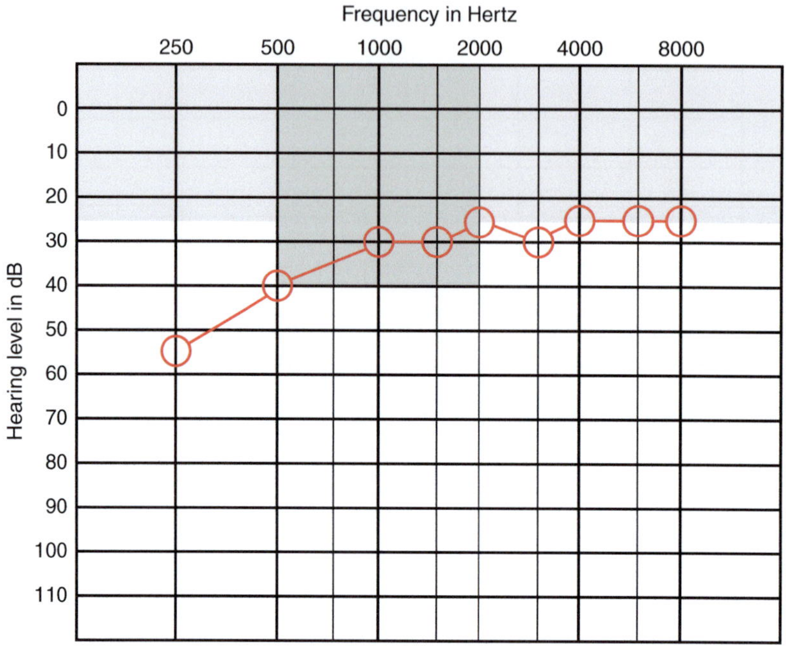

Fig. 10 Audiogram of a patient with a low-frequency hearing loss, suggestive of an early case of Menière's disease

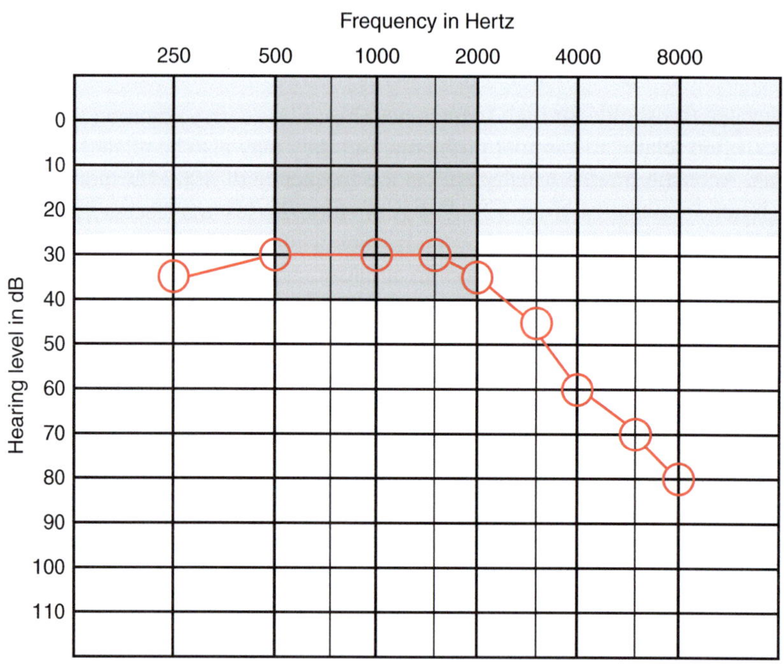

Fig. 11 Audiogram of a patient with a high-tone hearing loss, suggestive of vascular disorder

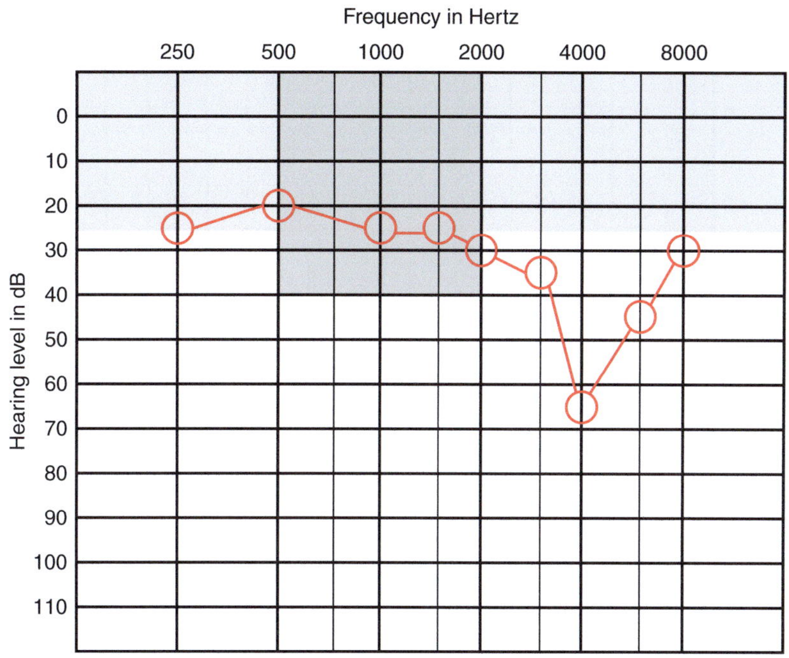

Fig. 12 Audiogram of a patient with a 4000 Hz peak, suggestive of acoustic trauma

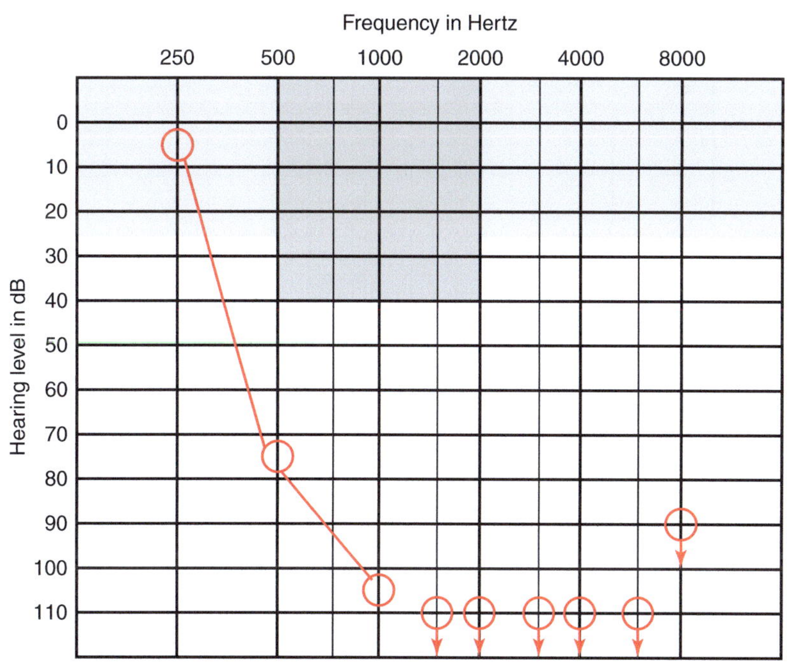

Fig. 13 Audiogram showing a "ski slope" high-frequency loss

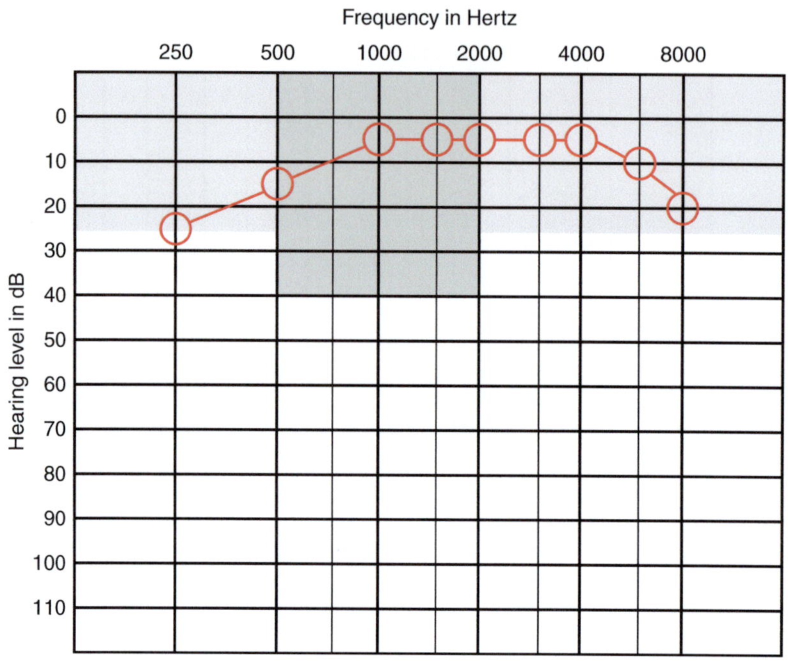

Fig. 14 An inverted U-shaped audiogram, commonly seen in patients with hyperinsulinemia or reactive hypoglycemia

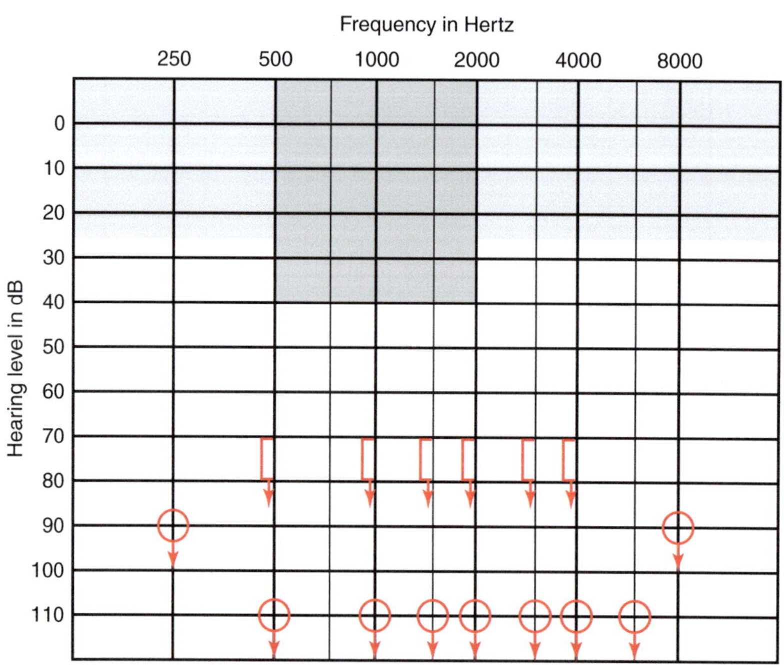

Fig. 15 A "no response" audiogram. The symbols are placed on the audiometer's high-intensity limits for each frequency. (See text)

that the audiogram is capable to produce. This audiogram usually represents a profound hearing loss, but it may represent a case of advanced otosclerosis, since the patient may have bone conduction thresholds in the area of the audiogram comprised between 70 and 120 dB that is impossible to be tested. The differential diagnosis is made through the clinical and/or familial history and by the fact that most of these patients have a surprisingly good result with hearing aids. A stapedectomy will improve these patients' hearing with the aid.

Air conduction thresholds of 90 dB or more characterize profound hearing loss, which is an indication for a cochlear implant.

Mixed Hearing Loss

A mixed hearing loss is usually a combination of a sensorineural hearing loss and a middle ear mechanical hearing loss. These patients usually have abnormal tympanic membranes, or perforations; or they have advanced otosclerosis, with a cochlear component.

But there are cases of *inner ear mixed hearing loss*, resulting, basically, from two sorts of conditions: perilymphatic hypertension or dehiscence of the anterior semicircular canal.

The perilymphatic hypertension syndrome is a congenital disorder that results from an enlarged cochlear aqueduct or a defect in the modiolus that allows the cerebrospinal fluid direct access to the cochlea [40, 41]. Anterior canal dehiscence is also a congenital defect but usually does not cause symptoms before the fourth decade of life [42]. The differential diagnosis is established by the clinical history and by the computerized tomography scans, which may be normal in the perilymphatic hypertension patients or may show enlarged cochlear aqueduct or modiolus, while it identifies the anterior canal fistula in the cases of canal dehiscence.

An important characteristic of the inner ear mixed deafness is that tympanic reflexes are present. This was described by one of us in 1992 [41]; it never happens in mixed hearing losses that possess a middle ear component.

Figure 16 shows the audiogram of a patient with a dehiscence of the right anterior semicircular canal.

The Role of Audiology in Differential Diagnosis

Tables 2, 3, 4, and 5 show the most common audiological findings in different vestibular disorders. It must be taken into consideration that patients with disorders that do not cause hearing losses may have previously unrelated hearing problems.

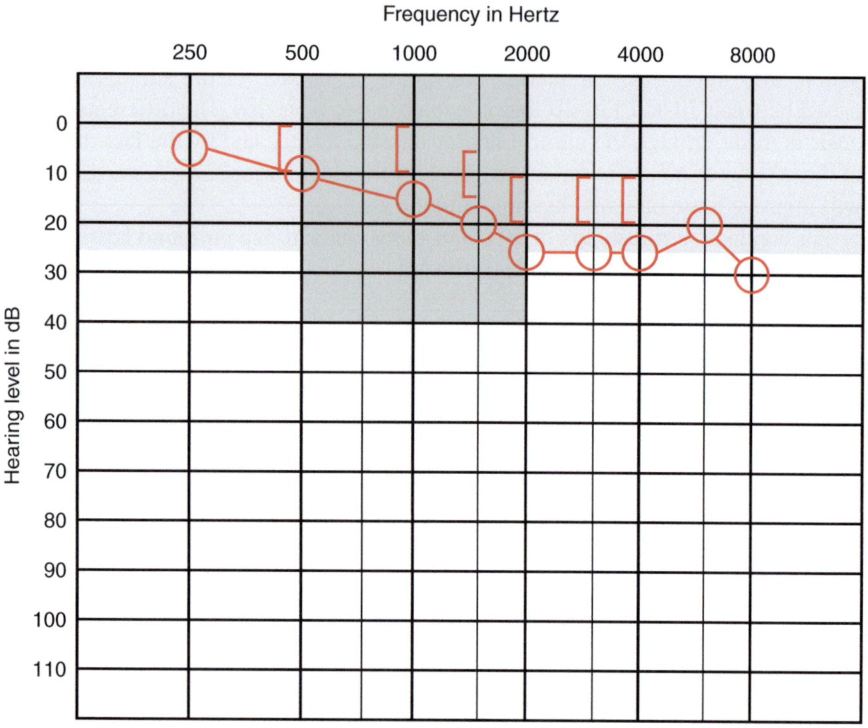

Fig. 16 The audiogram of a patient with dehiscence of the right anterior semicircular canal. The left ear was normal

Table 2 Patients with spontaneous episodic vertigo

Menière's disease	Fluctuant hearing loss, variable speech discrimination; recruitment
Vestibular migraine	Usually normal hearing
Hypoglycemia	Inverted U-shaped audiometric curves
Panic syndrome	Inverted U-shaped audiometric curves
Transient ischemic attack	Normal hearing
Cardiac arrhythmia	Normal hearing
Multiple sclerosis	ABR with long latencies

Table 3 Patients with positional episodic vertigo

Orthostatic hypotension	Normal hearing
Benign paroxysmal positional vertigo	Normal hearing; may have slight hearing loss
Central positional vertigo	Normal hearing

Table 4 Patients with acute or continuous spontaneous vertigo

Vestibular neuritis	May present sensorineural loss, often profound hearing loss
Bacterial or viral labyrinthitis	May present sensorineural loss, often profound hearing loss
Herpes zoster oticus	Sudden hearing loss accompanying facial paralysis
Cerebral vascular accident	May present sensorineural loss
Brainstem encephalitis	Usually normal hearing
Cerebellar infarct – AICA	Profound hearing loss
Cerebellar infarct – PICA	Normal hearing
Posterior fossa brain tumors	Sensorineural loss, frequent abnormal adaptation, frequent discrimination loss

Table 5 Patients with acute or continuous event-related vertigo

Drug intoxication	Sensorineural hearing loss
Physical or surgical trauma	May present sensorineural loss, sometimes profound loss
Acute acoustic trauma	Sensorineural loss
Carbon monoxide intoxication	Normal hearing
Wernicke's encephalopathy	Normal hearing

Final Comments

The inner ear is a system that responds to acceleration frequencies (from 0 to 16 Hz) and to sound frequencies (from 16 to 16,000 Hz), by means of very specialized ciliated receptor cells. There is a definite integration between the static and the acoustic parts. Therefore, the study of the acoustic system is an important complement to the study of the static receptors of the system.

Audiology, as a consequence, is an important part of neurotology.

References

1. Davis H, Walsh TE. The limits of improvement of hearing following the fenestration operation. Laryngoscope. 1950;60:273–95.
2. Shambaugh GE Jr. Pure tone and controlled speech tests in the election of cases for fenestration. Acta Otolaryngol. 1951–1952;40:199–210.
3. Sivian LJ, White SD. On minimal audible sound fields. J Acoust Soc Am. 1933;4:288–321.
4. Bárány R. A contribution to the physiology of bone conduction. 1932. Quoted by Hirsh IJ, The measurement of hearing. New York: McGraw-Hill; 1952.
5. von Békésy G. Experiments in hearing. New York: McGraw-Hill; 1960. p. 95–181.
6. Zwislocki JJ. In search of the bone conduction threshold in a free sound field. J Acoust Soc Am. 1957;29:795–804.

7. Fowler EP. Marked deafened areas in normal ears. 1928. Quoted by Hirsh IJ, The measurement of hearing. New York: McGraw-Hill; 1952.
8. Dix MR, Hallpike CS, Hood JD. Observations upon loudness recruitment phenomenon with especial reference to the differential diagnosis of disorders of the internal ear and 8th nerve. J Laryngol Otol. 1948;62:671–86.
9. Jerger JF. A difference limen recruitment test and its diagnostic significance. Laryngoscope. 1952;62:1316–32.
10. Jerger J, Carhart R, Lassman J. Clinical observations on excessive threshold adaptation. AMA Arch Otolaryngol. 1958;68(5):617–23.
11. Zwislocki JJ. Acoustic measurement of the middle ear function. Ann Otol Rhinol Laryngol. 1961;70:599–606.
12. Terkildsen K, Scott Nielsen S. An electroacoustic impedance measuring bridge for clinical use. Arch Otolaryngol. 1960;72(3):339–46. https://doi.org/10.1001/archotol.1960.00740010347009.
13. Metz O. Threshold of reflex contractions of muscles of middle ear and recruitment of loudness. AMA Arch Otolaryngol. 1952;55:536–43.
14. Kemp DT. Stimulated acoustic emissions from within the human auditory system. J Acoust Soc Am. 1978;64:1386–91.
15. Davis H. Principles of electric response audiometry. Ann Otol Rhinol Laryngol. 1976;85 Suppl 28:1–96.
16. Galambos R. Hallowell Davis: Father of the AER. In: Hirsh SK, Eldredge DH, Hirsh IJ, Silverman SR, editors. Hearing and Davis: Essays Honoring Hallowell Davis. Saint Louis, MO: Washington University; 1976.
17. Yoshie N, Oashi T. Clinical use of cochlear nerve action potential responses in man for differential diagnosis of hearing losses. Acta Otolaryngol. 1959;Suppl 252:71–87.
18. Sohmer H, Feinmesser M. Cochlear action potentials recorded from the external ear in man. Ann Otol Rhinol Laryngol. 1967;76(2):427–35.
19. Aram J-M, Le Bert G. Les réponses nerveuses cochléaires chez l'homme. Image du fonctionnement de l'oreille et nouveau test d'audiometrie objective. Rev Laryng (Bordeaux). 1968;89:361–78.
20. Schmidt PH, Eggermont JJ, Odenthal DW. Study of Menière's disease by electrocochleography. Acta Otolaryngol Suppl. 1974;316:75–84.
21. Ferraro JA, Tibbils RP. SP/AP area ratio in the diagnosis of Meniere's disease. Am J Audiol. 1999;8:21–8.
22. Devaiah AK, Dawson KL, Ferraro JA, Ator GA. Utility of area curve ratio electrocochleography in early Meniere's disease. Arch Otolaryngol Head Neck Surg. 2003;129(5):547–51.
23. Mangabeira-Albernaz PL, Fukuda Y, Ganança MM. Menière's disease. ORL J Otorhinolaryngol Relat Spec. 1980;42:91–100.
24. Jewett DL, Romano MN, Williston JS. Human auditory evoked potentials: possible brain stem components detected on the scalp. Science. 1970;167(3924):1517–8.
25. Hecox K, Galambos R. Brain stem auditory evoked responses in human infants and adults. Arch Otolaryngol. 1974;99:30–3.
26. Starr A, Achor J. Auditory brain stem responses in neurological disease. Arch Neurol. 1975;32:761–8.
27. Selters WA, Brackmann DE. Acoustic tumor detection with brain stem electric response audiometry. Arch Otolaryngol. 1977;103(4):181–7.
28. Don M, Kwong B, Tanaka C, Brackmann D, Nelson R. The stacked ABR: a sensitive and specific screening tool for detecting small acoustic tumors. Audiol Neurootol. 2005;10:274–90.
29. Teas DC, Eldredge DH, Davis H. Cochlear responses to acoustic transients: an interpretation of whole-nerve action potentials. J Acoust Soc Am. 1962;34:1438–59. https://doi.org/10.1121/1.1918366.
30. Lins OG, Picton TW. Auditory steady-state responses to multiple simultaneous stimuli. Electroencephalogr Clin Neurophysiol. 1995;96:420–32.

31. Goldstein R, Rodman LB. Early components of averaged evoked responses to rapidly repeated auditory stimuli. J Speech Hear Res. 1967;10:697–705.
32. Brackmann DE, Don M, Selters WA. Electric response audiometry. In: England GM, editor. Otolaryngology. Philadelphia: Lippincott Williams & Wilkins; 1998.
33. Davis H, Yoshie N. Human evoked cortical responses to auditory stimuli. Physiologist. 1963;6:164.
34. McCabe BF. Otosclerosis and vertigo. Trans Pac Coast Otoophthalmol Soc Annu Meet. 1966;47:37–42.
35. Davis H. A functional classification of auditory defects. Ann Otol Rhinol Laryngol. 1962;71:693–704.
36. Tonndorf J. Endolymphatic hydrops: mechanical causes of hearing loss. Arch Otorhinolaryngol. 1976;212:293–9.
37. Schuknecht H, Ishii T. Hearing loss caused by atrophy of the stria vascularis. Nihon Jibiinkoka Gakkai Kaiho. 1966;69:1825–33.
38. Kimura R, Perlman HB. Experimental obstruction of venous drainage and arterial supply of the inner ear. Ann Otol Rhinol Laryngol. 1957;66:537–46.
39. Mangabeira-Albernaz PL. Hearing loss, dizziness, and carbohydrate metabolism. Int J Otorhinolaryngol. 2016;20:261–70. https://doi.org/10.1055/s-0035-1558450.
40. Brown Farrior J, Endicott JN. Congenital mixed deafness: cerebrospinal fluid otorrhea. Ablation of the aqueduct of the cochlea. Laryngoscope. 1971;81:684–99.
41. Mangabeira-Albernaz PL, Hidal LBT, Iorio MCM. The perilymphatic hypertension syndrome. Acta Otolaryngol. 1992;112:306–10.
42. Minor LB, Solomon D, Zinreich J, Zee DS. Sound and/or pressure-induced vertigo due to bone dehiscence of the superior semicircular canal. Arch Otolaryngol Head Neck Surg. 1998;124:249–58.

The Vestibular Syndromes

All of the symptoms of vestibular system disorders, including dizziness, unsteadiness, vertigo, and oscillopsia, may be of peripheral or central origin. These symptoms have been clearly defined by a Bárány Society committee [1].

Conventionally, peripheral disorders are those that involve the inner ear and the vestibular nerve. Central disorders involve the vestibular nuclei and the vestibular pathways, all the way to the cerebral cortex. It is important to understand that the distinction into peripheral and central disorders is basically a classification. Actually, there are mixed entities, and some peripheral disorders may evolve to central disorders.

According to the Bárány Society, the vestibular syndromes can be classified in three groups [2]:

1. Episodic vestibular syndromes
2. Acute vestibular syndromes
3. Chronic vestibular syndromes

Many of these disorders may occur spontaneously or may be triggered by some kind of event. They will be discussed separately, in the manner proposed by Newman-Toker [3]. The mnemonic word that he suggested is TiTrATE: *Ti*ming, *Tr*iggers, *A*nd *T*argeted *E*xamination.

Episodic Spontaneous Syndromes

Patients with episodes of vertigo, dizziness, or unsteadiness may present Menière's disease, vestibular migraine, transient ischemic attacks, hypoglycemia, normal pressure hydrocephalus, or cardiac arrhythmia.

P. L. M. Albernaz et al., *The New Neurotology*,
https://doi.org/10.1007/978-3-030-11283-7_8

Menière's Disease

Patients with Menière's disease present fluctuant hearing loss and tinnitus and episodes of vertigo lasting from 20 minutes to 1 or 2 days. This entity is extensively discussed in a special chapter.

Vestibular Migraine

Vestibular migraine is getting to be recognized as a distinct clinical entity that accounts for a high proportion of patients with vestibular symptoms. This subject has also been carefully reviewed by a Bárány Society committee [4].

These patients have episodes of dizziness and vertigo, and also difficulties with quick head movements, and headache, photophobia, and phonophobia. The duration of attacks ranges from second to days. It is more frequently seen in female patients, in a proportion of five to one [5].

Physical examination and laboratory testing are usually normal in vestibular migraine but may be used to rule out vestibular disorders with overlapping symptoms.

The pathophysiology of vestibular migraine is not completely understood, but it may include neuroanatomical pathways to and from central vestibular structures and neurochemical modulation via the locus coeruleus and raphe nuclei [6].

The following criteria should be followed to establish the diagnosis of vestibular migraine [4]:

- At least five episodes with vestibular symptoms of moderate or severe intensity lasting between 5 minutes and 72 hours
- Current migraine or previous history of migraine with or without aura, according to the International Classification of Headache Disorders
- One or more migraine features with at least 50% of vestibular episodes:
  (a) Headache with at least two of the following characteristics:
  (b) One-side location, pulsating quality, moderate or severe pain intensity, aggravation by routine physical activity
  (c) Photophobia and phonophobia
  (d) Visual aura
- Not explained by other vestibular disorders

More data on vestibular migraine can be found in chapter "Vestibular Migraine".

Cerebellar Transient Ischemic Attacks

Transient ischemic attacks (TIA) are central vestibular disorders related to brief episodes of neurological disturbance caused by reduced blood supply to an area of the brain. As a rule they are milder than the cerebrovascular accidents (CVA), which are associated with longer-lasting neurological disturbances and permanent damage to the brain.

The risk factors for transient attacks are basically the same as those for CVA, including increasing age, male gender, race and family history, prior CVA or TIA, hypertension, diabetes, heart disease, carotid or peripheral vascular disease, obesity, high cholesterol, and physical inactivity.

Typically patients will present with one or a combination of motor symptoms, sometimes referred as the *deadly D's* of central dizziness [3]:

Deadly D's [3]
*D*iplopia
*D*ysarthria
*D*ysphagia
*D*ysphonia
*D*ysmetria
*D*ysesthesia
*D*rop attacks (without syncope)
*D*istortions (room tilt illusions)

The absence of these symptoms, however, does not exclude cerebellar TIA.

Among other variations, there are two important types of cerebellar TIAs, the AICA syndrome and the PICA syndrome.

The occlusion of the anterior inferior cerebellar artery (AICA) [7] may occur by embolism or thrombosis. There is a sudden episode of vertigo, usually accompanied by nausea and vomiting. After a few hours the patient presents deafness, facial paralysis, and cerebellar symptoms. These patients will show marked vestibular hyporeflexia on the side of the lesion. Table 1 shows the areas affected by the arterial occlusion and its corresponding clinical findings.

The occlusion of the posterior inferior cerebellar artery (PICA), also called *lateral medullary syndrome*, may also occur by embolism or thrombosis [7, 8]. The symptoms may develop gradually or suddenly. Hearing is not affected and the patient does not lose his consciousness. This disorder is rarely fatal but occurs in patients with vascular disorders that will eventually lead to other complications. Occlusion of the vertebral artery may account for similar symptoms.

Table 2 shows the areas affected by the PICA occlusion and its corresponding clinical findings.

Table 1 Involved areas and findings in AICA syndrome

Involved areas	Findings
Vestibular nuclei	Vertigo, nystagmus, vomiting
Ischemic necrosis of the labyrinth	Deafness, facial paralysis
Middle and inferior cerebellar peduncle	Contralateral analgesia and thermanesthesia of the trunk and extremities
Spinal tract of trigeminal nerve	Ipsilateral analgesia of the face

Table 2 Involved areas and findings in PICA syndrome

Involved areas	Findings
Vestibular nuclei	Vertigo, nystagmus, vomiting
Inferior cerebellar peduncle	Ataxia, dysmetria, dysdiadochokinesia
Nucleus ambiguus	Ipsilateral paralysis of the soft palate, pharynx, and larynx
Spinothalamic fibers	Contralateral analgesia and thermanesthesia of the trunk and extremities
Spinal tract of trigeminal nerve	Ipsilateral analgesia of the face
Descending hypothalamic sympathetic fibers	Ipsilateral Claude Bernard-Horner's syndrome – ptosis, enophthalmos, miosis, and facial anhidrosis

The HINTS protocol, described in chapter 4, is extremely useful for the diagnosis of cerebellar disorders in the emergency room [9, 10].

Other Episodic Spontaneous Peripheral Vestibular Disorders

Some patients have episodes of vertigo that last for only a few minutes and are not accompanied by hearing loss or tinnitus. They are found to have a unilateral or bilateral reduction of vestibular function. This disease was presented by Hallpike in a medical meeting in 1949 and published by Dix and Hallpike in 1952 [11], with the name of *vestibular neuronitis*. It is preferable to call it *unilateral or bilateral vestibular paresis*, to avoid confusion with *vestibular neuritis.*

This is a benign vestibular disorder that responds well to medical treatment and evolves to complete cure with vestibular compensation.

Other Episodic Spontaneous Central Vestibular Disorders

Intense hypoglycemia, cardiac arrhythmia, and panic syndrome may cause episodes of dizziness or unsteadiness. Their diagnosis is usually established by clinical history, clinical evaluation, and laboratory data.

Normal pressure hydrocephalus may cause episodes of unsteadiness but does not cause vertigo. Its diagnosis requires a cranial image, either computerized tomography or magnetic resonance, to be confirmed. These patients usually become asymptomatic with a ventriculoperitoneal low-pressure shunt [12].

- *Differential diagnosis* The differential diagnosis between vestibular migraine and TIA is mainly based on the clinical history. Migraine patients usually have a history of previous episodes, almost always refer visual or food triggers, and complain of visual aura and photophobia.

Migraine patients rarely present diplopia, or any of the other *deadly D's*. They also do not have sudden sustained pain in the posterior part of the neck.

A differential diagnosis must also be made between migraine and Menière's disease. Typical cases of Menière's disease may be diagnosed by clinical history. The distinction, however, may be difficult in atypical cases, and this situation is aggravated by the circumstance that the two diseases can be associated. Sometimes the diagnosis is accomplished only after a variable period of the patient's follow-up.

Episodic Positional Syndromes

As a rule the patients with episodes of vertigo triggered by head positions or motions present one of the following vestibular disorders:

1. Orthostatic hypotension
2. Benign paroxysmal positional vertigo (BPPV)
3. Central paroxysmal positional vertigo

Orthostatic Hypotension

Orthostatic hypotension, also called *postural hypotension*, is a sudden drop of arterial blood pressure that occurs when a person stands from a lying or sitting position. This is usually consequent to a delayed constriction of the blood vessels in the lower part of the body. In severe cases it may lead to falls or loss of consciousness. As a rule, the patient feels weak, sometimes tired, and vertigo or unsteadiness is common. Some patients report difficulty in concentrating and blurred vision.

Orthostatic hypotension may be caused by low blood volume, bleeding, and use of diuretics and/or beta-blockers, vasodilators, or other types of drugs, particularly in elderly people [12]. It may also be associated with other diseases, particularly neurological disorders.

The diagnosis is established when, on checking the vital signs, the patient's systolic pressure drops 20 or more mmHg or when the diastolic pressure drops 10 or more mmHg, when he gets up from a supine position.

Benign Paroxysmal Positional Vertigo (BPPV)

The name *benign paroxysmal positional vertigo (BPPV)* was proposed by Dix and Hallpike in 1952 [11], who defined its clinical characteristics. This is the most frequent vestibular disorder, related to displaced otoliths that stimulate mechanically one or more sensory areas in the semicircular ducts. There are many different types of BPPV that are discussed in a separate chapter.

Central Paroxysmal Positional Vertigo

While BPPV is a common peripheral disease, it must be carefully differentiated from central paroxysmal positional vertigo (CPPV). It is interesting to note that Nylén [13], in 1950, had already reported on patients with direction-changing positional nystagmus that were found to have tumors in the posterior cranial fossa. In 1960, Fernandez [14, 15] described positional nystagmus in cats after he practiced limited lesions in the nodulus of the cerebellar vermis, thus demonstrating that positional vertigo could have a central origin. In 1965 Riesco MacClure described two cases of CPPV due to tumors in the midline of the posterior fossa [16]. Other studies have emphasized the significance of this disease [17–19].

As a rule, CCPV indicates a disorder involving the loop between the vestibular nuclei and the archicerebellar structures in the vermis. The most likely explanation is that it is caused by a lack of inhibition of the vestibular reflexes to positional perception of the eyes or the head or trunk position [20].

The differential diagnosis between CPPV and BPPV can be difficult [21] and demands a high degree of suspicion on the part of the neurotologist, but there are some points that must be taken into consideration.

As a rule, CPPV is not accompanied by hearing loss or neurological symptoms.

Also, in CPPV, the positional nystagmus seen with the diagnostic maneuvers has no latency or presents a small period of latency. This nystagmus is usually vertical and may be downbeating (the most frequent) or upbeating. Rotatory nystagmus is less frequent. These types of nystagmus are persistent for longer times than those seen in BPPV, which are usually upbeating and last less than 1 minute. The sensation of vertigo is almost always of low intensity.

Obviously, CPPV does not respond to repositioning maneuvers.

Büttner et al., in 1999, revised the main differences between the peripheral and the central positional vertigos [22]:

1. Presence of other neurological symptoms or signs
2. Presence of nystagmus without dizziness or vertigo in the positional tests
3. Nystagmus with atypical direction in the positional tests
4. Nystagmus of long duration
5. Unsatisfactory responses to repositioning maneuvers
6. Frequently recurring symptoms

Magnetic resonance imaging is an absolute must in cases of suspected CPPV.

Acute Vestibular Syndromes

The term *acute vestibular syndrome* includes both peripheral and central disorders characterized by continuous dizziness, vertigo, or gait ataxia, lasting days or weeks, or even months, with nausea and vomiting, head motion discomfort, and nystagmus.

Unilateral Peripheral Acute Vestibular Syndrome

This is defined as a single intense episode of vertigo that results from a sudden unilateral loss of vestibular function. This nosological entity was described by Nylén, in 1924, with the name of *vestibular neuritis* [23]. It has also been called *sudden loss of vestibular function* (Lindsay & Hemenway [24]) or *vestibular paralysis of sudden onset* (Riesco MacClure [25] and Hart [26]).

The clinical symptoms are often dramatic. The patient has intense vertigo, with intense nystagmus beating to the side opposite to the lesion. Gait is difficult, with a tendency to fall to the side of the lesion. Neurovegetative symptoms – nausea, vomiting, and sudoresis – are usually present. Changes of the head position intensify the vertigo, causing the patient to remain immobile on his bed.

As days go by the symptoms gradually subside. It usually takes about 3 months for a complete recovery, which is obtained by means of vestibular compensation. The vestibular function of the affected side rarely returns.

Sudden sensorineural hearing loss may accompany the loss of vestibular function, but in the majority of the cases, there are only vestibular signs. It should be noted that sudden hearing loss, without vestibular symptoms, is more frequent than the peripheral acute vestibular syndrome and this is more common than the peripheral acute vestibular syndrome with associated sensorineural hearing loss.

Most of the cases seem to be of viral origin, but the evidences for this assumption are mainly circumstantial. The viruses most often considered as possible etiologies are herpes simplex, varicella, cytomegalovirus, Epstein-Barr, influenza A and B, parainfluenza 3, epidemic parotitis, rubella, and measles. Lyme's disease and histoplasmosis have been described as etiological factors in a smaller number of cases [27]. A recent clinical history of recent upper respiratory infection is very common. Occasionally there are many cases occurring more or less simultaneously, in epidemic fashion.

A more severe condition is caused by the varicella zoster virus when it reaches the geniculate ganglion. Herpes zoster oticus – Ramsay Hunt's syndrome – involves all of the nerves at the internal acoustic meatus, causing facial paralysis, vertigo, and hearing loss. Many patients require a total facial nerve decompression in view of the severity of the facial paralysis. The hearing gradually recovers in most patients, but sometimes it is permanent. The vestibular loss usually does not recover [28].

Peripheral acute vestibular syndromes, however, may be of vascular origin, most frequently in patients prone to vascular disorders. Most of the cases accompanied by sudden sensorineural hearing loss are of vascular origin.

One variation of the disease, the Lindsay-Hemenway syndrome, has been histologically proven to result from an obstruction of the anterior vestibular artery. Since this artery has no collaterals, its obstruction, besides inducing an intense episode of vertigo, also liberates utricular otoliths that reach the posterior semicircular canal, causing episodes of BPPV after the compensation of the sudden vertigo [24].

A complete neurotological examination is very difficult in the acute phase of the disease. The ear, nose, and throat examination is essentially normal. Audiological tests will be normal or may show unilateral sensorineural hearing loss. An intense horizontal spontaneous nystagmus, beating to the healthy ear, can be easily observed. The head impulse test (HIT) shows absent responses for the involved lateral semicircular canal. The video head impulse test may show reduced VOR in more than one semicircular canal [27]. The vHIT is very useful to confirm the diagnosis and to evaluate the patient's progressive compensation.

The prognosis is good in the cases without hearing loss. The vestibular symptoms gradually disappear by compensation, the completion of which may take several months. The sensorineural hearing loss, when present, rarely recovers.

- *Differential diagnosis* The peripheral acute vestibular syndrome must be distinguished from an initial attack of Menière's disease, the vertiginous episodes of which rarely extend to more than a few days. It also must be distinguished from the *central acute vestibular syndrome.*

Bilateral Peripheral Acute Vestibular Syndrome

Sometimes a peripheral acute vestibular symptom involves both ears. The degree of sensory loss is often asymmetrical. In most of these rare cases, a vestibular compensation will occur. When accompanied by hearing loss, some permanent loss may affect one or both ears.

Central Acute Vestibular Syndromes

The main causes of spontaneous acute vestibular syndrome of central origin are brainstem encephalitis; cerebral vascular accidents, both ischemic and hemorrhagic; degenerative central nervous system disorders (particularly multiple sclerosis); and brain tumors.

- *Viral encephalitis* Brainstem encephalitis of viral origin may give rise to symptoms that mimic peripheral disorders. Wennmo and Pyykkö, in 1982, described 6 cases of peripheral acute vestibular syndrome, of a group of 30 patients, who developed central symptoms and signs during the evolution of the disease [29]. The literature also mentions the epidemic occurrence of central vestibular involvement. The first observations were made by Barré and Reys in 1921 [30]; mentions of epidemic central vestibular disorders were also published by Pedersen [31], Merifield [32], Oosterveld et al. [33], and Baloh and Honrubia [34].

Patients with central vestibular syndromes of viral origin not related to epidemies have also been reported [35]. Central vestibular signs, of different kinds, were identified in these patients, allowing a precise diagnosis.

Unlike the peripheral acute vestibular syndrome that causes a permanent unilateral loss of vestibular function, these patients with viral encephalitis evolve to cure without sequelae. The clinical cure usually occurs in 4–6 weeks, but the vestibular examinations usually take 4–6 months to return to normal. The symptomatic treatment is done with corticosteroids; these patients feel worse when medicated with vestibular suppressors.

- *Bacterial brainstem encephalitis* Bacterial infection gives origin to the same basic symptoms of all acute vestibular syndromes, but the prognosis is definitely worse.

- *Episodic ataxia type 2* Familial episodic ataxias (EAs) are rare genetic diseases of autosomal dominant transmission. There are at least two well-defined varieties. Type 2 (EA 2) is characterized by recurrent attacks of dizziness and ataxia that are precipitated by physical activity, stress, or alcohol and usually last for hours. In between attacks, more than 90% of the patients have marked central oculomotor disturbances, often downbeat nystagmus. Episodic ataxia 2 is caused by mutations in the CACNA1A gene (PQ calcium channel gene) [36].

- *Cerebral vascular accident* Vertigo as a symptom of cerebrovascular disease (CVA) is not uncommon, either in ischemic or hemorrhagic events. Approximately 80% of the central acute vestibular syndromes are caused by CVAs, almost all ischemic.

When one or more of the three prominent central nervous system pathways – the spinothalamic, corticospinal, and dorsal column-medial lemniscus pathway – are affected, the patient may present hemiplegia, weakness of the facial muscles, and initial flaccidity, soon replaced by spasticity.

CVAs that involve the cerebral cortex result in aphasia, dysarthria, apraxia, and visual field and memory defects but are seldom accompanied by vertigo.

In brainstem CVAs the patients may complain of altered smell, taste, and hearing, total or partial loss of vision, ptosis, decreased sensation and muscle weakness of the face, altered breathing and heart rate, and balance problems and nystagmus.

If the cerebellum is involved, the patient will present vertigo and/or disequilibrium, altered gait, and eventually ataxia.

In patients with auditory symptoms, a differential diagnosis must be established with AICA obstruction.

- *Multiple sclerosis* Multiple sclerosis affects the vestibular system in 30% of the cases; in 5% the vestibular symptoms are the first manifestations of the disease [37]. There are rare cases with sudden hearing loss.

  The diagnosis is seldom achieved in the early cases.
  Other demyelinating diseases may also affect the vestibular system.

- *Brain tumors* Tumors of the cerebellopontine angle and its vicinity often compress the brainstem and may involve several cranial nerves. Vestibular schwannomas are the most frequent disorders of the cerebellopontine angle; the tumors that arise from the internal acoustic meatus produce hearing loss and may be diagnosed before the compression of the brainstem is established. Vertigo is rare, as automatic compensation will ensue with the slow growth of the tumor. The video head impulse tests will show decreased VOR responses on the side of the tumor.

On the other hand, the tumors arising in the cisterna may cause little or no hearing loss, and the vestibular tests may be normal. They are usually diagnosed by neurological signs of brainstem involvement or by involvement of other cranial nerves, particularly nerve V. Facial paralysis is rare, except in facial nerve schwannomas. Meningiomas and other types of tumors may cause similar symptoms. These patients may present unsteadiness. Spontaneous and direction-changing gaze nystagmus are usually the first sign of brainstem compression. Headaches and vomits not preceded by nausea will be seen in large tumors causing intracranial hypertension.

Bilateral vestibular schwannomas, characteristics of neurofibromatosis type 2, rarely produce episodes of vertigo but may show symptoms of central vestibular involvement.

Tumors of the midline of the posterior fossa do not cause hearing loss and do not cause changes in the peripheral vestibular system. Cerebellar signs are frequent, combined with central types of spontaneous and gaze nystagmus.

Ototoxicity

Many different drugs may cause inner ear intoxication. For some of them the toxic effects are reversible with the interruption of the medication; others cause permanent damage.

Ototoxicity by antibiotics of the aminoglycoside group is now less common than in the past, but they are still being used in treating patients with very serious infections and occasionally in patients submitted to transtympanic administration of gentamycin. Some chemotherapeutic drugs employed in patients with malignant tumors also have ototoxic effects.

The degrees of ototoxicity depend on the doses and length of treatment. The most serious condition is the bilateral loss of vestibular function that will be discussed in detail.

Cranial Trauma

Mild cranial trauma may cause transitory vestibular symptoms which usually evolve to spontaneous cure. More severe traumas may result in longer periods of disequilibrium and may be accompanied by hearing loss that may include mechanical components due to damage to the ossicular chain. Temporal bone fractures may cause profound hearing loss in the affected ear and vestibular symptoms similar to those of the vestibular neuritis. Some patients do not compensate and will require a labyrinthectomy that should not be performed less than 6 or more months after the trauma.

Wernicke's Encephalopathy

Wernicke's encephalopathy is a neurological disease caused by biochemical lesions of the central nervous system caused by lack of reserves of vitamins of the B group, particularly thiamine. The typical symptoms are ophthalmoplegia, ataxia, and mental confusion.

The ophthalmoplegia usually leads to eye movement disorders, the most common being a horizontal nystagmus. The ataxia may involve cerebellar signs. There is evidence that the medial vestibular nuclei may be involved [38].

Truncal Ataxia in Acute Vestibular Syndrome

The evaluation of a patient who consults for vertigo is a diagnostic challenge. We must in a short time define if the origin of its symptoms is a benign disorder or, on the contrary, what suffering can put your life at risk. In recent years we have witnessed great advances in the evaluation of patients with acute vestibular syndrome, not only in regard to diagnostic technology but also in recognizing the importance of the patient's report and physical examination. As demonstrated by Kattah [9], the physical examination is often more accurate than the neuroimaging in the diagnosis of injury at the level of the central vestibular system in the first hours of the event.

Since 2009 we have a new paradigm when evaluating patients with an acute vestibular syndrome: the HINTS protocol (see chapter "The Bedside Tests: Practical Key Strategies to the Diagnosis of Vestibular and Oculomotor Disorders"). It focuses on evaluating the presence or absence of altered head impulse test, the characteristics of nystagmus, and the presence or absence of ocular tilt (test of skew). The presence of a normal head impulse test and/or a nystagmus with central characteristics and/or the presence of skew forces us to suspect a central lesion as the origin of the symptoms.

This has improved diagnostic accuracy. Although its application seems simple, in practice it is not so much, since it requires a prolonged training to master the diagnostic maneuvers, in addition to the difficulties that arise when examining a patient who is with acute symptoms, which cause him an intense discomfort that interferes with the physical examination [39, 40].

There is a wide repertoire of signs that one can examine in a patient with vertigo, and in various studies some of them have been evaluated in the background [9, 41], but in others they have been the main objective [42]. One of them is the ataxia of the trunk. Lee et al. [41] defined it as a motor incoordination that makes walking difficult and established three grades:

- Grade 1: the patient has mild to moderate instability in the standing position but can walk without assistance.
- Grade 2: severe instability; the patient cannot roam without assistance.
- Grade 3: the patient is unable to be incorporated.

Babinski, in 1899 [43], evaluated ataxia by asking the patient, in a supine position, to get up without using his arms. If the patient was unable to do it, he called it a flexor asynergy, which was observed in both cerebellar syndromes and hemiparesis due to lesions of the pyramidal pathway. It can also be evaluated with the Romberg test and the tandem march.

The examination of the vestibular system is based on tests of its vestibulospinal and vestibulo-ocular connections, both under control of the cerebellum. Therefore, what we find in a patient with vertigo depends on the alterations in these connections or on the control that the cerebellum exerts on them. In the HINTS protocol, we evaluate head impulse test, nystagmus, and ocular tilt; these are alterations of the vestibulo-ocular connections and cerebellar control.

This protocol [9] has demonstrated high sensitivity (100%) and specificity (96%) when applied to patients with acute vestibular syndrome by trained examiners, even surpassing neuroimaging in the diagnosis of acute strokes that presents with vertigo as an isolated symptom. In fact, an abnormal HINTS may be the only manifestation in up to 20% of cases of strokes in vertebrobasilar territory, in the first 48 hours of the onset of the condition.

It has been pointed, however, that there are difficulties in its application, either because they do not have physicians with specific training in neurotology or because of the technical difficulties caused by the dramatic nature of the disease that produces such discomfort in the patient that makes it impossible to perform the diagnostic maneuvers as well as to properly interpret them [39, 40, 42].

Lee et al. [41], in 2006, published a study evaluating the symptoms and signs of stroke in the vertebrobasilar territory, where they found that grade 1 trunk ataxia was present in 29% of his patients, grade 2 in 4%, and grade 3 in the 65% of cases.

In the work of Kattah et al. [9], in which the foundations for the HINTS protocol were laid, severe trunk ataxia, defined as the inability of the patient to sit from the unassisted decubitus position, was present in 34% of the patients with central vestibular syndromes and was absent in the patients with peripheral vestibular disorders.

In 2016, we published [42] a retrospective study to evaluate whether trunk ataxia, defined by the criteria used by Lee et al. [41], was useful in the differential diagnosis of acute vestibular syndromes. We found that the presence of grade 2–3 trunk ataxia has a sensitivity of 92.9% and a specificity of 61.1% to discriminate between central and peripheral lesions. None of the patients with central lesions were free from ataxia, so its absence leads us to the diagnosis of a peripheral vestibular syndrome. None of the patients with vestibular neuritis presented grade 3 ataxia, so its finding will confirm an injury to the brainstem. We also found that Babinski's flexor asynergy was present in all patients with grade 3 ataxia and in all patients with grade 1 stroke and ataxia. In this study, the combination of two signs, such as grade 2–3 trunk ataxia and the characteristics of central type nystagmus, obtained a sensitivity of 100% with a specificity of 61.1%, making it impossible for a patient with a central vestibular syndrome to be classified as a patient with a peripheral lesion.

One has to be cautious when interpreting the ataxia of the trunk. Some patients with vestibular neuritis often deviate and/or fall to the injured side, when they walk; this can be further evidenced by the Romberg test [39]. But in general they are able to stand, sit, and walk without help.

Although our data were retrospectively collected and therefore subject to important biases, we believe that this is a study that presents vestibulospinal signs as potentially useful when evaluating a patient with a vestibular syndrome. These signs have the advantage of being easy to evaluate, not requiring too much training for their correct interpretation.

Chronic Vestibular Syndromes

These are vestibular diseases the symptoms of which can last for long periods of time. They can also be peripheral or central.

Bilateral Peripheral Vestibular Syndrome

The bilateral loss of vestibular function causes intense balance and vision problems, as a consequence of the loss of the multiple vestibular reflexes that maintain a person's equilibrium in different situations, like walking, standing, sitting, or swimming. The vestibular system makes us employ the eyes muscles to maintain accurate vision during our movements and controls the body muscular tonus. In patients with bilateral loss of vestibular function, all of these reflexes are lost [44–48].

These patients present disequilibrium, ataxic gait, hypersensitivity to head motions, and neurovegetative symptoms – sudoresis, nausea, vomits, and tachycardia. They do not have vertigo, spontaneous nystagmus, or auditory symptoms. They usually feel better, after the acute phase of the disease, when they are at rest, but have difficulties in performing movements. The main symptoms are disequilibrium and oscillopsia. Some vestibular compensation may occur, but it is never complete.

The main causes of bilateral loss of vestibular function are:

1. Ototoxicosis
2. Autoimmune ear disease
3. Infections – particularly meningitis

4. Bilateral peripheral acute vestibular syndrome (vestibular neuritis)
5. Intense cranial trauma
6. Bilateral vestibular schwannomas
7. Congenital inner ear malformations
8. Cochlear implants

Usually the patient comes to consultation supported by two persons, because of the severe gait ataxia. Some neurotologists employ a caloric test with iced water to confirm the bilateral loss, but some of the patients that do not respond to this stimulus do have residual vestibular function that helps in their rehabilitation. High-frequency rotatory tests are preferable [49], but there is one reported case of a patient that had no caloric responses and no responses for any of the semicircular canals on the Bárány chair and showed responses in vHIT [50].

The usual treatment of bilateral loss of vestibular function is rehabilitation, usually lengthy, with results that are quite variable. Some patients remain severely incapacitated [51].

Vestibular implants, still experimental, have been performed in patients with bilateral loss of vestibular function, with good results, stimulating the vestibular nerves with electric currents [52–54].

Some clinical details concerning these patients are discussed in chapter 13 (Ataxia).

Vestibular Paroxysmia

The term *vestibular paroxysmia* was introduced by Brandt and Dieterich in 1994 [55]. The patient refers to have short attacks of vertigo that generally last less than 1 minute and occur in a series of up to 30 or more per day. During the episodes that usually occur when the patient's head is in a certain position, hyperacusis or tinnitus may occur. Auditory and vestibular deficits are usually found.

Magnetic resonance imaging reveals a neurovascular compression of the eighth nerve in approximately 95% of the cases. The most frequent finding is a loop of the anterior inferior cerebellar artery [56].

Vestibular paroxysmia usually responds to clinical treatment with low doses of carbamazepine or oxcarbazepine. Surgical microvascular decompression of the eighth nerve is recommended only for medically intractable cases.

Persistent Postural-Perceptual Dizziness

Persistent postural-perceptual dizziness (PPPD) is a vestibular syndrome that persists for 3 or more months. The patient has symptoms of dizziness, unsteadiness, or non-spinning vertigo that are present on most days and become worse when he is standing or moving or is exposed to complex visual stimuli. This disorder used to be considered as a psychiatric disease and was named *phobic postural vertigo*.

PPPD may be precipitated by different conditions, including association with peripheral or central vestibular disorders, or other diseases, or stress. Anxiety is an integral part of this syndrome [57].

The pathophysiology of PPPD is still unknown. It probably arises from functional changes in postural control mechanisms, multisensory information processing, or cortical integration of spatial orientation and threat assessment [58].

Serotonin reuptake inhibitors are useful to change and regulate neural conduction through anxiety circuits and central vestibular neurons that respond to movement. A reduction of the symptoms can be obtained in approximately 70% of the patients. Vestibular rehabilitation can also be helpful [57].

The Bárány Society committees classified PPPD as a chronic vestibular disorder; it should not be considered as a structural or psychiatric condition [58].

References

1. Bisdorff A, Von Brevern M, Lempert T, Newman-Toker DE. Classification of vestibular symptoms: towards an international classification of vestibular disorders. J Vestib Res. 2009;19:1–13. https://doi.org/10.3233/VES-2009-0343.
2. Bisdorff A, Staab JP, Newman-Toker DE. Overview of the international classification of vestibular disorders. Neurol Clin. 2015;33:541–50. https://doi.org/10.1016/j.ncl.2015.04.010.
3. Newman-Toker DE, Edlow JA. TiTrATE: a novel, evidence-based approach to diagnosing acute dizziness and Vertigo. Neurol Clin. 2015;33(3):577–99,. viii. https://doi.org/10.1016/j.ncl.2015.04.011.
4. Lempert T, Olesen J, Furman J, Waterston J, Seemungal B, Carey J, Bisdorff A, Versino M, Eversi S, Newman-Toker DE. Vestibular migraine: diagnostic criteria. Consensus document of the Bárány Society and the International Headache Society. J Vestib Res. 2012;22(4):167–72. https://doi.org/10.3233/VES-2012-045.
5. Neuhauser H, Lempert T. Vestibular migraine. Neurol Clin. 2009;27(2):379–91. https://doi.org/10.1016/j.ncl.2008.11.004.
6. Furman JM, Marcus DA, Balaban CD. Vestibular migraine: clinical aspects and pathophysiology. Lancet Neurol. 2013;12(7):706–15. https://doi.org/10.1016/S1474-4422(13)70107-8.
7. D'Albora R, Castro L, Czizonas M. Síndromes vestibulares centrais de origem vascular. In: Zuma e Maia FC, Mangabeira-Albernaz PL, Carmona S, editors. Otoneurologia atual. Rio de Janeiro: Revinter; 2014. p. 259–73.
8. Merchant SN, Nadol JB Jr. Schuknecht's pathology of the ear. Shelton, CT: People's Medical Publishing House; 2010.
9. Kattah JC, Talkad AV, Wang DZ, Hsieh YH, Newman-Toker DE. HINTS to diagnose stroke in the acute vestibular syndrome: three-step bedside oculomotor examination more sensitive than early MRI diffusion-weighted imaging. Stroke. 2009;40(11):3504–10. https://doi.org/10.1161/STROKEAHA.109.551234.
10. Newman-Toker DE, Curthoys IS, Halmagyi GM. Diagnosing stroke in acute Vertigo: the HINTS family of eye movement tests and the future of the "Eye ECG". Semin Neurol. 2015;35(5):506–21. https://doi.org/10.1055/s-0035-1564298.
11. Dix MR, Hallpike CS. The pathology, symptomatology and diagnosis of certain common disorders of the vestibular system. Proc Royal Soc Med. 1952;45:341–54.
12. Mangabeira-Albernaz PL. Vertigo in elderly patients: a review of 164 cases in Brazil. Ear Nose Throat J. 2014;93(8):322–30.

13. Nylén CO. Positional nystagmus: a review and future prospects. J Laryng Otol. 1950;64:295–318.
14. Fernandez C, Alzate R, Linsay JR. Experimental observations on postural nystagmus in the cat. Trans Am Otol Soc. 1959;47:201–17.
15. Fernandez C, Lindsay JR, Alzate R. Postural nystagmus due to localized cerebellar lesions in the cat. Acta Otolaryngol. 1959;50(3–4):287–91.
16. Riesco MacClure JS. Nistagmus posicional en lesión comprovada de las estruturas de línea média de Fosa Posterior. Rev Otorrinolaringol (Chile). 1965;25:57–9.
17. Bertholon P, Bronstein AM, Davies RA, Rudge P, Thilo KV. Positional down beating nystagmus in 50 patients: cerebellar disorders and possible anterior semicircular canalithiasis. J Neurol Neurosurg Psychiatry. 2002;72:366–72.
18. Gregorius FK, Grandall PH, Baloh RW. Positional Vertigo with cerebellar astrocytoma. Surg Neurol. 1976;6:283–6.
19. Sakata E, Ohtsu K, Itoh Y. Positional nystagmus of benign paroxysmal type (BPPN) due to cerebellar vermis lesions, Pseudos-BPPN. Acta Otolaryngol (Stockh). 1991;111(Suppl 481):254–7.
20. Brandt T. Positional and positioning vertigo and nystagmus. J Nerol Sci. 1990;95:3–28.
21. Carmona S. Vertigem posicional central. In: Zuma e Maia FC, Mangabeira-Albernaz PL, Carmona S, editors. Otoneurologia atual. Rio de Janeiro: Revinter; 2014. p. 319–21.
22. Büttner U, Helmchen C, Brandt T. Diagnostic criteria for central versus peripheral positioning nystagmus and Vertigo: a review. Acta Otolaryngol (Stockh). 1999;119:1–5.
23. Nylén CO. Some cases of ocular nystagmus due to certain positions of the head. Acta Otolaryngol. 1924;6:106–19.
24. Lindsay JR, Hemenway WG. Postural vertigo due to unilateral sudden partial loss of vestibular function. Ann Otol Rhinol Laryngol. 1956;65:692–707.
25. Riesco MacClure JS. Lectures on the vestibular system. Saint Louis: Washington University; 1959.
26. Hart CWJ. Vestibular paralysis of sudden onset and probable viral etiology. Ann Otol Rhinol Laryngol. 1965;74:33–47.
27. Vaz Garcia F, Martins M. Neurite vestibular. In: Zuma e Maia FC, Mangabeira-Albernaz PL, Carmona S, editors. Otoneurologia atual. Rio de Janeiro: Revinter; 2014. p. 233–51.
28. Mangabeira-Albernaz PL, Ganança MM. Vestibular function and facial nerve paralysis. In: Fish U, editor. Facial nerve surgery. Amstelveen: Kugler; 1977. p. 165–73.
29. Wennmo C, Pyykkö I. Vestibular neuronitis. Acta Otolaryngol. 1982;84:507–16.
30. Barré JA, Reys L. L'encéphalite épidemique à Strasbourg. Sa forme labyrintique. Quoted by Mangabeira Albernaz PL, 1988.
31. Pedersen E. Epidemic vertigo. Clinical picture, epidemiology and relation to encephalitis. Brain. 1959;82:566–80.
32. Merified DO. Self-limited idiopathic vertigo (epidemic vertigo). Arch Otolaryngol. 1865;81:355–8.
33. Oosterveld WJ, James J, Boeles JF, Groen JJ, Jongkees LBW, Van Vliet AGM. Les Vertiges. Données fondamentales et cliniques sur l'équilibration. Paris: Doin; 1976.
34. Baloh RW, Honrubia V. Clinical neurophysiology of the vestibular system. Philadelphia: FA Davis; 1979.
35. Mangabeira-Albernaz PL, Ganança MM. Sudden vertigo of central origin. Acta Otolaryngol. 1988;105:564–9.
36. Strupp M, Brandt T. Diagnosis and treatment of vertigo and dizziness. Dtsch Arztebl Int. 2008;105(10):173–80.
37. Zeigelboim BS, Arruda WO, Mangabeira-Albernaz PL, Iório MC, Jurkiewicz AL, Martins-Bassetto J, Klagenberg KF. Vestibular findings in relapsing, remitting multiple sclerosis: a study of thirty patients. Int Tinnitus J. 2008;14(2):139–45.

38. Kattah JC, Guede C, Hassanzadeh B. The medial vestibular nuclei, a vulnerable target in thiamine deficiency. J Neurol. 2018;265(1):213–5. https://doi.org/10.1007/s00415-017-8670-1.
39. Venhovens J, Meulstee J, Verhagen WI. Acute vestibular syndrome: a critical review and diagnostic algorithm concerning the clinical differentiation of peripheral versus central aetiologies in the emergency department. J Neurol. 2016;263(11):2151–7.
40. Kerber KA, Meurer WJ, Brown DL, Burke JF, Hofer TP, Tsodikov A, Hoeffner EG, Fendrick AM, Adelman EE, Morgenstern LB. Stroke risk stratification in acute dizziness presentations. A prospective imaging-based study. Neurology. 2015;85(21):1869–78. https://doi.org/10.1212/WNL.0000000000002141.
41. Lee H, Sohn SI, Cho YW, Lee SR, Ahn BH, Park BR, Baloh RW. Cerebellar infarction presenting isolated vertigo. Frequency and vascular topographical patterns. Neurology. 2006;67(7):1178–83. https://doi.org/10.1212/01.wnl.0000238500.02302.b4.
42. Carmona S, Martínez C, Zalazar G, Moro M, Batuecas-Caletrio A, Luis L, Gordon C. The diagnostic accuracy of truncal ataxia and HINTS as cardinal signs for acute vestibular syndrome. Front Neurol. 2016;7:125. https://doi.org/10.3389/fneur.2016.00125.
43. Babinski J. De l'asynergie cérébelleuse. Rev Neurol (Paris). 1899;7:806.
44. Strupp M, Brandt T. Peripheral vestibular disorders. Curr Opin Neurol. 2013;26(1):81–9.
45. Kim S, Oh YM, Koo JW, Kim JS. Bilateral vestibulopathy: clinical characteristics and diagnostic criteria. Otol Neurotol. 2011;32(5):812–7.
46. Rinne T, Bronstein AM, Rudge P, Gresty MA, Luxon LM. Bilateral loss of vestibular function: clinical findings in 53 patients. J Neurol. 1998;245(6–7):314–21.
47. Mangabeira Albernaz PL. Arreflexia vestibular bilateral. In: Zuma e Maia FC, Mangabeira-Albernaz PL, Carmona S, editors. Otoneurologia atual. Rio de Janeiro: Revinter; 2014. p. 399–403.
48. Hain TC, Cherchi M, Yacovino DA. Bilateral vestibular weakness. Front Neurol. 2018;9:344. https://doi.org/10.3389/fneur.2018.00344.
49. Lucieer F, Duijn S, Van Rompaey V, Pérez Fornos A, Guinand N, Jean Philippe Guyot JP, Kingma H, van de Berg R. Full spectrum of reported symptoms of bilateral vestibulopathy needs further investigation – A systematic review. Front Neurol. 2018;9:352. https://doi.org/10.3389/fneur.2018.00352.
50. Mangabeira Albernaz PL, Cusin FS. The video head impulse test in a case of suspected bilateral loss of vestibular function. Int Arch Otorhinolaryngol. 2015;20:84–6. https://doi.org/10.1055/s-0034-1395999.
51. Sun DQ, Ward BK, Semenov YR, Carey JP, Della Santina CC. Bilateral vestibular deficiency: quality of life and economic implications. JAMA Otolaryngol Head Neck Surg. 2014;140(6):527–34. https://doi.org/10.1001/jamaoto.2014.490.
52. Guinand N, van de Berg R, Cavuscens S, Stokroos RJ, Ranieri M, Pelizzone M, Kingma H, Guyot JP, Perez-Fornos A. Vestibular implants: 8 years of experience with electrical stimulation of the vestibular nerve in 11 patients with bilateral vestibular loss. ORL J Otorhinolaryngol Relat Spec. 2015;77(4):227–40. https://doi.org/10.1159/000433554.
53. Valentin NS, Hageman KN, Dai C, Della Santina CC, Fridman GY. Development of a multichannel vestibular prosthesis prototype by modification of a commercially available cochlear implant. IEEE Trans Neural Syst Rehabil Eng. 2013;21(5):830–9. https://doi.org/10.1109/TNSRE.2013.2259261.
54. van de Berg R, Guinand N, Ranieri M, Cavuscens S, Khoa Nguyen TA, Guyot JP, Lucieer F, Starkov D, Kingma H, van Hoof M, Perez-Fornos A. The vestibular implant input interacts with residual natural function. Front Neurol. 2017;8:644. https://doi.org/10.3389/fneur.2017.00644.
55. Brandt T, Dieterich M. Vestibular paroxysmia: vascular compression of the eighth nerve? Lancet. 1994;343:798–9.

56. Brandt T, Strupp M, Dieterich M. Vestibular paroxysmia: a treatable neurovascular cross-compression syndrome. J Neurol. 2016;263(Suppl 1):S90–6. https://doi.org/10.1007/s00415-015-7973-3.
57. Bittar RSM, EMDvS L. Clinical characteristics of patients with persistent postural-perceptual dizziness. Braz J Otorhinolaryngol. 2015;81(3):276–82. https://doi.org/10.1016/j.bjorl.2014.08.012.
58. Staab JP, Eckhardt-Henn A, Horii A, Jacob R, Strupp M, Brandt T, Bronstein A. Diagnostic criteria for persistent postural-perceptual dizziness (PPPD): consensus document of the committee for the Classification of Vestibular Disorders of the Bárány Society. J Vestib Res. 2017;27(4):191–208. https://doi.org/10.3233/VES-170622.

Menière's Disease

On January 8, 1861, Prosper Menière presented at the Imperial Academy of Medicine, in Paris, his first description of the disease that bears his name [1]; the presentation was published in September of the same year in the Gazette Médicale de Paris [2].

In his paper he described patients with episodic vertigo and hearing loss and mentioned the postmortem examination of a young girl who experienced vertigo after a hemorrhage in the inner ear.

Before that time, vertigo was thought to be a cerebral symptom similar to epilepsy. Menière pointed out that vertigo frequently had a benign course. He was not attempting to define a disease or syndrome but rather to emphasize that vertigo originated from damage to the inner ear.

The disease that he described is still named after him. And he is praised by his precise clinical description of its symptoms. The French neurologists of that time, however, firmly believed that vertigo was a brain disorder. In fact, their belief was so intense that they attacked Menière in a vicious manner. These neurologists were renowned physicians, and their contribution to medical science was significant. But this time they were wrong. Menière wrote four papers in defense of his findings and did not write others because he died in 1862, less than 1 year after his famous monograph was published.

We also praise Menière for his use of basic sciences in his clinical approach – probably one of the first in the history of medicine. There is always a gap between medical researchers and clinicians, and at that time the gap was enormous; practically no interchange existed. And yet Menière was acquainted with the work of a pioneering neurophysiologist, Jean-Pierre Flourens, who had practiced destructions of the semicircular canals in pigeons, and this knowledge was essential to his conclusions.

Many years later, in 1914, the Nobel Prize in Medicine was given to Robert Bárány, the father of Neurotology. It is interesting to quote a small portion of Bárány's speech at the Karolinska Institute in Stockholm, when he received the prize in 1916 [3]:

P. L. M. Albernaz et al., *The New Neurotology*,
https://doi.org/10.1007/978-3-030-11283-7_9

> "As neither of these two great research scientists (Flourens and Purkinje) was able to find the solution to the mystery, it is small wonder that none of their contemporaries were able to do so either. Science stood still in this respect for nearly 40 years. Only in the year 1861 was a Frenchman, Menière, able to take a bold step forward."

> "Menière proceeded along totally different lines from his predecessors … He observed this kind of patient (patients with vertigo) for years and saw absolutely no symptoms of brain disease. Menière now had the idea that the vertigo phenomena were symptoms of disease in the semi-circular canal apparatus and he now succeeded, where Flourens and Purkinje had failed, in seeing through the confusing diversity of the vertigo manifestations in humans and in animals and recognizing that those animals whose semi-circular canals had been operated upon by Flourens had vertigo. This was the principal great achievement of the man who, unfortunately, did not survive to enjoy the fame of his discovery, since he died in the same year."

It should be noted that the term *Menière's syndrome* was employed until 1938. After that it began to be called *Menière's disease.* In 1995 the American Academy of Otolaryngology – Head and Neck Surgery proposed to separate the cases of idiopathic disease from those with established etiologies, which were called *Menière's syndrome*. In 2015 the Bárány Society, the Japan Society for Equilibrium Research, the European Academy of Otology and Neurotology, the Korean Balance Society, and also the American Academy of Otolaryngology – Head and Neck Surgery decided by consensus to use the term *Menière's Disease* for all cases, regardless of the establishment of an etiology.

This chapter follows these more recent and more accurate consensus criteria, which are shown in Table 1 [4].

Pathology

A German ophthalmologist and otologist, Hermann Jacob Knapp, suggested, in 1871, that the symptoms of Menière's disease might be due to an increase in labyrinthine pressure and compared it with the glaucoma in the eye [5].

Table 1 Diagnostic criteria for Menière's disease

Definite Menière's disease
A. Two or more spontaneous episodes of vertigo, each lasting 20 minutes to 12 hours
B. Audiometrically documented low- to medium-frequency sensorineural hearing loss in the affected ear on at least one occasion before, during, or after one of the episodes of vertigo
C. Fluctuating aural symptoms (hearing, tinnitus, or fullness) in the affected ear
D. Not better accounted for any other vestibular diagnosis
Probable Menière's disease
A. Two or more spontaneous episodes of vertigo, each lasting 20 minutes to 12 hours
B. Fluctuating aural symptoms (hearing, tinnitus, or fullness) in the affected ear
C. Not better accounted for any other vestibular diagnosis

The pathological confirmation of the increased pressure of endolymph – *endolymphatic hydrops* – was confirmed only in 1938 by Hallpike and Cairns, studying two temporal bones of patients who died after a section of the acoustic nerve through the posterior cranial fossa [6].

The presence of endolymphatic hydrops in Menière's disease has been confirmed by many authors, in many temporal bones. It is known, however, that endolymphatic hydrops may be presented in other inner ear diseases, such as tertiary syphilis and Mondini dysplasia.

The endolymphatic hydrops associated with Menière's disease is probably linked to faulty absorption of endolymph. It is different from the mild hydrops of patients with carbohydrate metabolism disorder, in whom there are changes in the chemical composition and density of endolymph.

The temporal bone studies have shown that some patients that had Menière's disease did not present hydrops; this has been attributed to the patient's death during a remission phase of the disease. On the other hand, hydrops has been described in temporal bones of persons that never had Menière's disease [7].

There are only rare atrophic changes in the organs of Corti, hair cells, and neural structures in most temporal bones of patient's with Menière's disease [8, 9].

Endolymphatic hydrops has been experimentally developed in laboratory animals – guinea pigs, cats, and rabbits – by obstructing the endolymphatic duct or destroying the endolymphatic sac [8, 9].

Etiology

The many attempts to determine the etiology of Menière's disease have not achieved significant facts.

Some of the proposed etiologies, as a psychosomatic origin, have been adequately excluded. There is much evidence that it may be a genetic disease; it has also been suggested that it may be linked to developmental problems of the inner ear or to autoimmune disorders. About one in three patients with Menière's disease has a first-degree relative that also has the disease.

It seems clear that a variation of Menière's disease, called *delayed endolymphatic hydrops*, is of viral origin, linked mainly to the virus of epidemic parotiditis [10]. Since the vestibular symptoms appear many years after the acute viral disease, it is quite possible that the typical cases of the disease may also evolve slowly from some past viral infection. There are also some pathologic data supporting a viral cause [11, 12]. Some cases of Menière's disease result from by physical or acoustic trauma [13].

It is also known that several astronauts developed Menière's disease after orbital flights, which means that exposure to different gravitational fields may act as an etiologic factor.

For the majority of the cases, the etiology cannot be established; these are usually labeled as idiopathic Menière's disease.

Symptoms and Signs

Clinical history is quite typical in most cases of Menière's disease, establishing an orientation as to the examinations that will confirm the diagnosis. There are, however, many different degrees regarding the morbidity of the disorder, and there are also atypical cases.

Menière, in his original paper, described three symptoms: hearing loss, usually fluctuant; tinnitus, and episodes of vertigo. In time one other symptom was added: the sensation of fullness or aural pressure.

Clinical History

An attack of vertigo, lasting 20 minutes or longer, is usually the first symptom referred by the patient. The first episode of vertigo is usually frightening, and the patient rarely pays attention to the hearing changes. As the episodes of vertigo recur, the patients begin to complain of hearing loss and aural pressure.

The frequency of the attacks is quite variable. There are patients that have two or three attacks each year, others that may have episodes of vertigo every day. Many patients have long intervals of remission of the symptoms.

The hearing loss may be unilateral or bilateral. In some bilateral cases, the hearing may be quite asymmetrical and commonly the patient only refers the hearing loss of the most affected ear.

Some patients come for consultation with cochlear symptoms only. They have fluctuant hearing losses and aural pressure, and their auditory tests are highly suggestive of Menière's disease but they do not have vertigo. This so-called *cochlear Menière's disease* almost always becomes a typical Menière's disease after a variable amount of time.

It has been suggested that some patients may have a *vestibular Menière*, with only vestibular symptoms. It is not infrequent to see patients with unilateral vestibular deficits who have episodic vertigo, but most of them have brief episodes; they rarely have vertiginous attacks during 20 or more minutes. Most of them get well by means of central compensation and do not develop cochlear symptoms.

Most patients with hearing losses present tinnitus, which also fluctuates according to the intensity of the hearing loss. For many patients the increase of the tinnitus loudness is an *aura* that indicates a forthcoming episode of vertigo.

After many years the patients' symptoms are changed. The hearing loss and the tinnitus tend to stabilize, and the episodes of vertigo become less intense and more frequent and no longer have auras [14]. This kind of *unbalanced* Menière's disease seems to result from the circumstance that the membranous labyrinth, after years of episodes of dilatation caused by the excess of endolymph, can no longer return to its original dimensions.

A rare type of Menière's disease is called *Lermoyez syndrome.* In these patients the hearing improves considerably immediately after an attack of vertigo.

Hearing Loss

The hearing loss in Menière's disease is sensorineural and varies with the intensity of the disease and with time. In early cases it is most frequently a low-tone loss. As the disease progresses, there will be some losses in high frequencies, configuring an inverted U-shaped audiogram. In advanced cases there is usually a more significant amount of hearing loss, with more elevated thresholds in the higher frequencies. Thresholds above 70 dB HL in most cases are suggestive of an irreversible hearing loss. Total loss is rare and probably results from rupture of the tectorial membrane.

Hearing loss in Menière's disease is fluctuant. In the early cases, the loss coincides with the episode of vertigo, and the hearing improves after the vertigo ceases. The recovery, however, is seldom complete, and the hearing loss progresses slowly. With the progression of the disease, the fluctuations occur at random, and the hearing loss eventually becomes constant, with very little fluctuations.

Intense loudness recruitment is a constant audiological finding in these patients, as first reported by Dix, Hallpike, and Hood [15]. Some patients refer diplacusis – a sensation of different sound frequencies in each ear.

Speech discrimination may be normal, but most patients have some discrimination loss. This loss, however, is smaller than that observed in tertiary syphilis and autoimmune deafness.

Figures 1, 2, and 3 show typical audiograms of patient with Menière's disease.

Immittance tests show normal tympanometric curves and tympanic reflexes with low thresholds, indicating the presence of loudness recruitment. This can also be shown by means of the Fowler test in unilateral cases or by the SISI tests. Auditory adaptation is absent.

Electrocochleography (ECochG) may show abnormal curves, caused by an increase in the amplitude of the summating potentials in relation to the action potentials [16]. These curves are not seen in patients with intense hearing losses. On the other hand, they are frequently seen in patients' better ears, indicating the occurrence of bilateral disease in apparently unilateral cases [17]. The ECochG curves in Menière's disease are different from the ones observed in patients with Mondini dysplasia [17, 18].

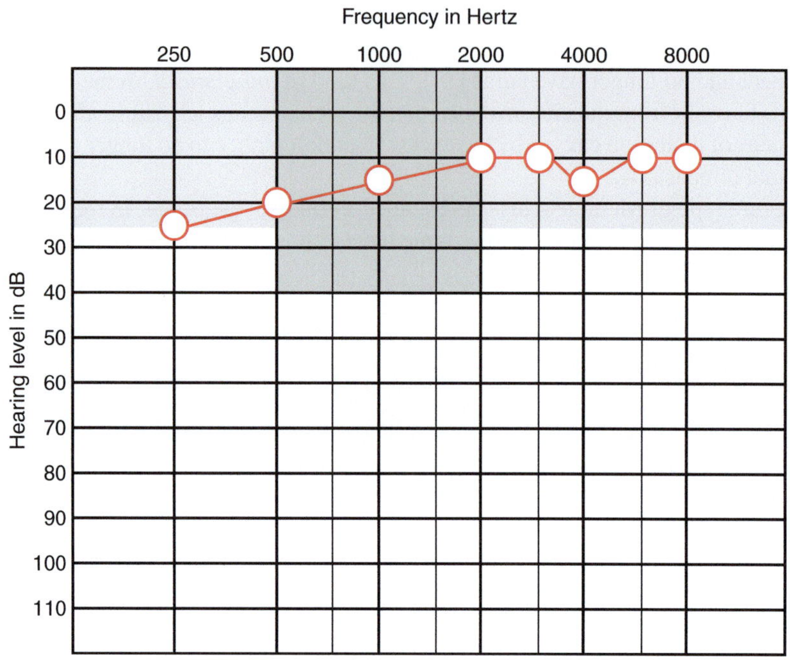

Fig. 1 Audiogram in an early case of Menière's disease

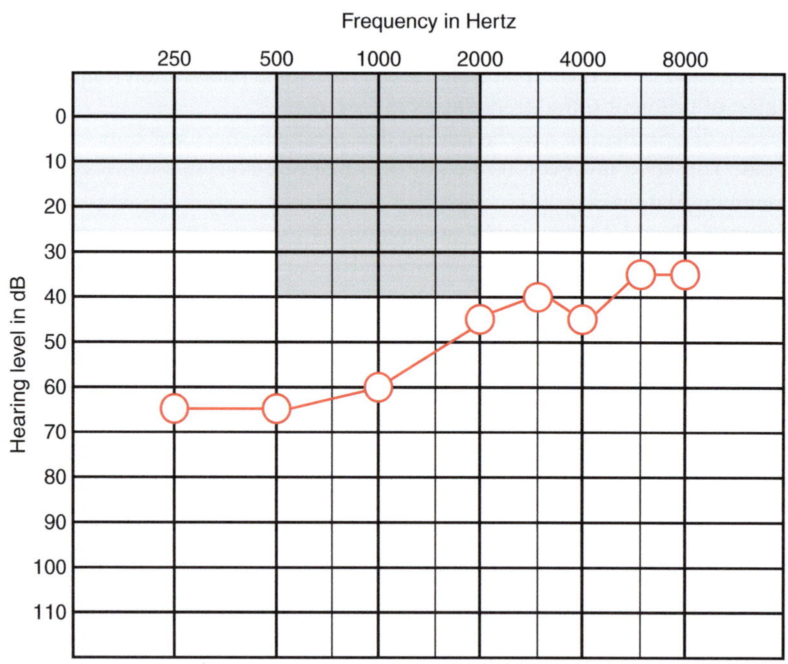

Fig. 2 Audiogram in a typical case of Menière's disease

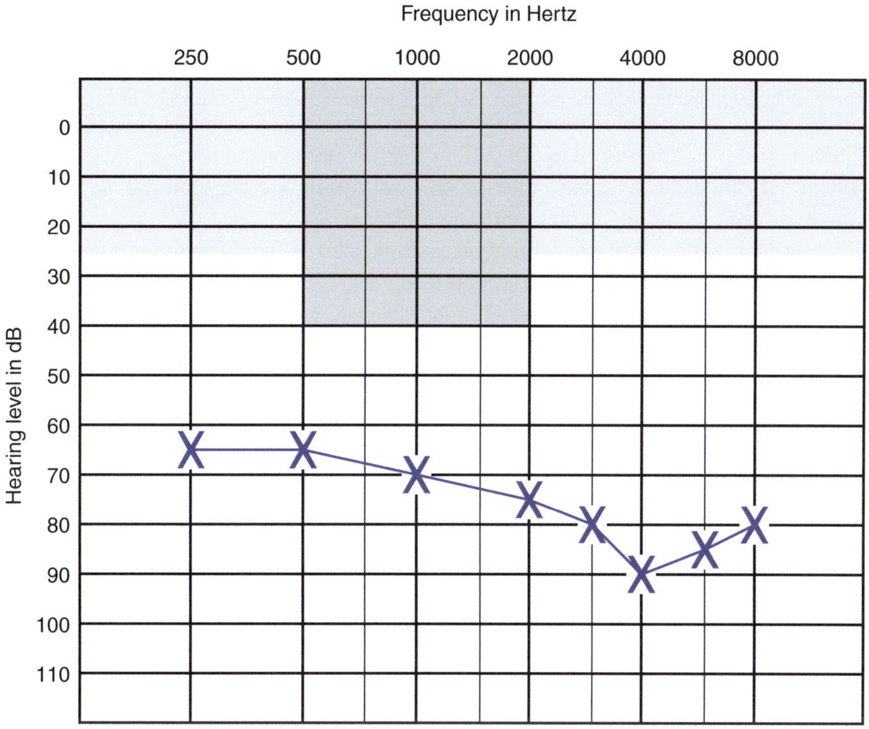

Fig. 3 Audiogram in a case of severe Menière's disease

Vertigo

The episodes of vertigo in Menière's disease are usually intense, and the patients seen during an attack have the usual signs of acute vestibular disorders, such as spontaneous nystagmus beating to the side opposite to the lesion and falling to the side of the lesion in the Romberg test.

When examined in a period between attacks, these signs are not seen.

The findings of the vestibular tests are variable. Spontaneous and gaze nystagmus are usually absent. Optokinetic and pursuit tests are also usually normal. For the caloric tests, the results may be normal, or there may be a directional preponderance of the post-caloric nystagmus, or there may be one hypoactive labyrinth. As a rule, directional preponderance precedes hypoactive responses in the evolution of the disorder. It has been recently demonstrated that the changes in the caloric tests may derive from a reduction of convective fluid movement due to the endolymphatic hydrops [19, 20].

The video Head Impulse tests, on the other hand, are almost always normal.

The vestibular electric myogenic potentials (cervical VEMP and ocular VEMP) are sensitive vestibular tests for Menière's disease. These electric responses are frequently altered by the changes in the saccule and utricle, structures that are also distended by the excessive volume of endolymph. Both cVEMP and oVEMP may be employed to detect early cases of endolymphatic hydrops [21, 22].

Imaging

Recently developed techniques [23, 24] allow for adequate images of the endolymphatic space by means of magnetic resonance imaging. A contrast media, usually gadolinium, is administered to the patient 2 hours previous to the examination or is injected through the tympanic membrane. The results are very similar, so that the transtympanic technique is now seldom employed.

Routine magnetic resonance imaging is important in the differential diagnosis of the disease. Tumors of the endolymphatic sac may mimic Menière's disease; they are usually a result of Von Hippel–Lindau disease, a genetic disorder caused by a mutation in the Von Hippel–Lindau tumor suppressor gene. Meningiomas that reach the endolymphatic sac area can also mimic Menière's disease.

Episodic vertigo in patients with vestibular schwannomas is rare but may be occasionally seen. It would be advisable to order a MRI in patients that will be subjected to surgery for Menière's disease, as well as in all atypical cases.

Bilateral and Unilateral Cases

There are many controversies regarding the percentage of bilateral cases of Menière's disease. It has been shown in long-term follow-up studies that there is a definite increase in bilateral cases [25].

It should be added that ECochG tests often show altered summating potentials in apparently normal ears [16, 17]. The available data suggest that at least 50% of the cases become bilateral in the course of the disease.

Treatment

Vertigo Episodes

Several medications can be used to provide relief for the attacks of vertigo. Dimenhydrinate and meclizine are often used as a symptomatic medication for vertigo, sometimes associated with ondansetron, when nausea and vomiting are present. When dimenhydrinate and meclizine are ineffective to control the vertigo, chlorpromazine or droperidol may be employed. Droperidol is the most effective vertigo-suppression drug but requires hospitalization and the help of an anesthesiologist, in view of the serious side effects that include extrapyramidal reactions; therefore it is used only when other medications fail. Tranquilizers may be added, depending on the patient's degree of anxiety in relation to the attack. There are very few publications related to the use of corticosteroids, but many physicians use them as an attempt to reduce the length of time of the episodes.

Treatment Between Attacks of Vertigo

Unfortunately the clinical treatments for chronic Menière's disease yield variable results. Several medications have been empirically used and provide relief in a percentage of cases. Good results have been reported with the long-term use of betahistine. Small doses of clonazepam that liberate neurotransmitters, primarily GABA, have been found helpful in some cases. Diuretics are often used; it must be understood, however, that they do not reduce the volume of endolymph; they just intoxicate the stria vascularis. Corticosteroids are also being used, either orally or by transtympanic injections, equally with variable results.

Approximately 5% of the patients will need transtympanic injections of gentamicin or surgical treatment. These treatments will be discussed in a separate chapter.

Final Comments

In spite of having been described in 1861, and of generating an enormous number of clinical and research studies, Menière's disease still constitutes a challenge to the neurotologist. Many physicians have discussed it in numerous medical meetings, but many of its aspects remain obscure.

References

1. Menière P. Sur une forme de surdité grave dépendant d'une lésion de l'oreille interne. Bulletin de l'Académie Impériale de Médecine. 1861;t. XXVI:241.
2. Menière P. Mémoire sur des lésions de l'oreille interne donnant lieu à des symptômes de congestion cérébrale apoplectiforme. Gazette Médicale de Paris. 1961;série 3(16):597.
3. Bárány R. Nobel lecture: some new methods for functional testing of the vestibular apparatus and the cerebellum. Nobelprize.org. Nobel Media AB 2014. Web. 9 Dec 2016. Retrieved from http://www.nobelprize.org/nobel_prizes/medicine/laureates/1914/barany-lecture.html.
4. Lopez-Escamez JA, Carey J, Chung WH, Goebeld JA, Magnusson MM, Newman-Toker DE, Strupp M, Suzuki M, Trabalzini F, Bisdorff A. Diagnostic criteria for Menière's disease. J Vestib Res. 2015;25:1–7. https://doi.org/10.3233/VES-150549.
5. Knapp HJ. A clinical analysis of the inflammatory affections of the inner ear; 1871. Quoted by Shambaugh GE, Jr. Surgery of the Ear. Philadelphia: Saunders; 1959.
6. Hallpike CS, Cairns H. Observations on the pathology of Ménière's syndrome: (section of otology). Proc R Soc Med. 1938;31(11):1317–36.
7. Rauch SD, Merchant SN, Thediner BA. Meniere's syndrome and endolymphatic hydrops: double blind temporal bone study. Ann ORL. 1989;98(11):873–83.
8. Schuknecht HF. Pathology of the ear. Cambridge: Harvard University; 1974.
9. Merchans SN, Nadol JB Jr. Schuknecht pathology of the ear. 3rd ed. Shelton, CT: People's Medical Publishing House; 2010.
10. Mangabeira-Albernaz PL. Unusual cases of delayed endolymphatic hydrops. Acta Otolaryngol. 2007;127(4):355–9.

11. Gacek RR, Gacek MR. Meniere's disease as a manifestation of vestibular ganglionitis. Am J Otolaryngol. 2001;22(4):241–50.
12. Linthicum F. Herpes simplex virus DNA in endolymphatic sacs in patients with Meniere's disease. The National Temporal Bone Registry Newletter, Winter 2001/2002, Vol 9, #2.
13. Paparella MM, Mancini F. Trauma and Meniere's disease. Laryngoscope. 1983;93:1004–12.
14. House WF. Fisiopatologia da doença de Menière. In: Mangabeira Albernaz PL, Ganança MM, House WF, editors. Surdez neuro-sensorial. São Paulo: Moderna; 1978.
15. Dix MR, Hallpike CS, Hood JD. Observations upon loudness recruitment phenomenon with especial reference to the differential diagnosis of disorders of the internal ear and 8th nerve. J Laryngol Otol. 1948;62:671–86.
16. Gibson WP, Moffat DA, Ramsden RT. Clinical electrocochleography in the diagnosis and management of Menière's disorder. Audiology. 1977;16(5):389–401.
17. Mangabeira-Albernaz PL, Fukuda Y, Ganança MM. Ménière's disease. ORL (Basel). 1980;42(1–2):91–100.
18. Mangabeira-Albernaz PL, Fukuda Y, Chammas F, Ganança MM. The Mondini dysplasia – a clinical study. ORL (Basel). 1981;43(3):131–52.
19. Welgampola MS, Akdal G, Halmagyi GM. Neuro-otology – some recent clinical advances. J Neurol. 2017;264:188–203. https://doi.org/10.1007/s00415-016-8266-1.
20. Choi JE, Kim Y-K, Young SC, Lee K, Park HW, Yoon SH, Kim H-J, Chung W-H. Morphological correlation between caloric tests and vestibular hydrops in Ménière's disease using intravenous Gd enhanced inner ear MRI. PLoS One. 2017;12(11):e0188301. https://doi.org/10.1371/journal.pone.0188301.
21. de Waele C, Huy PT, Diard JP, Freyss G, Vidal PP. Saccular dysfunction in Meniere's disease. Am J Otol. 1999;20(2):223–32.
22. Taylor RL, Wijewardene AA, Gibson WP, Black DA, Halmagyi GM, Welgampola MS. The vestibular evoked-potential profile of Ménière's disease. Clin Neurophysiol. 2011;122(6):1256–63. https://doi.org/10.1016/j.clinph.2010.11.009.
23. Nakashima T, Naganawa S, Sugiura M, Teranishi M, Sone M, Hayashi H, Nakata S, Katayama N, Ishida IM. Visualization of endolymphatic hydrops in patients with Meniere's disease. Laryngoscope. 2007;117(3):415–20. https://doi.org/10.1097/MLG.0b013e31802c300c.
24. Pyykkö I, Zou J, Poe D, Nakashima T, Naganawa S. Magnetic resonance imaging of the inner ear in Meniere's disease. Otolaryngol Clin N Am. 2010;43(5):1059–80. https://doi.org/10.1016/j.otc.2010.06.001.
25. Stahle J, Friberg U, Svedberg A. Long-term progression of Meniere's disease. In Huang T-S (ed), Meniere's disease. Proceedings of the Satellite Bárány Society Meeting, Taipei, 1990. Acta Otolaryngol. 1991;Suppl 485:78–83.

Vestibular Migraine

In 2004 the Headache Classification Subcommittee of the International Headache Society defined *migraine headache* as an intermittent headache, recurrent, unilateral, gravitational and disabling, associated with nausea and vomiting, and sensible to sound and light.

One of the most frequent *associations* of migraine are *vestibular symptoms*. Vestibular migraine (VM, also called "migraine vertigo," "headache vertigo," "vertigo migraine," or "recurrent benign vertigo") is, in our experience, the first cause of recurrent vertigo. Vestibular symptoms occur as a part of the migraine crisis more than as a comorbid disorder [1].

In 2012 the Bárány Society established the criteria for Vestibular Migraine, ending the confused nosology that existed until that moment [2]:

Definite vestibular migraine requires recurrent attacks with vestibular symptoms of moderate or severe intensity, a history of migraine according to the International Classification of Headache Disorders, and migraine symptoms during at least half of the vertigo attacks (included in the Third Edition of the ICHD).

For *probable vestibular migraine*, the patients must have recurrent vestibular symptoms of moderate or severe intensity, with either a history of migraine or migraine symptoms accompanying the attack (it will be included when more evidence is obtained).

Clinical Picture

Typically, the patient feels vertigo, or instability, of sudden onset, usually accompanied by nausea and vomiting, intolerance to changes in position and to cephalic movement. The headache – when present – can precede, accompany, or follow the vertigo. Just as the pain in the migraine crisis, the symptoms may last for hours to days.

P. L. M. Albernaz et al., *The New Neurotology*,
https://doi.org/10.1007/978-3-030-11283-7_10

Motion sickness is highly prevalent in these patients and must be considered in the patient's clinical history. It is present in approximately 50% of the migraine sufferers, and it is even higher in patients that have vestibular migraine [3].

Family history is also highly prevalent (see below in Pathophysiology).

The clinical findings in the moment of the crisis – *essential to make the diagnosis* – can be divided into:

1. A harmonic peripheral vestibular syndrome, not distinguishable from the one that can be found in other disorders.
2. A central vestibular syndrome where the axial ataxia is almost always present (95% of the cases) and we will find a central nystagmus (vertical, upbeating or downbeating, rotatory or horizontal), or a central positional nystagmus [4]. These findings that can be seen during a period of 24–72 hours following the crises (up to a week in some cases) must show a remission, to configure the status of an episodic condition.

Migraine and Hearing Symptoms

The relationship between migraine and vertigo has been mentioned by Prosper Menière himself. Many patients report a sensation of blocked ears or fullness, tinnitus, and even hearing impairment during the crisis [5]. In a recent work, we found an incidence of 41% of these symptoms in a group of 92 patients with confirmed VM diagnosis.

We are convinced that this is a particular *subtype* of migraine in which:

1. The prevailing peripheral symptoms are associated with one of the ears.
2. The crisis lasts less time than in the central forms.
3. There seems to be an association between sudden deafness, homolateral to the affected ear and labyrinth, greater than in the general population [6, 7].

Pathophysiology

1. Migraine with aura seems to be the clinical expression of the "spreading depression," and vertigo is the most common aura in basilar migraine. Spreading depression affecting the brainstem structures can be the cause of the brief episodes of VM [8].
2. The vasospasm of the internal auditory artery could explain the vestibular and auditory symptoms in migraine, similar to the retinal vasospasm observed in retinal migraine [9].
3. Functional imaging studies using PET during the acute migraine crisis have identified activation of the brainstem regions in projection of the locus coeruleus and the dorsal raphe nuclei, suggesting that those neural structures are involved

in the start of the migraine attacks. As the vestibular nuclei ceases to receive adrenergic projections from the locus coeruleus [10] and serotoninergic input from the nuclei of the dorsal raphe [11], it is assumed that the activation of those structures can affect the central vestibular process. The CGRP (calcitonin gene-related peptide) that is released during the migraine crisis has a neuromodulator role over the peripheral and central vestibular system.

4. Relationships between the trigeminal ways and the vestibular system:

   (a) *Central vestibular system*: the excitation of the central vestibular ways increases the visually induced motion sickness in migrainous patients [12]; other authors expressed that the trigeminal stimulus produces a vestibular asymmetry that is manifested as nystagmus [13]. The reciprocal connections among the medial, inferior, and lateral vestibular nuclei and the caudal trigeminal spinal nucleus can be the basis by which a vestibular signal may influence the trigeminal vascular system [14].

   (b) *Peripheral vestibular system*: there is an important sensory innervation of the stria vascularis and of the modiolus vessels and the dark cells of the crista ampullaris [15]. Powerful vasodilators such as the P substance and neurokinin A (NKA) are present in the eight nerve terminals and can be released by vestibular and auditory activation [16]. CGRP is also present in the cochlear and vestibular epithelium [17].

A channelopathy can explain the peripheral and central dysfunction, and it seems to be the most promising hypothesis for VM. Other paroxysmal disorders that are also present with migraine vertigo are the result of gene mutations of the calcium channel CACNA1A, as the family hemiplegic migraine and the episodic ataxia type 2 [18, 19].

In 2001 Oh et al. [20] studied 24 families with what they called "recurrent benign vertigo" (RBV) and concluded that it is a hereditary migraine syndrome in a dominant autosomal way with a decrease of penetrance in males. It has many things in common with the EA-1 (disease of K+ channels) and EA-2 (involvement of the Ca++ channels), mainly with the latter, suggesting that it represents a hereditary channelopathy.

Diagnosis

There are no universally accepted criteria for this pathology. In our opinion VM must be suspected when there is an episode of vertigo lasting minutes, hours, or even days in which a central or peripheral vestibular syndrome can be clinically confirmed when:

1. The patient is young or middle aged (with higher incidence in women).
2. The patient had previous similar episodes or has a family history of headache.
3. The headache usually follows precipitating factors (alcohol, stress, lack of sleep, hormonal changes).

4. The patient may not have headaches during or after the crisis.
5. There are no associated symptoms: auditory (except fullness), neurologic (except the usual ones during the vertigo or headache episodes – photo- and phonophobia, anorexia, nausea, and vomiting).

The clinical experience shows that the VM must always be an *exclusion diagnosis.*

The diagnosis vestibular migraine diagnosis may be maintained in those cases with normal or discrete unilateral hyporeflexia and normal audiometry. If the vestibular evaluation shows a central condition, it does not invalidate the diagnosis but requires MRI scans to rule out other disorders.

As in Menière's disease, the patient's follow-up is often necessary to reach a definitive diagnosis.

Differential Diagnosis

The following diseases must be taken in consideration in the differential diagnosis of VM:

1. *Menière's disease*: at some point in its evolution, auditory symptoms and constant hearing loss will be detected.
2. *Vertiginous epilepsy*: within the spectrum of temporal lobe epilepsy, pure vertigo is rare; according to Wieser's classification, it is present only in opercular-insular crises, associated with auditory hallucinations, borborygmus, eructation, vegetative signs, unilateral facial spasm, paresthesias, and olfactory and gustatory hallucinations.
3. *Transient ischemic accidents of the posterior fossa*: they usually occur in middle age or old patients, always associated with other symptoms, like blurred vision, diplopia, dysarthria, dysphagia, hemibody or alternate paresthesias, and drop attacks.

Grad and Baloh, in 1989 [21], published a series of 84 patients with pure vertigo of abrupt onset and minutes of duration who suffered labyrinthine infarcts, demonstrating its special vulnerability within the vertebrobasilar system, a fact which forces the performance of neurotologic studies.

Treatment

VM's treatment does not differ, in essence, from that of other types of headaches, and may be separated into symptomatic and prophylactic.

Symptomatic Treatment

It usually employs medications commonly used in common headaches.

Ergotamine, sumatriptan, and zolmitriptan are not very effective for vertigo [22]. Promethazine is more useful, given its antivertiginous effects. Ondansetron or metoclopramide can be used for nausea and vomit.

Prophylactic Treatment

We have studied and followed up a group of patients treated with topiramate, in daily doses of 50–100 mg, during 9 months in average, with very good results. This drug appears to be especially useful in those patients with vestibular migraine and auditory symptoms [7, 23–25]. Other drugs of standard use for the treatment of migraine headache seem to be effective also in the treatment of vertigo [26]. Reploeg and Goebel [27] used a diagram which began with a diet free of tiramide, with which they achieved only a 16% reduction in the crises, and then added tricyclic antidepressants and beta-blockers and calcium channel blockers increasing the efficiency to 95%. The improvement in headaches and crises of vertigo occurred together. Bisdorff [28] demonstrated the use of lamotrigine, and we have positive experience with gabapentin at a daily dose of 600–1200 mg/day.

A new era is starting now with the use of the monoclonal antibodies to block the CGRP. The vast majority of these compounds are delivered through subcutaneous injection once per month. Since its use is very new, there is little experience in VM. For headache, erenumab showed 7 fewer days in a 3-month study vs placebo for chronic migraine and 3–4 fewer days in episodic migraine in a 6-month study [29].

There is little experience with physical therapy [30], but vestibular rehabilitation is recommended in some cases, particularly when the crises are far apart or have been stabilized with prophylactic treatment.

Benign Paroxysmal Vertigo of Childhood and Benign Paroxysmal Torticollis of Childhood

Benign paroxysmal vertigo (BPV) of childhood is quite frequent and is the first cause of vertigo in early childhood. Its prevalence is approximately 2.6% [31], and the incidence is the same in both sexes.

Clinical Picture

Typically, the crises begin between ages 1 and 4, rarely after 10. The child suffers an attack of vertigo, with ataxic gait, gets scared, and tries to grab a person or object nearby. The symptoms are always associated with paleness and sweating, and sometimes there is nausea and vomiting. During the crisis, nystagmus and divergent strabismus can be seen. The episode lasts seconds or minutes, rarely hours.

Natural History

The attacks occur with variable frequency, from many times a week to once a year. They gradually disappear. At an adult age, almost 100% of the patients have headaches.

Pathophysiology

This entity is believed to be a variety of vertiginous migraine.

Treatment

In most of the cases, it is sufficient to tranquilize the patients and the parents. Medical treatment is usually restricted to patients with very frequent crises or when there is intense family anxiety. It is usually performed with calcium channel blockers, with good results.

Snyder, in 1969 [32], described a paroxysmal torticollis that starts around the age of 1 and disappears near the age of 5. Its recurrence, duration, and association with migraine remind of paroxysmal vertigo in childhood. It is believed that this last one is a dysfunction of the vestibular postmedullar nuclei, while in the case of torticollis, the mesencephalic segment near the zona incerta and the nucleus interstitial of Cajal would be compromised.

Motion Sickness

The expression *motion sickness* is defined as the presence of autonomic and cognitive signs that occur with the exposure to certain movements, either real (car or airplane traveling, for instance) or virtual (simulation stimuli) [1].

Motion sickness shares certain features with migraine. Women are more susceptible, and it is known that the risk of migraine aura without headache is greater in adults with a history of motion sickness in childhood (odds ratio = 2.7).

It is empirically known that motion sickness responds to antihistamines and anticholinergics, so histamine, acetylcholine, and noradrenaline have been proposed as symptom mediators.

When the episodes are sporadic and related to specific stimuli, such as a trip, symptomatic treatment is the best choice. In those patients in whom motion sickness has a negative impact on their daily life, vestibular rehabilitation strategies have been successful, mainly in adolescents.

References

1. Neuhauser H, Leopold M, von Brevern M, Arnold G, Lempert T. The interrelations of migraine, vertigo, and migrainous vertigo. Neurology. 2001;56(4):436–41.
2. Lempert T, Olesen J, Furman J, Waterston J, Seemungal B, Carey J, Bisdorff A, Versino M, Eversi S, Newman-Toker D. Vestibular migraine: diagnostic criteria. J Vestib Res. 2012;22(4):167–72. https://doi.org/10.3233/VES-2012-0453.
3. Furman JM, Marcus D. Migraine and motion sensitivity. Continuum Neuro-otology. 2006;12(4):116–34.
4. Von Brevern M, Zeise D, Neuhauser H, Clarke AH, Lempert T. Acute migranous vertigo: clinical and oculographic findings. Brain. 2005;128:365–74.
5. Rassekh CH, Harker LA. The prevalence of migraine in Ménière's disease. Laryngoscope. 1992;102:135–8.
6. Carmona S, Bruera O. Migraine – vertigo with auditory symptoms a definite subtype of migraine? Proceedings of the XXV Bárány Society Meeting, 2008; p. 173.
7. Carmona S, Bruera O. Prophylatic treatment of migraine and migraine clinical variants with topiramate: an update. Ther Clin Risk Manag. 2009;5:661–9.
8. Dieterich M, Brandt T. Episodic vertigo related to migraine (90 cases): vestibular migraine? J Neurol. 1999;246:883–92.
9. Baloh R. Neurotology of migraine. Headache. 1997;37:615–21.
10. Schuerger RJ, Balaban CD. Organization of the coeruleo-vestibular pathway in rats, rabbits and monkeys. Brain Res Rev. 1999;30:189–217.
11. Halberstadt AL, Balaban CD. Organization of projections from the raphe nuclei to the vestibular nuclei in rats. Neuroscience. 2003;120:573–4.
12. Drummond PD, Granston A. Facial pain increases nausea and headache during motion sickness in migraine sufferers. Brain. 2004;127:526–34.
13. Marano E, Marcelli V, Di Stasio E, Bonuso S, Vacca G, Manganelli F, Marciano E, Perretti A. Trigeminal stimulation elicits a peripheral vestibular imbalance in migraine patients. Headache. 2005;45(4):325–31.y col.
14. Buisseret-Delmas C, Compoint C, Delfini C, Buisseret P. Organization of reciprocal connections between trigeminal and vestibular nuclei in the rat. J Comp Neurol. 1999;409:153–68.
15. Vass Z, Shore SE, Nuttal AL, Miller JM. y col.Direct evidence of trigeminal innervation of the cochlear blood vessels. Neuroscience. 1998;84:559–67.
16. Scarfone E, Ulfendahl M, Lundbert T. The cellular localization of the neuropeptides substance P, neurokinin A, calcitonin gene-related peptide and neuropeptide Y in guinea-pig vestibular sensory organs: a high resolution confocal microscopy study. Neuroscience. 1996;75:587–600.

17. Kong WJ, Scholtz AW, Hussl B, Kammen-Jolly K, Schrott-Fischer A. Localization of efferent neurotransmitters in the inner ear of the homozygous Bronx waltzer mutant mouse. Hear Res. 2002;167:136–55.
18. Baloh R, Jen J. Genetics of familial episodic vertigo. Ann N Y Acad Sci. 2002;956:338–45.
19. Ophoff RA, Terwindt GM, Vergouwe MN, van Eijk R, Oefner PJ, Hoffman SM, Lamerdin JE, Mohrenweiser HW, Bulman DE, Ferrari M, Haan J, Lindhout D, van Ommen GJ, Hofker MH, Ferrari MD, Frants RR. Familial hemiplegic migraine and episodic ataxia type-2 are caused by mutations in the Ca2+ channel gene CACNL1A4. Cell. 1996;87:543–52.
20. Oh AK, Lee H, Jen JC, Corona S, Jacobson KM, Baloh RW. Familial benign recurrent vertigo. Am J Med Genet. 2001;100(4):287–91.
21. Grad A, Baloh RW. Vertigo of vascular origin: clinical and electronystagmographic features in 84 cases. Arch Neurol. 1989;46(3):281–4.
22. Neuhauser H, Radtke A, von Brevern M, Lempert T. Zolmitriptan for treatment of migranous vertigo: a pilot randomized placebo-controlled trial. Neurology. 2003;60:882–3.
23. Carmona S, Settecase N. Use of topiramate (Topamax) in a subgroup of migraine vertigo patients with auditory symptoms. Ann N Y Acad Sci. 2005;1039:517–20.
24. Carmona S. Topiramate in migraine vertigo. Proceedings of the XXIV Bárány Society Meeting. Uppsala, 2007.
25. Gode S, Celebisoy N, Kirazli T, Akyuz A, Bilgen C, Karapolat H, Sirin H, Gokcay F. Clinical assessment of topiramate therapy in patients with migrainous vertigo. Headache. 2010;50:77–84.
26. Baier B, Winkenwerder E, Dieterich M. Vestibular migraine: effects of prophylactic therapy with various drugs. A retrospective study. J Neurol. 2009;256:436–42.
27. Reploeg MD, Goebel JA. Migraine-associated dizziness: patient characteristics and management options. Otol Neurotol. 2002;23:364–71.
28. Bisdorff AR. Treatment of migraine related vertigo with lamotrigine: an observational study. Bull Soc Sci Med Grand Duche Luxemb. 2004;2:103–8.
29. Goadsby PJ, Reuter U, Hallström Y, Broessner G, Bonner JH, Zhang F, Sapra S, Picard H, Mikol DD, Lenz RA. A controlled trial of erenumab for episodic migraine. N Engl J Med. 2017;377(22):2123–32. https://doi.org/10.1056/NEJMoa1705848.
30. Whitney SL, Wrisley DM, Brown KE, Furman JM. Physical therapy for migraine-related vestibulopathy and vestibular dysfunction with history of migraine. Laryngoscope. 2000;110:1528–34.
31. Abu-Arafeh I, Russel G. Paroxysmal vertigo as a migraine equivalent in children: a population-based study. Cephalalgia. 1995;15:22–5.
32. Snyder CH. Paroxysmal torticollis in infancy. Am J Dis Child. 1969;117:458–60.

Benign Paroxysmal Positional Vertigo

Benign paroxysmal positional vertigo (BPPV) is the most frequent type of vertigo. It was reported by Alfred Adler in 1897 and by Robert Bárány in 1922, but it was only described in detail by Hallpike in 1952. Overall, its prevalence ranges from 10.7 to 64 per 100,000 individuals; it is more frequent in women and has a peak incidence in the 50–60-year age group [1–3].

It is due to a mechanical disorder of the labyrinth which is characterized by brief and violent crises of spinning sensation showing brisk onset and rapid decrease – *paroxysmal vertigo*. Each crisis usually lasts from 15 to 60 seconds and is related to head position changes with respect to gravity – *positional vertigo*. It usually has a favorable course and therefore is defined as *benign*; however BPPV can occasionally be very disabling because of a high recurrence rate and/or a low response to the physical therapy, so that some authors prefer to omit the term benign [4].

BPPV usually occurs spontaneously. Sometimes it can be associated with triggering mechanical events causing otoconial detachment. Such a causal relationship can be hypothesized in case of minor head trauma occurring within the last 24–72 hours (domestic injuries, sports injuries, school injuries, dental care), while only a possible or probable relationship can be assumed with viral or vascular illness. A higher BPPV incidence is reported in patients with vestibular migraine or Menière's disease.

The labyrinthine mechanical disorder which causes BPPV is due to the presence of otoconial debris detached from the utricular macula and free floating inside the semicircular canals (*canalolithiasis*) or attached to the ampullary cupula (*cupulolithiasis*). Both of the previous conditions transform the ampullary cupula of the involved canal from a detector of angular accelerations into a detector of linear accelerations, thus becoming *gravity sensitive*. According to the canalolithiasis theory, the otoconial conglomerate gravitates inside the canal because of head movements and in so doing pushes the endolymphatic column. In this way, the otoconial bolus, working like a piston, provokes a hydrodynamic drag on the endolymph, which deflects the ampullary cupula, thus generating an excitatory or an inhibitory stimulus which causes the paroxysmal vertigo.

P. L. M. Albernaz et al., *The New Neurotology*,
https://doi.org/10.1007/978-3-030-11283-7_11

According to the cupulolithiasis theory, the otoliths are attached to the cupula which becomes heavier than the surrounding endolymph and gravity sensitive (heavy cupula). In our experience cupulolithiasis is much less frequent than canalolithiasis.

Rajguru et al. [5] developed a mathematical tridimensional model to quantify the biomechanical origin of the gravity-induced responses of the semicircular canals in the presence of canalolithiasis. This model predicts the latency and intensity of the nystagmus resulting from the Dix-Hallpike maneuver. It was observed that the latency peaks, which are related to the length of time taken by the particles to move from the ampulla to the posterior apex of the canal, were essentially dependent on the size and number of the particles. Small particles were correlated to long latencies and large particles to small intensities and reduced cupula displacements. Groups of small particles yielded short latencies. The intensity of the responses was essentially dependent on the number of particles. In spite of the fact that this study was focused on biomechanics, according to the authors, the model can be applied to the clinical interpretation of eye movements, complementing these results with the role of the vestibulo-ocular reflex system.

The BPPV diagnosis s*hall be always based on the evoked nystagmus and not on the kind of maneuver which provokes positional vertigo*. In fact, both excitatory and inhibitory stimuli of each semicircular canal are linked to a typical nystagmus, as every vestibular stimulus triggered by each ampullary cupula deflection provokes the contraction of a couple of extrinsic ocular muscles, thus generating a specific and characteristic eye movement in response to each ampullary nerve input. Therefore, there are maneuvers suggested to diagnose every single type of BPPV, but the pathognomonic nystagmus for a specific subtype of BPPV is sometimes evoked performing the maneuver recommended to diagnose a different BPPV subtype. Thus it is the evoked nystagmus and not the kind of the performed maneuver that allows us to properly diagnose which one is the involved semicircular canal [6].

From clinical experience, it is also known that BPPV is a transient phenomenon that, as a rule, recovers spontaneously in about 2–6 weeks. Sometimes, however, positional vertigo episodes are recurrent or persistent. Zucca G et al. [7] suggest that the spontaneous remission of BPPV episodes is chiefly due to the fact that endolymph, owing to its low content of ionized calcium (20 μM), is able, by itself, to dissolve dislodged otoconia, thus producing a progressive attenuation, up to disappearance, of BPPV symptoms. Horii et al. [8] performed three-dimensional T2 magnetic resonance reconstructions in 13 untreatable patients and observed that the stenosis of the SCC or its closing by a mass of otoconia (jam) was the cause for the failure of the therapeutic procedures.

The pharmacological treatment of BPPV has been disappointing. Literature does not show any evidence that vestibular suppressive drugs are effective in BPPV or as a substitute for repositioning maneuvers [9, 10].

The combination of evocative anamnesis with the results of positional tests, which should be performed under Frenzel lenses or devices that suppress ocular fixation, is usually sufficient for diagnosing BPPV.

The most used classification of types of BPPV observed in clinical practice is based on the involved canal, as reported in Table 1.

Table 1 Classification of BPPVs according to Asprella-Libonati

Classification of BPPVs		
Involved canal	Affected side	Variants
Posterior semicircular canal (PSC BPPV)	Left Right Bilateral	Geotropic (typical) Apogeotropic
Lateral semicircular canal (LSC BPPV)	Left Right Bilateral	Geotropic Apogeotropic
Anterior semicircular canal (ASC BPPV)	Left Right Bilateral	
Multicanal involvement (Multicanal BPPV)	Simultaneous involvement Unilateral Bilateral Non-simultaneous involvement Post-maneuver canal conversion Unilateral	

Posterior Semicircular Canal BPPV (PSC BPPV)

Posterior semicircular canal (PSC) BPPV is the most common form of BPPV, accounting for about 80% of all BPPV cases.

The patient usually experiences his first PSC BPPV attack getting up in the morning, but vertigo recurs when the head is moved in the PSC plane. The patient suffers a new attack every time he flexes or extends his head while upright or when he lies down on the bed or even when he turns toward the affected ear while supine. Vertigo is generally brief and violent and can be associated with more or less intense neurovegetative symptoms. Each attack lasts from 15 to 30 seconds, but the patient often reports longer discomfort due to nausea and vomiting.

Free-floating debris inside the posterior semicircular canal modify the cupula's sensitivity to accelerations, according to the canalolithiasis mechanism, and so doing the PSC cupula becomes sensitive to linear accelerations (i.e., gravity) and to accelerations provoked by brisk head movements on the same plane of the involved PSC (inertial accelerations).

BPPV is defined "secondary" if any inner ear disease is recognized as possible cause of the otoconia detachment. The mechanism of the otoconia detachment is not completely explained; in most of the BPPV cases, the cause of debris detachment is unknown, so these are defined as idiopathic.

Secondary PSC BPPV may be the delayed result of acute labyrinthine damage which caused a crisis of severe vertigo that gradually resolved itself within a few weeks. PSC BPPV sometimes follows an acute episode of vertigo within a variable, usually short delay; this sequence of symptoms is named "Lindsay-Hemenway syndrome" (Hemenway and Lindsay 1956) [11]. It is usually described as a delayed effect of the anterior vestibular artery ischemia which causes a selective labyrinthine damage localized in the crista ampullaris of both anterior semicircular canal (ASC) and lateral semicircular canal (LSC) and in the utricular macula. Such partial vestibular damage is ascribed likewise to a neuritis of the superior vestibular nerve. It is sometimes possible to detect the simultaneous occurrence of PSC BPPV and acute vertigo due to sudden vestibular damage (Asprella-Libonati 2012) [4]. This association of concurrent symptoms is usually missed, because the positioning tests, such as the Dix-Hallpike maneuver, are not routinely performed in patients suffering from acute vertigo with spontaneous nystagmus or, at least, they are not performed at the right moment. If they were regularly done, the typical PSC BPPV nystagmus would be found as a possible concurrence with the spontaneous horizontal nystagmus due to acute unilateral vestibular loss (Asprella-Libonati 2012) [4].

The PSC BPPV diagnosis is made by identifying the typical nystagmus of PSC canalolithiasis. It is evoked by an ampullofugal (excitatory) flow of the debris caused by the positioning tests. All its typical features are shown in Table 2.

Observing the PSC BPPV nystagmus, we should pay particular attention to the eyes' position in the orbit; in fact, the torsional component of the eyes' movements is more evident if the patient looks toward the affected ear, and the vertical one is more evident if the patient looks toward the unaffected ear.

It is easier to make the correct diagnosis examining the patient after a short delay from the vertiginous symptoms onset, when the typical BPPV nystagmus is more

Table 2 Nystagmus features of PSC BPPV canalolithiasis

Quick phase	Torsional component: geotropic Counterclockwise for right PSC Clockwise for left PSC Vertical component: upbeating
Nystagmus is dissociated	Torsional component More evident in the ipsilateral eye Vertical component More evident in the contralateral eye
Nystagmus is paroxysmal	Rapid increase to a plateau and a more gradual decrease Short duration: 15/60 sec.
Nystagmus' latency	3–15 second period of latency after the evocative maneuver and prior to the onset of nystagmus
Nystagmus' fatigue	The repetition of the positioning test reduces nystagmus' intensity
Nystagmus' direction	Nystagmus reverses its direction when the patient sits up after being in the head-hanging position Usually this nystagmus has a lower intensity than the nystagmus evoked by Dix-Hallpike maneuver, because it is caused by an inhibitory stimulus, which evokes a response smaller than the one consequent to an excitatory stimulus, according to Ewald's second law Sometimes its direction spontaneously reverses while staying in the head-hanging position This last condition is more frequent if the nystagmus intensity is very strong

easily and clearly evoked by the diagnostic maneuvers; we define this phase as *the active period.*

The so-called diagnostic maneuver or diagnostic tests are specific movements that were found to be most efficient in eliciting the typical PSC BPPV nystagmus. The most known diagnostic maneuver is the *Dix-Hallpike maneuver* (D-Hm).

Figure 1 illustrates the Dix-Hallpike maneuver for left side [1] and for the right side [2].

The patient sits on the examination bed. The examiner, keeping the patient's head between his/her hands, rotates it 45° toward the examined ear. The patient is then rapidly and gently brought down to the head-hanging position, getting supine with the head still rotated 45° toward the tested ear and hyperextended approximately 20° off of the headrest. After a variable delay, between 3 and 15 seconds, due to nystagmus latency, the typical paroxysmal PSC BPPV nystagmus appears, caused by otoconial debris floating away from the ampulla.

The consequential ampullofugal deflection of the ampulla generates an excitatory discharge of the ipsilateral posterior vestibular nerve and the resulting paroxysmal nystagmus. A reversal nystagmus is observed when the patient returns to the sitting position. Cupulolithiasis should be suspected in cases that do not exhibit fatigability [12].

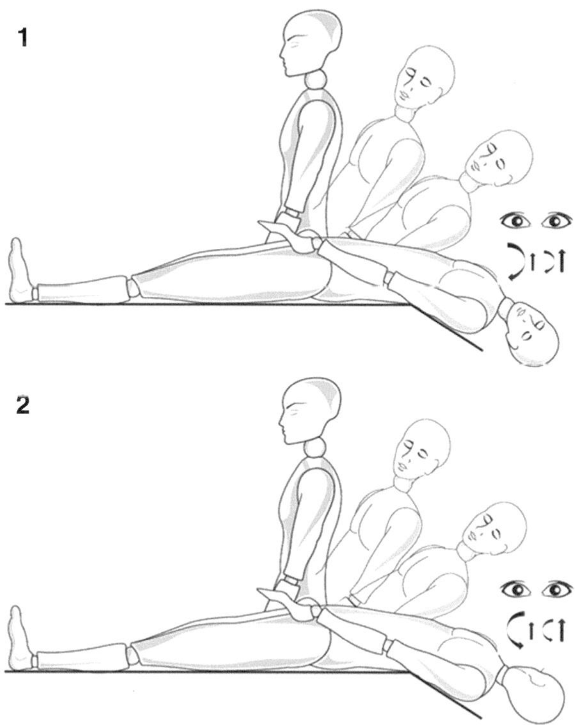

Fig. 1 Dix-Hallpike maneuver

Both PSCs may be affected, but there seems to be a predominance of the right side, because there is a general preference for sleeping in a right lateral decubitus position [13]. Shim et al. [14] found a statistically significant correlation between the head-lying side during sleep and the side affected by BPPV. The simultaneous involvement of both PSCs is less frequent.

The treatment of BPPV consists in removing the otoconia from the canal to which they have moved to and reposition them in the utricle, regardless of the affected SCC. The PSC BPPV therapy is usually performed immediately after the identification of the affected side and is based on rehabilitation procedures. The most popular therapeutic techniques are the *canalith repositioning procedure (CRP)* or *Epley's maneuver* and the *Semont's maneuver*.

Epley's Maneuver

Epley's canalith repositioning procedure, or Epley's maneuver (Fig. 2), is absolutely the most frequently used technique for PSC BPPV therapy all around the world.

The patient initially sits in the middle of the examination bed (S). Then the patient is brought back keeping his/her head turned 45° toward the target ear and finally lies down with the head extended 20° below the table, reaching the 1st position [1]. Particles gravitate in ampullofugal direction, thus generating an excitatory discharge of the ampullary nerve and the typical PSC BPPV nystagmus: clockwise with vertical upbeating component for left PSC BPPV.

Then, still keeping the head extended 20°, it is turned 45° to the contralateral side, 2nd position, so that particles approach the apex and an excitatory nystagmus like the previous one appears once again [2]. On the contrary, if the nystagmus reverses its beating direction, this is a sign that the debris are coming back along the canal (flowchart 1). After that, the patient rolls on to his/her shoulder getting face-down 135°: 3rd position. Particles now enter the common crus, and a purely vertical downbeating nystagmus is usually observed [3]. The patient finally comes back upright, head still turned: 4th position. Particles gravitate through the common crus

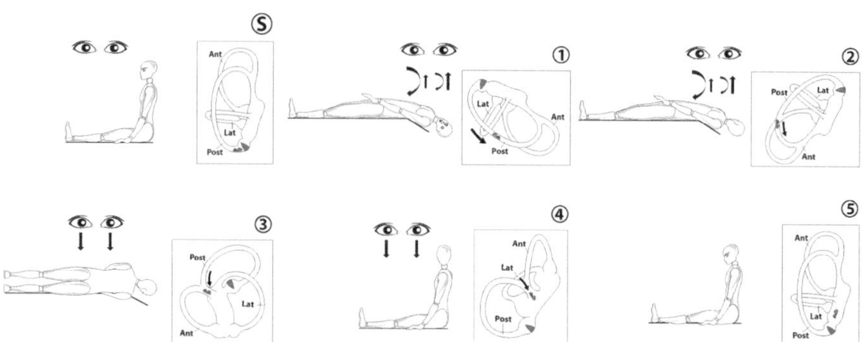

Fig. 2 Epley's maneuver

now, and the downbeating nystagmus is still beating [4]. Finally, the head is straightened and tilted forward 20°: 5th position [5]. Particles drop into the utricle. Now we are ready to start another cycle, if necessary.

According to our experience, it is more natural and correct to directly continue with the CRP when a positive diagnostic Dix-Hallpike maneuver has been observed, without coming back to the sitting position. In so doing, we evoke less vertigo episodes, less neurovegetative symptom, and better treatment tolerance according to "the strategy of the minimum stimulus" (Asprella-Libonati 2003–2005) [15, 16]. A nystagmus-based approach was suggested in monitoring whether or not ampullofugal progression of the debris in the canal occurs by the real-time observation of the evoked nystagmus during each step of the liberatory technique.

Semont's Maneuver

Semont's liberatory maneuver [17] (Fig. 3) starts with a triggering maneuver (D-Hm). For this purpose, the patient is seated on the edge of the examination table. The patient is then laid down laterally so that the head is turned 45° upward.

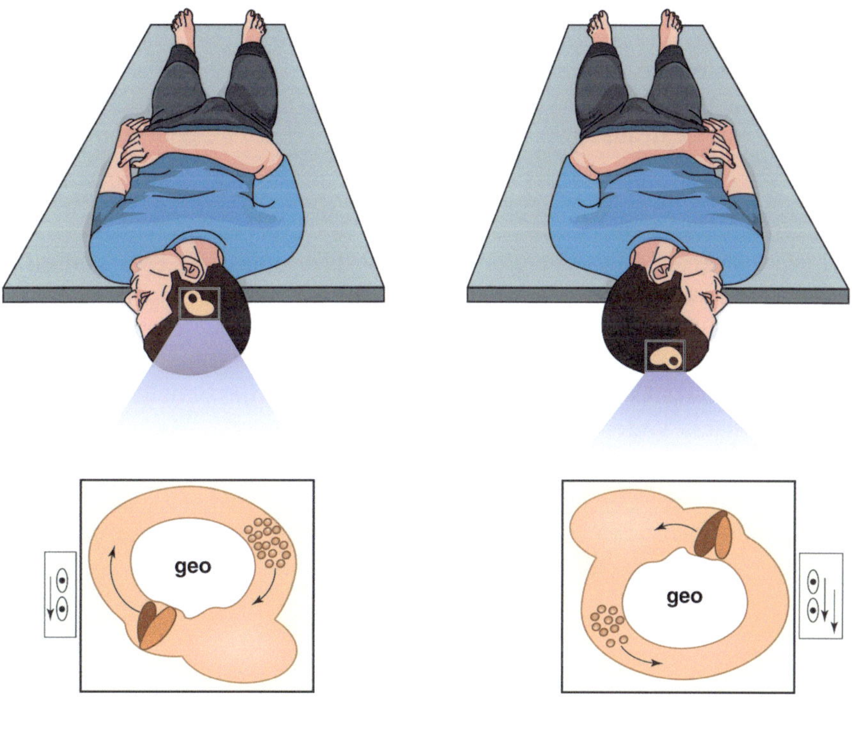

Fig. 3 Semont's maneuver

The head is maintained in this position for up to 5 minutes. Then the patient's trunk is moved quickly so that the head makes a 180° arch while passing the vertical position. This movement is stopped abruptly before the patient's face touches the opposite extremity of the examination bed, and the head is maintained in the 45° downward turn, with the side of the nose touching the table. A few seconds after being in this position, the patient reports his vertigo, and we can observe a nystagmus beating toward the opposite direction (relative to the Hallpike maneuver). After another 4–5 minutes, the patient is slowly returned to the seated position, and the patient remains immobilized for another 4–5 minutes. Sometimes when the patient is in the seated position, he reports an intense vertigo and feels as if he were being pushed back. This is when the particles move from the *crus communis* to the utricle. The key to a successful maneuver is the abrupt deceleration of the head's movement, and the indicator of that success is the inversion of the direction of the nystagmus after deceleration. Semont recommends that patients sleep with their heads elevated (45°) for the first two nights, and they should wear a cervical collar during the first 2 days. They should also be told not to sleep on the affected side until the follow-up visit.

We usually perform the post-maneuver control after about 20–30 minutes or later, checking again the affected side by the Dix-Hallpike maneuver. We could have a "false-negative" control test waiting for a too short time due to a fatigue effect.

Positive signs observed in performing the post-maneuver control are:

- No nystagmus: the treatment has been effective.
- A slight no paroxysmal downbeating nystagmus: the treatment has been effective.
- No vertigo: the treatment has been effective (only if associated with one of the previous signs).

Negative signs observed in performing the post-maneuver control are:

- Typical paroxysmal nystagmus of CSP BPPV: the treatment has been ineffective (repeat the same therapeutic maneuver, add mastoid vibrator, change maneuver if BPPV doesn't resolve).
- Horizontal paroxysmal nystagmus: canal conversion, the debris have migrated from the posterior semicircular canal to the lateral one (perform the therapy for lateral canal BPPV).

The role of post-maneuver postural restrictions on successful treatment and BPPV's recurrence rates isn't definitely established yet. Notwithstanding some recent control studies that state that there is no significant effect of post-maneuver postural restrictions on either successful treatment or recurrence rates, our experience suggests us to invite our patients to slowly and carefully move their head avoiding to tilt it front and back. In addition, we usually suggest them to sleep keeping down the unaffected ear on a double pillow for 4–5 days after the treatment, and finally we advise our patients of the possibility of increased dizziness after the maneuver, so that they could feel like being on a boat for a few days.

Apogeotropic Variant of PSC BPPV

Vannucchi et al. [18] described the apogeotropic variant of PSC BPPV in 2009 and in 2012 published a description of six patients affected by this BPPV variant [19]. All of their patients showed a positional downbeating nystagmus with absent or poor torsional components which was typically suggestive of an ASC BPPV, but a typical nystagmus of contralateral PSC BPPV appeared after the liberatory maneuver for ASC BPPV was performed. Thus, the authors supposed that this was a canalolithiasis of PSC caused by otoconial debris, free floating along the non-ampullary PSC arm close to the common crus, that can mimic the contralateral ASC BPPV.

In fact, when the debris inside the PSC is close to the common crus, it gravitates toward the PSC ampullary arm during the Dix-Hallpike maneuver, thus generating an ampullopetal endolymphatic current and the consequential cupular deflection toward the utricle. The resulting nystagmus has the same features as the one generated by excitatory stimulation of the contralateral ASC.

A positional downbeating nystagmus evoked by the Dix-Hallpike maneuver, with poor or absent torsional components and without clinical evidence of CNS dysfunction, is generally ascribed to an ASC BPPV, but such a nystagmus observed in patients with a history suggesting BPPV may be the sign of a PSC VPPB variant, caused by an otoconial mass originally located close to the common crus.

For disabling conditions that do not respond to any of the repositioning maneuvers and that are fortunately few, surgical procedures have been described, such as neurectomies of the posterior ampullary nerve and occlusion of the PSC [20].

Lateral Semicircular Canal BPPV (LSC BPPV)

The second most common type of BPPV is HSC LPPV, accounting for 15–25% of all BPPV cases.

The patient usually experiences his first LSC BPPV attack turning sideways while sleeping. The violent vertigo abruptly awakes the patient and is generally associated with very intense neurovegetative symptoms. Each attack lasts from 30 to 60 seconds, sometimes longer. Vertigo recurs when the head is moved in the LSC's plane. It is more intense when the head is rotated from side to side while supine, but the patient can suffer from mild vertigo every time the otoliths inside the affected lateral canal begin to gravitate because of head movements, e.g., by rotating the head to the upright position, by lying straight down or on one side. The presence of neurovegetative symptoms and dizziness while walking is usually more intense in the course of LSC BPPV than in PSC BPPV.

The pathophysiology of LSC BPPV is most frequently ascribed to free-floating debris inside the lateral semicircular canal, modifying the cupula's sensitivity to accelerations, according to the canalolithiasis theory. Therefore, the LSC cupula becomes sensitive to linear accelerations, i.e., gravity and accelerations provoked by brisk head movements on the same plane of the involved LSC. Two LSC canalolithiasis variants are known:

1. Geotropic LSC BPPV, about 75% of all LSC BPPV, is due to debris floating along the LSC non-ampullary posterior arm.
2. Apogeotropic LSC BPPV, about 25% of all LSC BPPV, is due to debris floating close to the LSC ampulla (anterior arm) or attached to the cupula, either on the canal or on the utricular side [21].

Pathophysiology of the geotropic variant: shortly after rotating the patient's head to the impaired side while supine, the otoliths gravitate toward the ampulla along the LCS posterior arm, generating an ampullopetal excitatory endolymphatic current, and a geotropic nystagmus beating to the impaired ear. When the patient's head is turned to the healthy side, the otoliths float along the LSC posterior arm toward its utricular orifice, generating an ampullofugal inhibitory endolymphatic current. As a result, the nystagmus will be geotropic once again beating to the healthy side (Fig. 4).

Pathophysiology of the apogeotropic variant: when the patient lies on the impaired side, the debris in the ampullary segment of the LSC will move away from the cupula, resulting in an inhibitory ampullofugal endolymphatic current, which causes an apogeotropic nystagmus beating toward the healthy ear. When the head is turned to the opposite side, the otoliths will drop toward the ampulla with an excitatory discharge, and an apogeotropic nystagmus beating toward the affected side will be observed (Fig. 5).

The diagnosis is performed identifying the LSC BPPV canalolithiasis nystagmus whose typical features are reported in Table 3.

The typical paroxysmal nystagmus is sometimes evoked only after repeating the diagnostic HSC BPPV maneuver again and again. This could happen in patients

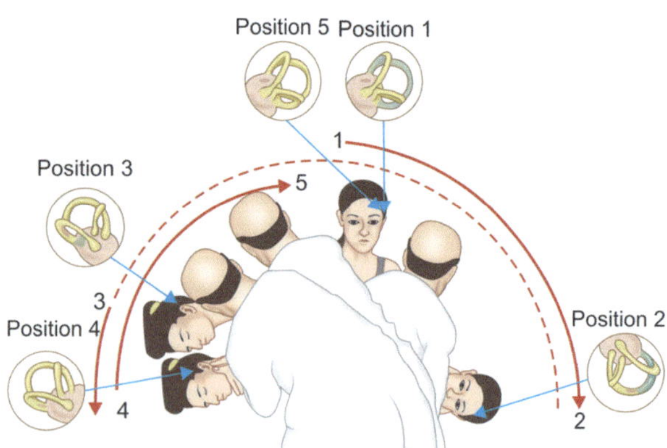

Fig. 4 Geotropic lateral semicircular canal BPPV pathophysiology, right side

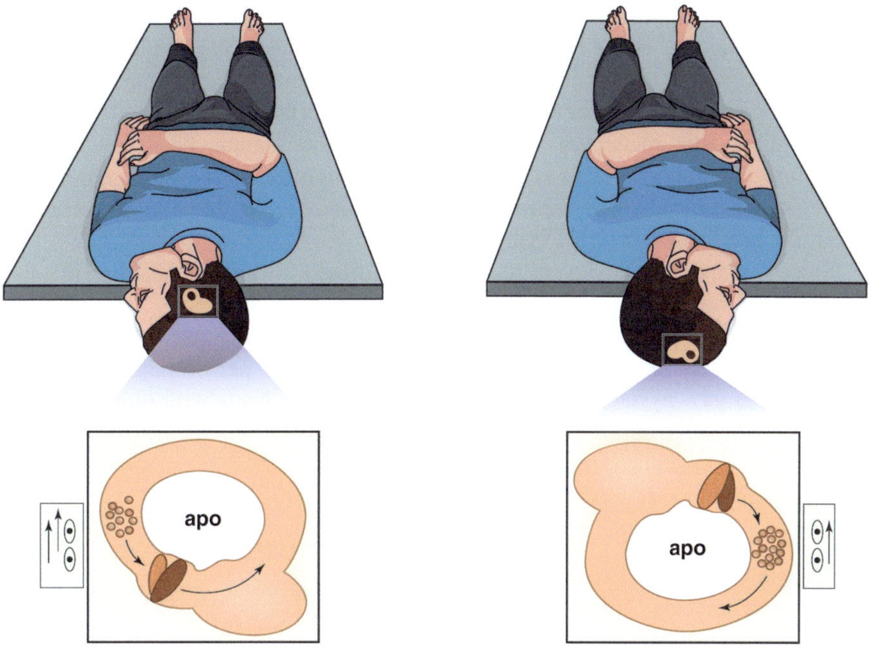

Fig. 5 Apogeotropic lateral semicircular canal BPPV pathophysiology, right side

Table 3 HSC BPPV canalolithiasis nystagmus features

Nystagmus' quick phase	It is a direction-changing, bidirectional, bi-positional purely horizontal nystagmus Geotropic variant: nystagmus beats toward the ground Apogeotropic variant: nystagmus beats away from the ground
Nystagmus is paroxysmal	It very rapidly increases, reaches a so-called plateau, and then slowly decreases It has a longer duration than the PSC BPPV one: 30/60 sec., sometimes longer
Nystagmus' latency	Its latency is shorter than the PSC BPPV one: 2/3 sec., sometimes no latency
Nystagmus' fatigue	Repetition of the positioning test induces less nystagmus fatigue than the PSC BPPV one. Actually, it is often impossible to proceed with retesting to determine how much the nystagmus is really fatigable because of violent associated neurovegetative symptoms
Nystagmus' direction	Sometimes its direction spontaneously reverses while keeping the head in the evocative position This last condition is more frequent if the nystagmus intensity is very strong It occurs more frequently turning the patient on the affected ear in the geotropic variant It is sometimes observed turning the patient on the unaffected ear in the apogeotropic variant

with a delayed diagnosis, because the otoliths are initially spread inside the LSC. In fact, the movement of the otoliths results in a deflection of the cupula only when they are conglomerated, acting like a piston. The repeated head rotations move the debris by congregating them due to the forces of superficial adhesion.

The diagnostic maneuver for LSC BPPV is the "supine head roll test" or "McClure-Pagnini test." This is performed by turning the head 180° to either side while supine. Since it is performed on the yaw plane, it should be more correct to call it the head yaw test (HYT) while supine.

Since therapeutic maneuvers should be performed toward the healthy side, the diagnosis of the affected side is critical for a successful treatment.

The first clinical sign that was described in order to identify the impaired side in LSC BPPV is the intensity of the nystagmus evoked by performing HYT while supine: head yaw nystagmus. The head yaw nystagmus beats with more intensity toward the impaired ear, according to Ewald's second law, which postulates that the response to an excitatory stimulus is always more intense than the one following an inhibitory stimulus, so that:

- In the geotropic variant, the affected side is the one on which the nystagmus is more intense in HYT.
- In the apogeotropic variant, the affected side is the one on which the nystagmus is less intense in HYT.

New clinical signs to diagnose the HSC BPPV affected side have been described in the last few years. All of them show non-paroxysmal long-lasting nystagmus, which generally are of low intensity (Table 4).

A nystagmus evoked by bringing the patient down from a sitting position was first described in 2005 [15]. This is evoked by the seated supine positioning test (SSPT). When the patient lies supine, having the head flexed 30°, the LSC is on a vertical plane; therefore, due to gravity, the otoliths are pushed downward: when they are in the posterior arm, geotropic variant, they float away from the ampulla. When they are near the cupula, apogeotropic variant, they float toward the ampulla. Therefore, the SSPT evokes a nystagmus beating toward the healthy side in the geotropic variant and toward the affected side in the apogeotropic variant: seated supine positioning nystagmus (SSPN) (Fig. 6, Table 4).

A nystagmus observed in an upright position has been described in patients suffering from LSC BPPV. It could be mistaken for a "spontaneous" nystagmus, but it is a direction-changing nystagmus because it is strongly modulated by head position; therefore it has been most properly defined as a "pseudo-spontaneous nystagmus" (PSN). It beats toward the healthy side in geotropic LSC BPPV and toward the affected side in apogeotropic HSC BPPV. It increases if the head is bent 30° backward, disappears when the head is bent 30° forward (neutral position), and reverses its direction if the head is additionally inclined forward to 60° (Fig. 7, Table 4). It is sometimes useful to slowly rotate the patient's head horizontally, because such a maneuver evokes the PSN when it is not evident yet while the head is erect.

A single theory was postulated to explain both the pseudo-spontaneous nystagmus observed in the upright position, with its modifications induced by

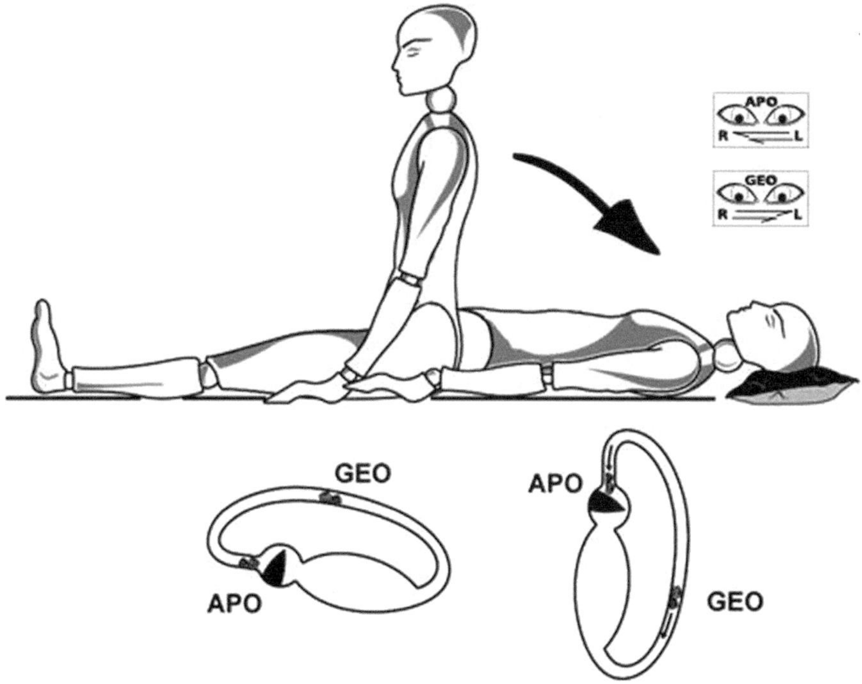

Fig. 6 Lateral semicircular canal BPPV seated supine positional nystagmus, right side

Table 4 LSC BPPV: rules to diagnose the affected side

1. The direction of the more intense nystagmus in the *head yaw test while supine* is toward the affected ear
2. The direction of both the *pseudo-spontaneous nystagmus* and the *seated supine positioning nystagmus* is toward the unaffected ear in the geotropic LSC BPPV
3. The direction of both the *pseud- spontaneous nystagmus* and the *seated supine positioning nystagmus* is toward the affected ear in the apogeotropic LSC BPPV

slowly flexing and extending the head (head pitch test, HPT), and the nystagmus induced by the seated supine positioning test. Both should be considered as the biological response to a single physical phenomenon: the otoliths gravitate along the inclined plane of the lateral semicircular canal (Asprella-Libonati 2008–2010) [22]. The only variable is the gravity vector size which is active in displacing the otoliths along the LSC. Thus, the acceleration due to gravity on the debris varies from zero (neutral point) when the LSC is orthogonal to the gravity axis (head flexed 30° forward in upright position) to the maximum when the LSC is parallel to the gravity vector (supine position, with the head straight and bent about 30° forward).

The pseudo-spontaneous nystagmus sometimes is very intense. This last condition is more frequent in patients observed with a very short delay after the symptom

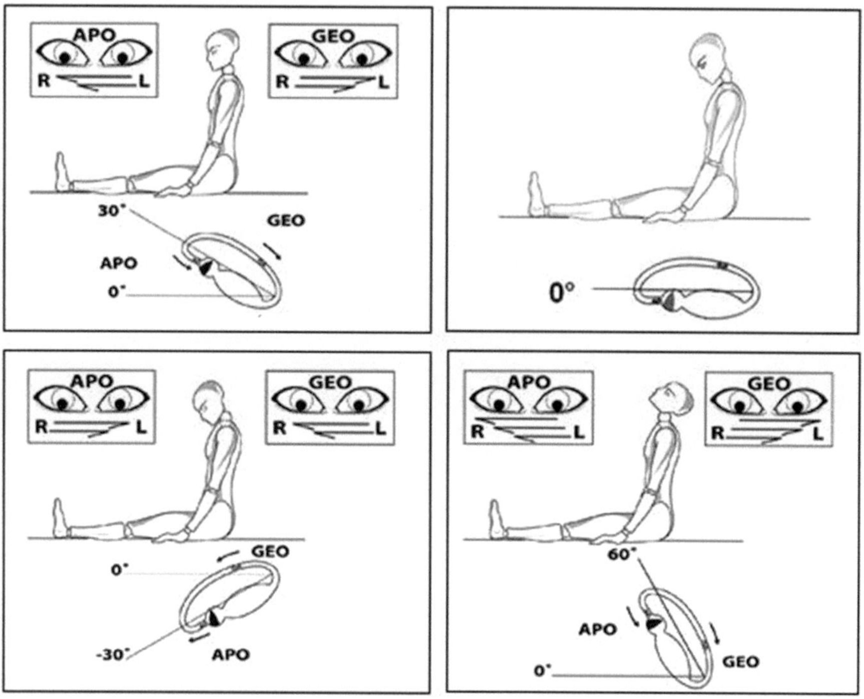

Fig. 7 Pseudo-spontaneous nystagmus, right side

onset, less than 12 hours. It can cause the misdiagnosis of acute unilateral vestibular loss (vestibular neuritis (VN)). The differential diagnosis is based on two points:

1. PSN shows poor or no torsional component.
2. PSN reverses its beating direction by flexing and extending the patient's head while sitting: positive head pitch test.

The horizontal nystagmus should be checked in all patients suffering from acute vertigo by performing the HPT while sitting: if the nystagmus doesn't change its beating direction, it is a direction-fixed nystagmus due to VN, and if the nystagmus reverses its beating direction, it is a direction-changing nystagmus due to HSC BPPV (PSN).

Many therapeutic techniques have been proposed for LSC BPPV, all of them aiming to achieve the ampullofugal endocanalar progression of the otoconial debris (Table 5).

The *barbecue rotation techniques* work by negative inertia. They are done performing abrupt rotations of the patient's head in steps of 90° toward the healthy side while supine, thus moving the debris in the direction opposite to the head rotation. According to Lempert, the head is rotated three times toward the healthy side, thus applying an overall 270° rotation (Fig. 8).

Table 5 LSC BPPV liberatory techniques

Type of applied acceleration	Maneuver
Angular acceleration Negative inertia	Barbecue rotation: Lempert (270°) Baloh (360°) Vannucchi-Asprella (450° or more)
Linear acceleration Positive inertia	Gufoni's maneuver
Gravitational sedimentation	Forced prolonged position (Vannucchi)
Angular and linear accelerations plus gravity action (mixed maneuver)	Asprella's maneuver
Angular accelerations	Barbecue rotation techniques, Vannucchi-Asprella's maneuver
Gravitational sedimentation	Vannucchi forced prolonged position (FPP)
Linear accelerations	Gufoni's liberatory maneuver

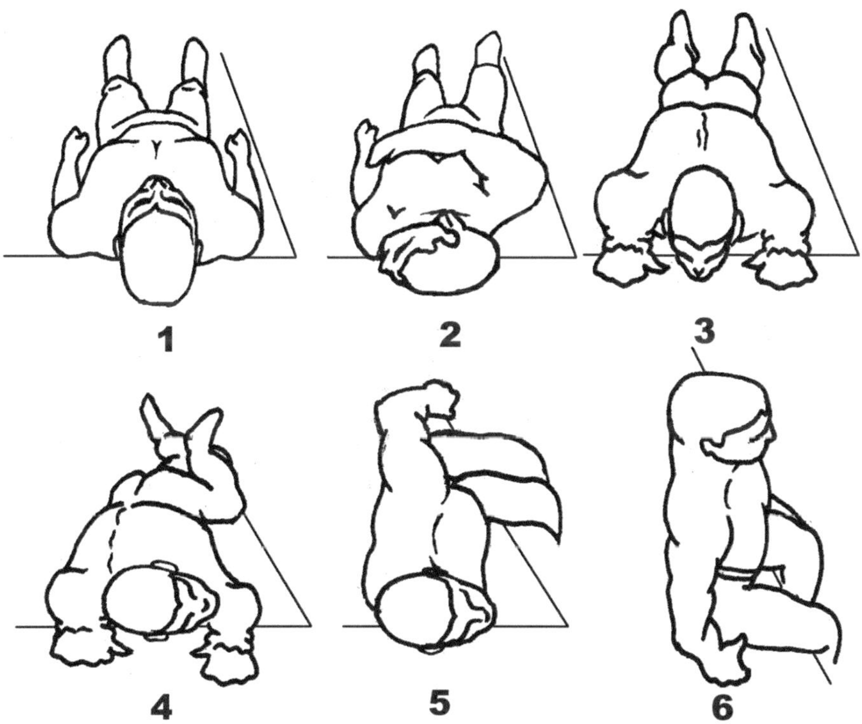

Fig. 8 Barbecue maneuver

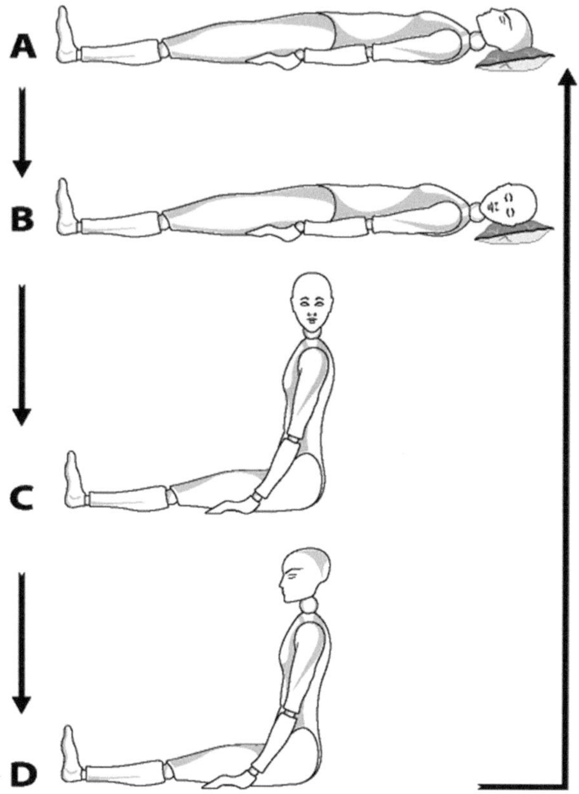

Fig. 9 Asprella's maneuver

The *Vannucchi-Asprella's maneuver* (Fig. 9) is a variant of the barbecue maneuvers. It can at once solve both geotropic and apogeotropic forms, as well as sometimes converting apogeotropic into geotropic forms. In addition, it is easier to be performed than any other barbecue maneuver. In fact, it avoids movements from supine to prone and vice versa. As in the typical barbeque maneuver, the patient's head is quickly rotated 90° toward the healthy side, while supine, and then keeping the head turned in this way, he/she sits up and slowly brings the head back in line with the body. This sequence of movements is repeated five times or more, as long as it does not provoke nystagmus or vertigo. It is important to perform this maneuver under videonystagmoscopic (VNS) monitoring in order to check if the nystagmus is still beating toward the healthy side immediately after each step. Such a nystagmus denotes that the otolithic mass is moving toward the utricle. A nystagmus beating toward the affected ear means the debris are floating toward the ampulla, so the maneuver is being ineffective. The absence of nystagmus finally suggests that the canal has been rid of debris.

Vannucchi forced prolonged position (FPP): in the geotropic LSC BPPV, the patient is instructed to lie overnight, approximately 12 hours, on the healthy side, one or more times. In this position the affected ear is the uppermost one, with debris in the downward-facing non-ampullary arm (Fig. 10). Due to gravity, the

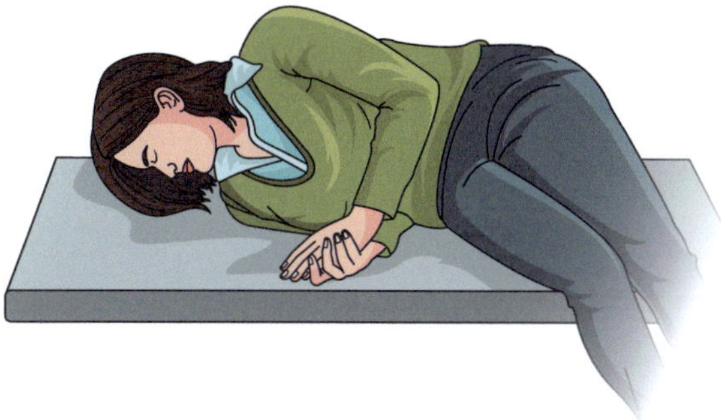

Fig. 10 Vannucchi forced prolonged position (FPP). The patient is instructed to lie overnight, approximately 12 hours, on the healthy side

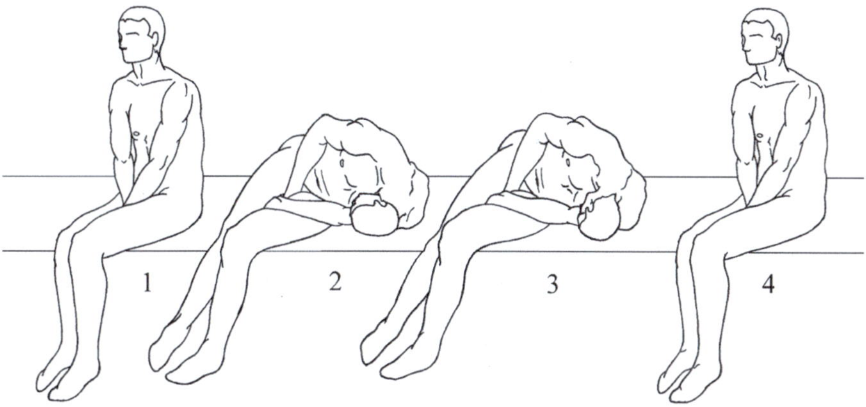

Fig. 11 Gufoni's maneuver

debris gradually moves into the utricle. FPP can be used in the apogeotropic form, but in this case the patient must lie on the affected side; in this way the debris move from the anterior to the posterior arm of the canal, changing from apogeotropic to geotropic form. The patient must then lie on the healthy side to become symptom-free.

Gufoni's maneuver: it works by positive inertia. The maneuver consists of the following steps:

1. The patient sits on the edge of the bed.
2. The patient suddenly lies down on one side which is the healthy one for geotropic LSC BPPV and the affected one in the apogeotropic form.
3. The head is rotated 45° downward and so kept for 2–3 minutes. In this position the outlet of the LSC in the geotropic form and the ampulla in the apogeotropic one are vertically oriented favoring the debris to gravitate down.
4. The patient finally returns to the sitting position (Fig. 11).

The transformation of the nystagmus from apogeotropic into geotropic is usually observed during the course of canalolithiasis therapy. A geotropic nystagmus can be

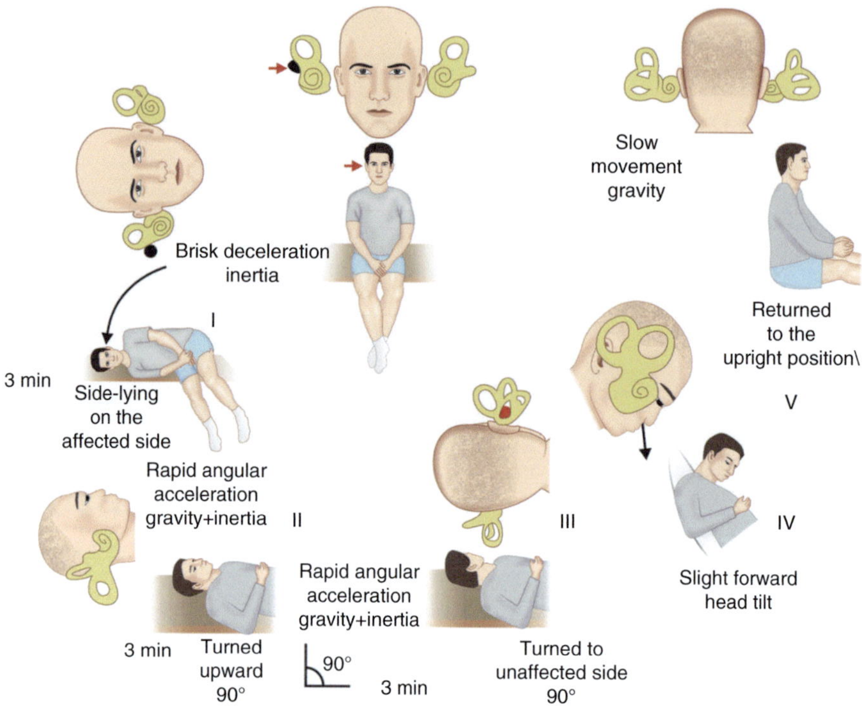

Fig. 12 Zuma's maneuver

transformed into an apogeotropic one if the maneuver is performed toward the affected ear by mistake. Both these conversions are explained by the migration of the otoconial mass from the anterior LSC arm into the posterior one and in the opposite direction, respectively.

Recently Zuma e Maia [23] proposed a new strategy for the apogeotropic LSC BPPV aiming to detach the debris from the anterior arm and also those that are attached to the utricular side of the cupula. Briefly: this maneuver is performed with patients in the sitting position. First, the patient is asked to quickly lie down on the affected side (step I) and is held in this position for 3 minutes. Then, the patient's head is rotated 90° toward the ceiling (step II) and held in this position for another 3 minutes. After 3 minutes, the patient moves the body into dorsal decubitus, and the head is turned 90° toward the unaffected side (step III) and held in this position for another 3 minutes. Finally, the patient's head is tilted slightly forward (step IV), followed by a slow return of the patient to the sitting position (step V) (Fig. 12).

Anterior Semicircular Canal BPPV (ASC BPPV)

The incidence of BPPV of the anterior canal is considered rare by almost all authors. However, Jackson et al. [24] described a frequency of 21.2%, which is higher than that reported for horizontal BPPV (11.9%).

The patient usually experiences his/her ASC BPPV attack while moving the head in the sagittal plane. The patient suffers a new attack every time he/she flexes or extends the head while upright or even by rotating toward the affected ear while supine. Vertigo isn't generally violent and is associated with dizziness when walking.

ASC BPPV is more frequently observed in post-traumatic BPPV with multiple canal involvement.

The pathophysiology of ASC BPPV is more frequent due to canalolithiasis: free-floating debris inside the anterior semicircular canal make its cupula sensitive to linear accelerations, i.e., gravity and accelerations provoked by brisk head movements on the same plane of the involved ASC.

The diagnosis is performed identifying the ASC BPPV canalolithiasis nystagmus. It is evoked by an ampullofugal thus excitatory flow of the debris caused by positioning tests. ASC BPPV nystagmus shows a quick phase with a geotropic torsional component, which is counterclockwise for right ASC and clockwise for left ASC. The vertical component is always downbeating. Actually, often the torsional component is poor or not evident, and ASC nystagmus rarely appears as a real paroxysmal one.

The diagnostic test for ASC BPPV is the Dix-Hallpike maneuver (D-H). When this maneuver is performed on one side, the opposite side ASC is checked: i.e., right D-H checks left ASC, and left D-H checks right ASC.

The ASC BPPV diagnosis is sometimes difficult, as the ASC involvement of one side can show a nystagmus provoked by a bilateral Dix-Hallpike and also by straight head-hanging positioning. The differential diagnosis should be made with other canalolithiasis variants and particularly with the PSC BPPV apogeotropic variant.

In this regard it is useful to perform the diagnostic tests repeatedly, monitoring both eyes by videonystagmography, with one camera for each eye. The diagnosis of ASC BPPV is confirmed when the positional downbeating nystagmus, with or without a torsional component, recovers completely after the therapeutic maneuvers.

A new ASC BPPV therapeutic maneuver has been proposed by Yacovino et al. in 2009 [25]. It consists of four steps with intervals of 30 seconds (Fig. 13). The same maneuver can be used for the left and right side. In fact, it does not require to previously identify which one is the affected side, thus simplifying the immediate treatment. Casani et al. in 2011 obtained an elevated percentage of success by using a variant of the Yacovino's maneuver which differs only for a longer time waiting after each step, 3 minutes instead of 30 seconds.

Atypical Paroxysmal Positional Vertigo

In 2015 a Committee of the International Classification of Vestibular Disorders (ICVD) of the Bárány Society issued a consensus document of the diagnostic criteria for benign paroxysmal positional vertigo (BPPV) [26]. The characteristics of the different types of BPPV – canalolithiasis and cupulolithiasis of the posterior, lateral, and anterior semicircular canals – were defined and established. The consensus also

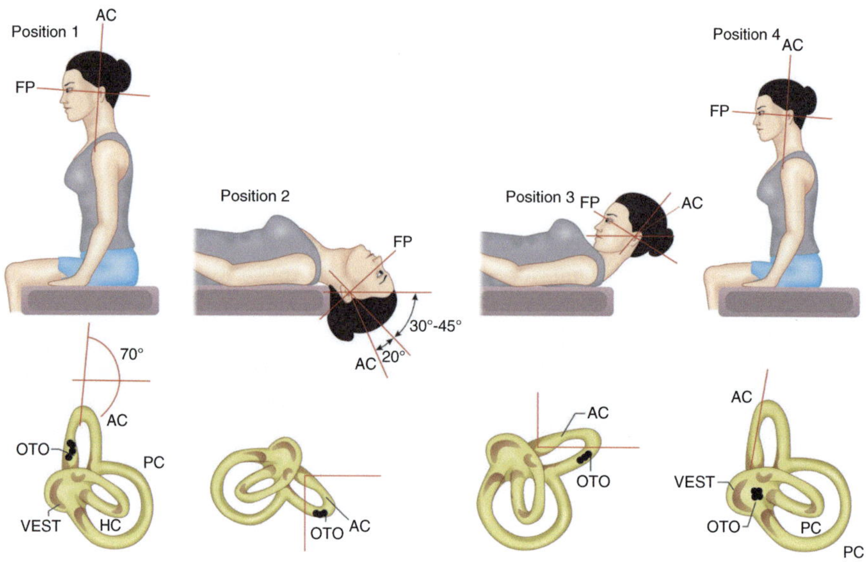

Fig. 13 Yacovino's maneuver

included a category of *possible BPPV* for the cases in which it is not possible to establish an etiology.

Occasionally we see patients with postural vertigo whose examinations do not show the typical established characteristics. These patients demand a greater magnitude of suspicion and must be thoroughly investigated.

Some illustrating cases will be discussed.

Atypical Lateral Canal BPPV

A 62-year-old woman complained of episodes of positional vertigo in the last 3 months. When submitted to the roll test, she presented a short latency, direction-changing geotropic nystagmus that lasted for 10 minutes in the left position and 7 minutes in the right. The position on the left caused more discomfort, and the one on the right showed a more intense nystagmus. She was suspected of having a lateral canal BPPV and was submitted to a repositioning maneuver that produced no results. Taking into consideration the atypical long-duration nystagmus and the lack of responses with the repositioning maneuver, she was submitted to a MRI scan that showed a right vestibular schwannoma [27].

A 14-year-old girl presented episodes of positional vertigo that lasted for a few seconds. In the roll test she presented a short latency, direction-changing geotropic nystagmus, more intense in the left position. The repositioning maneuvers were of little help. During one of the return consultations, she complained of headache and presented a downbeat vertical nystagmus. The MRI showed an image compatible with a cavernous hemangioma adjacent to the cerebellar vermis on the right side [28].

Atypical Posterior Canal BPPV

We recently published a series of cases of 30 patients with a complaint of positional vertigo who presented a downbeat vertical nystagmus, with or without a torsional component, during the Dix-Hallpike maneuver. They were submitted to neuroimaging studies and did not have central lesions. They were then diagnosed as cases of anterior canal BPPV. They did not, however, respond to the anterior canal repositioning maneuvers. Some of these patients afterward developed a nystagmus suggestive of posterior canal BPPV. When treated with posterior canal repositioning maneuvers, they became asymptomatic. Most probably they presented an apogeotropic variation of posterior canal BPPV, in agreement with hypotheses proposed by other authors [29, 30].

Vestibular Neuritis with Positional Nystagmus

An 18-year-old young man with an acute vestibular syndrome. Following the acute phase of the disease, he complained of episodes of positional vertigo. The examination showed a downbeat vertical nystagmus with a latency of 30 seconds and simultaneous vertigo, during the Dix-Hallpike maneuver, suggestive of a BPPV of the posterior canal, or its apogeotropic variation. The video head impulse test showed a pronounced reduction of the left posterior canal VOR (gain = 0.46). In all probability the downbeat nystagmus was due to the relative hyperfunction of the contralateral anterior canal [31].

Comments

The cases that were presented are a sample of the atypical cases that can be found in the clinical practice.

At the present moment, there is no precise definition of what can be considered an "atypical BPPV." It may be used to describe the cases that do not fit into the classical categories, like the apogeotropic type of posterior canal BPPV or the lateral canal BPPV accompanied by unidirectional positional nystagmus. But the word "atypical" may also be employed for the cases in which the possibility of central disorders must be investigated, in view of examination results that do not fit into the established varieties of BPPV.

See Chap. 8 for a description of central paroxysmal positional vertigo and its differential diagnosis.

References

1. Asprella Libonati G, Gufoni M. Vertigine Parossistica da CSL: manovre di barbecue ed altre varianti. In: XVI Giornate Italiane dOtoneurologia. Revisione critica di venti anni di vertigine parossistica posizionale benigna. Sorrento, NA: Formenti; 1999. p. 321–36. 2.
2. Mizukoshi K, Kobayashi H, Ohashi N, et al. Quantitative analysis of the visual vestibuloocular reflex using sinusoidal rotation in patients with peripheral vestibular disorders. Acta Otolaryngol Suppl. 1984;406:178–81.
3. Froehling DA, Silverstein MD, Mohr DN, et al. Benign positional vertigo: incidence and prognosis in a population- based study in Olmsted County, Minnesota. Mayo Clin Proc. 1991;66:596–601.
4. Asprella Libonati G. Benign paroxysmal positional vertigo and positional vertigo variants. Int J Otorhinolaryngol Clin. 2012;4(1):25–40.
5. Rajguru SM, Ifediba MA, Rabbitt RD. Three-dimensional biomechanical model of benign paroxysmal positional vertigo. Ann Biomed Eng. 2004;32:831–46.
6. Asprella Libonati G. Vertigem Posicional Paroxística Benigna. In Otoneurologia Atual. Zuma e Maia F, Mangabeira Albernaz PL, Carmona S. Rio de Janeiro, Revinter; 2014.
7. Zucca G, Valli S, Valli P, et al. Why do benign paroxysmal positional vertigo episodes recover spontaneously? J Vestib Res. 1998;8(4):325–9.
8. Horii A, Kitahara T, Osaki Y, et al. Intractable benign paroxysmal vertigo: long-term follow-up and inner ear abnormality detected by three-dimensional magnetic resonance imaging. Otol Neurotol. 2010;31:250–5.
9. Hain TC, Uddin M. Pharmacological treatment of vertigo. CNS Drugs. 2003;17:85–100.
10. Hain TC, Yacovino D. Pharmacologic treatment of persons with dizziness. Neurol Clin. 2005;23:831–53.
11. Hemenway WG, Lindsay JR. Postural vertigo due to unilateral sudden partial loss of vestibular function. Ann Otol Rhinol Laryngol. 1956;65(3):692–706.
12. Gans RE, Harrington-Gans PA. Treatment efficacy of benign paroxysmal positional vertigo (BPPV) with canalith repositioning maneuver and Semont liberatory maneuver in 376 patients. Semin Hear. 2002;22(2):598–604.
13. von Brevern M, Seelig T, Neuhauser H, et al. Benign paroxysmal positional vertigo predominantly affects the right labyrinth. J Neurol Neurosurg Psychiatry. 2004;75:1487–8.
14. Shim DB, Kim JH, Park KC, et al. Correlation between the head-lying side during sleep and the affected side by benign paroxysmal positional vertigo involving the posterior or horizontal semicircular canal. Laryngoscope. 2012;122(4):873–6.
15. Asprella-Libonati G. Diagnostic and treatment strategy of the lateral semicircular canal canalolithiasis. Acta Otorhinolaryngol Ital. 2005;25:277–83.
16. Asprella-Libonati G, Gagliardi G, Cifarelli D, Larotonda G. "Step by step" treatment of lateral semicircular canal canalolithiasis under videonystagmoscopic examination. Acta Otorhinolaryngol Ital. 2003;23:10–5.
17. Semont A, Freyss G, Vitte E. Curing the BPPV with a liberatory maneuver. Adv Otorhinolaryngol. 1988;42:290–3.
18. Vannucchi P, Giannoni B, Pecci R. "Labirintolitiasi: la variante apogeotropa della VPP del CSP". Oral communication presented at XXXII National Meeting of Società Italiana di Audiologia e Foniatria. Firenze – Oct. 2009.

19. Vannucchi P, Pecci R, Giannoni B. Posterior semicircular canal benign paroxysmal positional vertigo presenting with torsional downbeating nystagmus: an apogeotropic variant. Int J Otolaryngol. 2012;2012:413603.
20. Hawthorne M, el-Naggar M. Fenestration and occlusion of posterior semicircular canal for patients with intractable benign paroxysmal positional vertigo. J Laryngol Otol. 1994;108(11):935–9.
21. Cakir BO, Ercan I, Cakir ZA, et al. What is the true incidence of horizontal semicircular canal benign paroxysmal positional vertigo? Otolaryngol Head Neck Surg. 2006;134(3):451–4.
22. Asprella Libonati G. Benign paroxysmal positional vertigo. Chap. In: Carmona S, Asprella-Libonati G, editors. Neuro-otology. 3rd ed. 2011; Buenos Aires, Akadia ed.
23. Zuma e Maia FC. New treatment strategy for apogeotropic horizontal canal benign paroxysmal positional vertigo. Audiol Res. 2016;6:163.
24. Jackson LE, Morgan B, Fletcher JC Jr, et al. Anterior canal benign paroxysmal positional vertigo: an underappreciated entity. Otol Neurotol. 2007;28(2):218–22.
25. Yacovino DA, Hain TC, Gualtieri F. New therapeutic maneuver for anterior canal benign paroxysmal positional vertigo. J Neurol. 2009;256(11):1851–5.
26. von Brevern M, Bertholon P, Brandt T, Fife T, Imai T, Nuti D, Newman-Toker D. Benign paroxysmal positional vertigo: diagnostic criteria. J Vestib Res. 2015;25(3–4):105–17. https://doi.org/10.3233/VES-150553.
27. Carmona S, Salazar R, Zalazar G. Atypical benign paroxysmal positional vertigo in a case of acoustic neuroma. J Otolaryngol ENT Res. 2017;8(5):00261. https://doi.org/10.15406/joentr.2017.08.00261.
28. Carmona S, Grinstein G, Weinschelbaum R, Zalazar G. Benign paroxysmal positional vertigo: differential diagnosis in children. Biomed J Sci &Tech Res. 2018. BJSTR.MS.ID.000711.;2(1) https://doi.org/10.26717/BJSTR.2018.02.000711.
29. Carmona S, Zalazar G, Weisnchelbaum R, Grinstein G, Breinbauer H, Asprella Libonati G. Downbeating nystagmus in benign paroxysmal positional vertigo: an apogeotropic variant of posterior semicircular canal. Curr Opin Neurol Sci. 2017;1(6):301–5.
30. Büki B, Mandalà M, Nutib D. Typical and atypical benign paroxysmal positional vertigo: literature review and new theoretical considerations. J Vestib Res. 2014;24(5–6):415–23. https://doi.org/10.3233/VES-140535.
31. Carmona S, Grinstein G, Weinschelbaum R, Zalazar G. Topodiagnosis of the inner ear: illustrative clinical cases. Ann Otolaryngol Rhinol. 2018;5(1):1201.

Bilateral Vestibulopathy

The progressive loss of vestibular function is often overlooked, in view of the superimposition of the different systems related to the sense of balance. These patients complain of instability and oscillopsia when they walk, and these symptoms become more intense at night. They have no auditory or neurological disorders, and their examinations indicate a pure vestibular ataxia.

The video head impulse tests may be bilaterally positive, but this is rather infrequent, probably due to VOR compensation; when present, however, these findings are quite useful to establish a diagnosis of bilateral vestibular deficit.

The clinical suspicion is based on three simple tests:

1. A bilateral positive vHIT test.
2. A decreased performance in dynamic visual acuity (DVA) tested with head rotation.
3. A positive Romberg test when performed over a foam block [1]

One must take into consideration the fact that, particularly in elderly patients with a complaint of instability or unsteadiness, the vestibular evaluation may indicate a unilateral vestibular hypo- or areflexia. Most probably this results from an inability to achieve vestibular compensation linked to a deterioration of the other systems related to the sense of balance.

The patients with symmetrical bilateral reduction or absence of vestibular function will have small responses to caloric stimulation, in terms of frequency, amplitude, and duration. In cases with responses, the peak slow-phase velocities do not exceed 5°o/s. Sometimes no responses can be observed, even with ice water stimulation.

The torsion swing rotational tests also show symmetrical reduced responses. The vestibular autorotation test (VAT) is particularly useful for demonstrating a constant pattern of decrease in VOR gain, accompanied by an advancement in its phase. It

P. L. M. Albernaz et al., *The New Neurotology*,
https://doi.org/10.1007/978-3-030-11283-7_12

should be noted that the caloric test results may be doubtful in patients with external or middle ear problems.

Epidemiology

In a series of patients with bilateral vestibulopathy, 51% were found to be idiopathic; 27% caused by gentamicin ototoxicity, 8.9% by bilateral vestibular neuritis, 4.7% by tobramycin ototoxicity, 3.8% by cranial trauma, 3.3% by autoimmune vestibulopathy, 1.9% by Menière's disease, and 1.4% by streptomycin ototoxicity; and 0.9% congenital [2].

In another study [3], 31% of the cases were found to be idiopathic, and only 47% had a clearly defined etiology; the most frequent causes were genetical disorders (17%), Menière's disease (16%), otoxicicity (12%), infectious diseases (6%), and neurodegenerative disorders (4%); in 22% of the patients, a clear etiology could not be determined.

In other series the following etiologies have been reported: idiopathic (51%), toxic or metabolic (13–21%), infectious (3.8–2%), and autoimmune (10%); other etiologies were less frequent [3].

In our experience, ototoxicity, most frequently with gentamicin, is the most common bilateral vestibulopathy, but there are patients in whom a precise etiology cannot be determined. These findings were corroborated in other studies [2, 3].

The age of these patients varies mainly from 38 to 57 years [4], with a minimum of 20.

Baloh [5] divided this class of patients into two groups:

1. Sequential – patients with vertiginous attacks lasting from hours to days, impossible to distinguish from a vestibular neuritis, for a period of time before the establishment of the bilateral vestibulopathy
2. Progressive – patients with the occurrence of the bilateral vestibulopathy without any preceding symptoms

In cases with unestablished etiologies, family history may be important, since some patients present autosomal recessive inherited diseases [6, 7].

Differential Diagnosis

Ototoxicity

These are the most frequent cases in all series. Gentamicin is the most common agent because of its vestibular selectivity [8]. The patient's age and renal disorders seem to be the main predisposing factors [9]. Streptomycin and gentamicin strike mainly the vestibular hair cells, while kanamycin, tobramycin, and neomycin are more destructive to the cochlear hair cells [8]. Both types of cells can be ephemerally damaged by high doses of furosemide and salicylates [10].

Sequential Vestibular Loss

There is a possibility that a patient will have a vestibular neuritis in each ear, occurring at different times. The endpoint is a bilateral loss of vestibular function that may be considered by some authors as idiopathic.

Autoimmune Inner Ear Disease

These patients present bilateral fluctuant hearing loss with loss of speech discrimination. This will be the key to their diagnosis.

Primary Cerebellar Atrophy

Posterior cerebral artery syndrome (PCA) and olivopontocerebellar atrophy (OPCA) may cause bilateral loss of vestibular function. The first one is of vascular origin, OPCA is hereditary, but the genetical factors involved are not known. In these cases, there are always cerebellar signs, such as dysmetria and dysarthria, and oculomotor disorders that clearly establish the neurological origin of the problem. Both in PCA and in Friedreich's ataxia, however, the peripheral vestibular system is bilaterally involved.

Otosclerosis

Patients with extensive otospongiotic bone extending into the cochlea may present unsteadiness and episodic crises of vertigo. These symptoms have been attributed to bony compression of the vestibular nerve or the semicircular ducts [11].

Bone Dysplasias

Vestibular atelectasis [12], new bone formation in Paget's disease, and Camurati-Engelmann disease may cause uni- or bilateral progressive loss of vestibular function.

Other Diseases Related to Vestibular Disorders

1. Polyneuropathies and cranial neuropathies, including auditory neuropathy.
2. Meningitis, most often causing hearing losses, may also affect the vestibular function.
3. Neoplasms, like bilateral vestibular schwannomas (neurofibromatosis type II), non-Hodgkin's lymphoma, leptomeningeal metastases, and cranial base infiltration.
4. Cochlear implants may lead to loss of vestibular function; it has been advised that the side to be chosen for the operation should be the one with worse vestibular responses [13, 14].
5. Recently one of us [15–17] and other authors [18] demonstrated that Fabry disease may cause uni- or bilateral auditory and/or vestibular disorders. Enzyme replacement therapy has been found to be effective for treating this disease.
6. Alport syndrome (interstitial nephritis with sensorineural hearing loss) may cause loss of vestibular function, as well as Waardenburg syndrome, bilateral Mondini dysplasia, Usher syndrome (hereditary hearing loss and retinitis pigmentosa), labyrinthitis ossificans, mitochondrial diseases, macroglobulinemia, and vertebral artery dolichoectasia.

Diagnostic Criteria

In 2017, Strupp et al. [19] published the following diagnostic criteria for both definite and probable bilateral vestibulopathies, according to the International Classification of Vestibular Disorders (ICVD).

Diagnostic Criteria for Bilateral Vestibulopathy

(a) Chronic vestibular syndrome with the following symptoms:

   1. Unsteadiness when walking or standing plus at least one of 2 or 3
   2. Movement-induced blurred vision or oscillopsia during walking or quick head/body movements
   3. Worsening of unsteadiness in darkness and/or on uneven ground

(b) No symptoms while sitting or lying down under static conditions

(c) Bilaterally reduced or absent angular VOR function documented by:

   - Bilaterally pathological horizontal angular VOR gain <0.6, measured by the video-HIT or scleral-coil technique
   - Reduced caloric response (sum of bithermal max. peak SPV on each side $<6°/s$)

– Reduced horizontal angular VOR gain <0.1 upon sinusoidal stimulation on a rotatory chair (0.1 Hz, Vmax = 50°/sec) and a phase lead >68°o (time constant <5 s)

(d) Not better accounted for by another disease

Diagnostic Criteria for Probable Bilateral Vestibulopathy

(a) Chronic vestibular syndrome with the following symptoms:

1. Unsteadiness when walking or standing plus at least one of 2 or 3
2. Movement-induced blurred vision or oscillopsia during walking or quick head/body movements
3. Worsening of unsteadiness in darkness and/or on uneven ground

(b) No symptoms while sitting or lying down under static conditions
(c) Bilaterally pathological horizontal bedside head impulse test
(d) Not better accounted for by another disease

References

1. Petersen J, Straumann D, Weber K. Clinical diagnosis of bilateral vestibular loss: three simple bedside tests. Ther Adv Neurol Disord. 2013;6(1):41–5. https://doi.org/10.1177/1756285612465920.
2. Hain TC, Cherchi M, Yacovino DA. Bilateral vestibular weakness. Front Neurol. 2018;9:344. https://doi.org/10.3389/fneur.2018.00344.
3. Lucieer F, Vonk P, Guinand N, Stokroos R, Kingma H, van de Berg R. Bilateral vestibular hypofunction: insights in etiologies, clinical subtypes, and diagnostics. Front Neurol. 2016;7:26. https://doi.org/10.3389/fneur.2016.00026.
4. Vibert D, Liard P, Hausler R. Bilateral idiopathic loss of peripheral vestibular function with normal hearing. Acta Otolaryngol (Stockh). 1995;115:611–5.
5. Baloh RW, Jacobson K, Fife T. Familial vestibulopathy: a new dominantly inherited syndrome. Neurology. 1994;44:20–5.
6. Verhagen WI, Huygen PL, Horstink MW. Familial congenital vestibular areflexia. J Neurol Neurosurg Psychiatry. 1987;50(7):933–5.
7. Baloh RW, Jacobson K, Honrubia V. Idiopathic bilateral vestibulopathy. Neurology. 1989;39:272–5.
8. Schuknecht HF. Pathology of the ear. Cambridge: Harvard University Press; 1974.
9. Barza M, Lauermann M. Why monitor serum levels of gentamycin? Clin Pharmacokin. 1978;3:202–15.
10. Myers E, Bernstein J, Fostiropolous G. Salicylate ototoxicity. A clinical study. N Engl J Med. 1965;273:587–90. https://doi.org/10.1056/NEJM196509092731104.
11. Thomas JE, Cody DT. Neurologic perspectives of otosclerosis. Mayo Clin Proc. 1981;56:17–21.
12. Merchant SN, Schuknecht HF. Vestibular atelectasis. Ann Otol Rhinol Laryngol. 1988;97:565–76.

13. Valentin NS, Hageman KN, Dai C, Della Santina CC, Fridman GY. Development of a multichannel vestibular prosthesis prototype by modification of a commercially available cochlear implant. IEEE Trans Neural Syst Rehabil Eng. 2013;21(5):830–9. https://doi.org/10.1109/TNSRE.2013.2259261.
14. Mangabeira Albernaz PL. Areflexia vestibular bilateral. In: Zuma e Maia FC, Mangabeira-Albernaz PL, Carmona S, editors. Otoneurologia atual. Rio de Janeiro: Revinter; 2014. p. 399–403.
15. Carmona S, Pardal A, Marchesoni C, Salvatico N, Reisin RC, Romero C, Meli F, Sevlever G, Yañez P, Vazquez S. Neuro otologic abnormalities in patients with Fabry disease. Neurology. 2008;70(Suppl 1):A263.
16. Carmona S, Salvático N, Marchesoni C, Pardal A, Romero C, Melli F, Reisin R. Neuro-otology of the Fabry disease. Proceedings of the XXV Bárány Society Meeting, Kyoto, 2008; p. 388.
17. Carmona S, Weinschelbaum R, Pardal A, Marchesoni C, Zuberbuhler P, Acosta P, Caceres G, Kisinovsky I, Bayón L, Reisin R. Neuro-otological and peripheral nerve involvement in Fabry disease. Audiol Res. 2017;7:176. https://doi.org/10.4081/audiores.2017.176.
18. Palla A, Hegemann S, Widmer U, Straumann D. Vestibular and auditory deficits in Fabry disease and their response to enzyme replacement therapy. J Neurol. 2007;254:1433–42. https://doi.org/10.1007/s00415-007-0575-y.
19. Strupp M, Kim JS, Murofushi T, Straumann D, Jen JC, Rosengren SM, Della Santina CC, Kingma H. Bilateral vestibulopathy: diagnostic criteria consensus document of the Classification Committee of the Bárány Society. J Vestib Res. 2017;27(4):177–89. https://doi.org/10.3233/VES-170619.

Ataxia

Introduction

The word *ataxia*, in Greek, means "out of order." From a clinical point of view, it is a degenerative disorder that affects the movement coordination and execution, in terms of velocity, range, direction, and duration. It also affects the sustained muscle contraction, both reflex and voluntary, necessary to maintain a posture and/or balance, in the absence of paresis or sensory disorders. This classical definition, however, has an exception that will be discussed further on in the text.

It should be noted that, in ataxia, the movements involve the correct body parts and the correct motor plan and sequencing, but it presents disruptions in relation to how easily they are performed. This is different from apraxia, which is characterized by a failure of the movement sequence and its conceptual organization [1–4].

This lack of coordination indicates a disorder or dysfunction in the cerebellum or in the connection between the cerebellum and other areas of the central nervous system.

There is another type of loss of coordination, due to a lack of proprioceptive information, which is called *sensory ataxia*, sometimes referred to as *spinal ataxia*. This is just a sensory ataxia due to damage to the tracts that carry proprioceptive information. Sensory ataxia may be caused by an impairment of the dorsal root ganglion, a very rare disorder called *ganglionopathy*, or sensory neuropathy [2].

In classical texts, one may find a reference to frontal lobe ataxia, which is not a real ataxia, but a gait apraxia, as it is an inability to produce and execute a motor plan [2].

Signs and Symptoms

Patients may consult due to "instability," "dizziness," frequent falls, and "motor clumsiness." When questioning these patients, it is important to collect data as to the onset of the condition, its duration, evolution, aggravating or mitigating factors, and family history.

P. L. M. Albernaz et al., *The New Neurotology*,
https://doi.org/10.1007/978-3-030-11283-7_13

There are three elements that must be taken into consideration when we evaluate ataxia: *dyssynergia*, *dysmetria*, and *dysdiadochokinesia*.

Dyssynergia is the system's inability to generate a coordinated contraction of different muscles to perform a precise movement. Dysmetria refers to the system's inability to reach a targeted object by estimating the right distance to it. This, in turn, makes it possible to coordinate the necessary movements to reach the object. Finally, dysdiadochokinesia is the system's inability to easily perform alternating movements. Though each one of these elements is altered in different types of ataxia, many times they are not altered in the same way, and the alteration is more marked in some of them than in others. It should also be mentioned that these elements, which are predominantly but not exclusively controlled by the cerebellum, may be altered in other central nervous system disorders, as many areas and structures that, to a certain extent, may modify them are involved in the execution of every motor plan (i.e., dysdiadochokinesia may be present in basal ganglia lesions). The medical history and the physical examination many times make it possible to assess whether these alterations are produced by lesions in the cerebellum or its connections or by lesions in other structures.

Each of these two types of ataxia, apart from the alterations they have in common, has associated symptoms and signs that make it possible to correctly differentiate them. Yet, in some occasions, there are certain conditions that combine both types of ataxia, which makes this differentiation more difficult [1–4].

Cerebellar Ataxia

Gait and Posture Alteration

The patient usually refers instability, dizziness, difficulty when riding a bike, and unsure gait. The lack of axial muscle coordination results in gait and posture alterations. This is called *truncal ataxia*. We will see a widened base of support in the standing position, as well as an increase in trunk oscillations in every direction. Romberg test is usually positive, though not so clearly as in vestibular or proprioceptive alterations. Gait is performed with a widened base of support and in an irregular manner similar to that of a drunken person.

Limb Ataxia

The patient may refer clumsiness in writing, picking up objects, or performing slow movements. Upper limb ataxia may be assessed by means of the index finger-to-nose test or the index finger-chasing test. In these cases of cerebellar ataxia, we may find an action tremor that may be assessed by asking the patient to maintain his or her index fingers 1 centimeter apart at chest height. Diadochokinesia may be assessed by alternating pronation and supination hand movements on the person's tights or by tapping the foot on the floor or the index finger on the thumb. In the case of the lower limbs, the heel-knee test and the finger-toe test are the usual maneuvers used. These patients usually show intention tremor, which becomes evident with the same maneuvers used to assess ataxia.

Dysarthria and Bulbar Symptoms

Speech is assessed by listening to how words are produced and by the repetition of phrases. The voice shows slow and slurred speech, hesitation, and incorrectly stressed syllables. Moment-by-moment pitch and loudness variations when speaking are characteristic, due to inappropriate respiratory control *(scanning speech).* Dysphagia may be present.

Visual Symptoms and Oculomotor Findings

Some patients refer oscillopsia and blurred vision. We may also find nystagmus, abnormalities in slow pursuit, saccades and in the vestibulo-ocular reflex.

Sensory Ataxia

In patients with sensory ataxia, we will not find dysarthria, bulbar symptoms, or visual or oculomotor manifestations; they will present symptoms such as paresthesias and numbness. The physical examination will show a deficit in proprioceptive information, and the ataxia is worse when the patients are examined with the eyes closed, as compared to the test with open eyes; they are clearly visually dependent.

Semiologic Maneuvers

From a semiological point of view, ataxia may be classified as axial or appendicular, depending on the affected muscle group, and as static or dynamic, depending on the type of muscle activity. Each one has specific maneuvers that we must know to appropriately address our patient's condition.

Maneuvers for Static Ataxia

1. Station: we assess whether the patient, in order to maintain a standing position, needs to widen the base of support to show trunk or head oscillations.
2. Romberg test: the patient is asked to stand with his feet together, arms on each side, and eyes closed. This maneuver may be even more sensitive when patient is asked to put one foot in front of the other.
3. Barany's pointing test: patient is asked to outstretch both arms with stretched index fingers.

Maneuvers for Dynamic Ataxia

1. Finger-to-nose test: the patient is asked to touch the tip of the nose with the index finger, stretch the arm, and repeat the process, first with the eyes opened and then with the eyes closed. Patients with cerebellar lesions show the same difficulty at performing both tests, while patients with sensory ataxia improve their performance with eyes opened (as they correct their coordination mistakes with vision) and worsen with eyes closed.
2. Index finger-to-nose test: the patient is asked to touch the tip of the nose with his or her index finger and then with the examiner's index finger.
3. Index finger-chasing test: patient is asked to touch the examiner's index finger with his or her finger; the examiner changes the position of his or her finger, and the patient has to touch it in the new position.
4. Heel-knee test: the patient, lying supine, is asked to touch the knee on one side with the opposite heel and then to pass the heel slowly down the front of the shin to the ankle. As in the finger-nose test, this test is performed first with eyes closed and then with eyes open, and it is interpreted in the same way.
5. Babinski's asynergy: the patient, lying supine, is asked to sit down with arms crossed across the chest. The individual with ataxia is not able to do this and bends the arms on the pelvis.

Following Lee et al.'s proposal [5], we have assessed and classified truncal ataxia according to the patient's ability to walk and/or maintain a standing or sitting position.

Grade 1 – when the patient has mild to moderate instability in the standing position but can walk without assistance

Grade 2 – when the patient has severe instability and cannot walk without assistance

Grade 3 – when the patient cannot sit up

Our results show that the presence of grades 2 and 3 truncal ataxia has a 92.9% sensitivity and a 61.1% specificity to differentiate between central and peripheral lesions in patients who consult due to acute vertigo. None of the patients with peripheral vestibular lesions presented grade 3 ataxia; thus this finding always indicates a central lesion. We have also found that Babinski's flexion asynergy was present in all patients with grade 3 ataxia and in all patients with stroke and grade 1 ataxia, but none of the patients with peripheral vestibular lesions.

When assessing a patient with ataxia, we may find the axial, or the appendicular or both types of ataxia, to be altered. When the cerebellum is involved, one ataxia will have predominance over the other, depending on the topography of the lesion. In a global cerebellar condition, the patient will present with both axial and appendicular ataxia manifestations. In cases with conditions that cause sensory ataxia, the clinical manifestations will depend on the site of the lesion.

Etiology

There are many causes of ataxia. It is not the intention of this chapter to discuss all the known etiologies in an exhaustive manner. We will discuss those conditions which, given their frequency or importance, shall be known by every physician who treats a patient with dizziness or vertigo. We believe that the important conduct is to be able to recognize the ataxic syndrome in itself, so as to make a proper differential diagnosis, specially emphasizing those causes that require urgent care [3, 6].

One way of approaching the study of a patient with ataxia is to differentiate between acquired and hereditary types, a differentiation that is complemented with the age of onset. Another way is to consider the progression of the symptoms: episodic, acute, subacute, and chronic. The acute cases are caused by rapidly progressing diseases, like cerebrovascular accidents and infections. The subacute ones may be caused by brain tumors and autoimmune or degenerative diseases. The chronic ones may be genetical or metabolic disorders, which account for a gradual loss of cerebellar neurons.

Table 1 shows the main etiologies related to subacute or chronic ataxia.

Table 2 classifies the ataxia according to the age of onset.

These etiologies will be discussed, except for those related to vascular disorders, demyelinating diseases, structural malformations, and cerebellar tumors.

Alcoholic Cerebellar Degeneration

This type of ataxia is a consequence of a large amount of alcoholic beverages consumed during a long period of time [3, 7]. It is attributed to a direct toxic effect of the alcohol on the cerebellar cells, but a deficiency of vitamin B1 is also a possible factor.

Table 1 Etiological classification

Acquired	Genetical
Degenerative ataxia Multisystemic atrophy Idiopathic late-onset cerebellar ataxia Acquired ataxia CVA (hemorrhagic or ischemic) Toxic Alcohol Drugs – anticonvulsants, lithium, chemotherapeutics, metronidazole, cyclosporin Heavy metals Solvents Immunomediated Infectious – abscess, cerebellitis Trauma Cerebellar tumors or metastases Metabolic – hypothyroidism Structural defects – Arnold-Chiari, agenesia, dysplasias	Autosomal dominant – spinocerebellar ataxia, episodic ataxia Autosomal recessive – Friedreich's ataxia, type C Niemann-Pick, vitamin E deficiency, Wilson's disease, etc. X-linked – fragile X-associated tremor/ataxia syndrome Mitochondrial – mitochondrial encephalopathy, lactic acidosis, and stroke-like episodes (MELAS) syndrome, myoclonic epilepsy with ragged red fibers (MERRF) syndrome, Leigh's syndrome

Table 2 Ataxia according to age of onset

Age of onset	Acquired	Genetical
Infancy	Ataxic cerebral palsy Other intrauterine injuries	Congenital hereditary ataxia (Joubert, Gillespie)
Childhood	Acute cerebellitis; cerebellar abscess; posterior fossa tumors (ependimomas, gliomas); arteriovenous malformations; congenital anomalies (Arnold-Chiari, etc.); anticonvulsants; opsoclonus; myoclonus	Friedreich's ataxia; other recessive ataxia; episodic syndromes; mitochondrial syndromes; spinocerebellar ataxia types II, VII, and XIII; dentatorubral-pallidoluysian atrophy
Young adults	Abscess; human immunodeficiency virus (HIV); space-occupying lesions (meningiomas, gliomas, etc.); arteriovenous malformations; multiple sclerosis, Arnold-Chiari malformation; hypothyroidism; toxic (alcohol, anticonvulsants)	Friedreich's ataxia; ataxia due to genetic metabolic disorders; spinocerebellar ataxia; hereditary tumor syndromes (von Hippel-Lindau syndrome)
Elderly persons	Same as young adults plus: idiopathic ataxia, immunomediated ataxia (anti-glutamate decarboxylase, gluten ataxia)	Benign spinocerebellar ataxia, like type VI

The degeneration involves particularly the superior portion of the cerebellar vermis, and for this reason, the ataxia is predominant in relation to the lower limbs, being mainly axial, rather than appendicular. These patients have intense difficulty in walking, with little involvement of the extremities. Nystagmus is rare.

The treatment requires alcohol restriction, vitamin B1, and vestibular rehabilitation.

Toxic Ataxia

Several medications may exert toxic effects on the cerebellum, with consequent cerebellar atrophy and ataxia. Among them are phenytoin, lithium, amiodarone, and some chemotherapeutic agents, like 5-fluorouracil. Some heavy metals, like mercury and thallium, may also intoxicate the cerebellum [8].

Paraneoplastic Cerebellar Degeneration

Cerebellar degeneration may be related to a paraneoplastic phenomenon associated with different types of tumors, particularly small cell lung cancer, ovarian and breast cancers, and Hodgkin's lymphoma. It is believed to be a consequence of the production of antibodies against the cerebellum. The ataxia is subacute and often occurs before the diagnosis of the tumor. The study of antibodies like anti-HU (present in lung cancer) and anti-YO (present in ovarian and breast cancer) may be useful. The magnetic resonance scans may be normal; the cerebellar atrophy may not be visible in the early stages [9, 10].

The treatment is that of the tumor that gives rise to the cerebellar disease. Immunological treatment with human intravenous immunoglobulin may be of help for the ataxia.

Autoimmune Ataxia

Gluten ataxia is an autoimmune disease triggered by the ingestion of gluten. It causes a loss of Purkinje cells in the cerebellum. People with gluten ataxia usually present gait abnormality or incoordination and tremor of the upper limbs. Gaze-evoked nystagmus and other ocular signs of cerebellar dysfunction are common. Myoclonus, palatal tremor, and opsoclonus may also appear [11].

Early diagnosis and treatment with a gluten-free diet seem to improve the ataxia and prevent its progression. The diagnosis usually relies on antibody studies and intestinal biopsy, since most of the patients have no gastrointestinal symptoms.

Ataxia Related to Anti-GAD Antibodies

These patients present a pluriglandular autoimmune syndrome, with positive anti-glutamic acid decarboxylase antibodies (anti-GAD antibodies). Besides the ataxia, they also have a type I diabetes mellitus [12].

The treatment requires corticosteroids or intravenous human immunoglobulin.

Ataxia Related to Hashimoto's Encephalopathy

Hashimoto's encephalopathy, also known as *steroid responsive encephalopathy associated with autoimmune thyroiditis (SREAT)*, is a neurological condition characterized by encephalopathy and thyroid autoimmunity. It is associated with Hashimoto's thyroiditis. Ataxia is present in 65% of the cases: it is a subacute type associated with cognitive changes [13].

This disease has good clinical response to corticosteroids.

Multiple System Atrophy (MSA)

This is a neurodegenerative disease, with two different subtypes: MSA-p, or parkinsonian subtype (approximately 80% of the cases), and MSA-c, or cerebellar dysfunction subtype (20%). The cerebellar subtype usually begins its progression after age 55 [3].

MSA is characterized by the following symptoms, which can be present in any combination:

1. Autonomic dysfunction
2. Parkinsonism
3. Ataxia
4. Orthostatic hypotension
5. Urinary incontinence
6. Erectile dysfunction

The advance of the atrophy, which occurs in the olivopontocerebellar area, can be estimated by magnetic resonance imaging.

There is no treatment for this disorder.

Vitamin Deficiency

The deprivation of thiamine (vitamin B1) and other vitamins of the B group may cause Wernicke's encephalopathy, associated with ophthalmoplegia and a confusional syndrome. This disease is found in patients with alcoholism.

The deprivation of vitamin B12 may determine intestinal malabsorption syndromes, like atrophic gastritis, pernicious anemia, and others. These syndromes are accompanied by a sensitive ataxia, brought forth by damage of the posterior tracts of the spinal cord, with involvement of the pyramidal tracts causing pyramidal signs and sometimes peripheral neuropathy.

The diagnosis is established by the low amount of vitamin B12 in the patient's plasma. The treatment is accomplished by restoring the vitamin B12 normal blood levels [3, 7].

Idiopathic Late-Onset Cerebellar Ataxia (ILOCA)

The clinical presentations of ILOCA are characterized by late ages at onset, slow progression, and cerebellar ataxia. The coordination of the upper limbs is relatively preserved. There is no dysautonomia. Additional neurological signs may be present, such as pyramidal signs, mild dementia, supranuclear ophthalmoplegia, optic atrophy, dysphagia, parkinsonism, sphincter disturbances, or hypopallesthesia. The neuroimages only demonstrate the cerebellar atrophy [3].

Episodic Ataxia

These are hereditary autosomal dominant neurological diseases. They are infrequent and are responsible for paroxysmal crises of ataxia and vertigo. The ataxia is progressive. These patients may also have migraine-like headaches, and a differential diagnosis must be established with vestibular migraine. They may also have epileptic seizures and dystonia [1, 3].

The mutations are linked to neuronal potassium and calcium channel genes. Although these channels are well distributed in the central nervous system, they are particularly numerous in the cerebellum.

Six subtypes have been described; EA1 and EA2 are the most frequent.

Infections

Some chronic central nervous system infectious diseases may lead to progressive ataxia. The classical example is tabes dorsalis, or syphilitic myelopathy, that is now rare, caused by demyelination in patients with advanced tertiary syphilis.

Whipple's disease is a systemic infectious disease caused by a bacterium, *Tropheryma whipplei*. The patients have elevated temperature, weight loss, diarrhea, abdominal pain, and arthritis. Cerebellar ataxia is seen in approximately one half of the Whipple's disease patients that have neurological symptoms.

HIV-positive patients may present ataxia, usually due to focal cerebellar lesions caused by opportunistic infection or CNS lymphomas. In rare cases the cerebellar lesions may be directly produced by the HIV; in these cases the ataxia begins with a subacute episode and evolves to disabling intensity in a few months [3, 14].

The infection with JC virus, called progressive multifocal leukoencephalopathy, can also account for progressive ataxia.

Creutzfeldt-Jakob disease leads to rapidly progressive ataxia followed by dementia. In the sporadic variation of the disease (sCJD), the dementia precedes the ataxia [15].

Mitochondrial Diseases

Ataxia is one of the frequent manifestations of CNS involvement in mitochondrial illnesses. Sporadic ataxia in adults is often found in MERRF (myoclonic epilepsy with ragged red fibers) syndrome, mitochondrial myopathy, MELAS (mitochondrial encephalopathy, lactic acidosis, and stroke-like episodes) syndrome, and NARP (neuropathy, ataxia, and retinitis pigmentosa) syndrome [3].

Spinocerebellar Ataxia

This is a hereditary type that can be inherited in an autosomal dominant, autosomal recessive, or X-linked manner. Many different types have been described.

An autosomal dominant variety may be found as sporadic ataxia in adults. The most frequent type is SCA6, due to a mutation in gene CACNA1A [16].

Autosomal Recessive Ataxia

Some varieties of autosomal recessive ataxia are more benign and usually begin in adults. This group includes Friedreich's ataxia and several variations of lysosomal storage diseases, like Krabbe disease, Niemann-Pick disease, and Tay-Sachs disease [17].

References

1. Carmona S, Kattah J, editors. Manejo del Síndrome Vestibular Agudo. Buenos Aires: Akadia; 2017.
2. Campbell WW. De Jong's the neurologic examination. 7th ed. Philadelphia: Wolters Kluver, Lippincott Williams & Wilkins; 2013.
3. Klockgether T. Sporadic ataxia with adult onset: classification and diagnostic criteria. Lancet Neurol. 2010;9(1):94–104. https://doi.org/10.1016/S1474-4422(09)70305-9.
4. Carmona S, Asprella-Libonati G. Neuro-otología. 3rd ed. Buenos Aires: Akadia; 2018.

5. Lee H, Sohn SI, Cho YW, Lee SR, Ahn BH, Park BR, Baloh RW. Cerebellar infarction presenting isolated vertigo. Frequency and vascular topographical patterns. Neurology. 2006;67(7):1178–83. https://doi.org/10.1212/01.wnl.0000238500.02302.b4.
6. Akbar U, Ashizawa T. Ataxia. Neurol Clin. 2015;33:225–48. https://doi.org/10.1016/j.ncl.2014.09.004.
7. Kril JJ. Neuropathology of thiamine deficiency disorders. Metab Brain Dis. 1996;11:9–17.
8. Alekseeva N, McGee J, Kelley RE, Maghzi AH, Gonzalez-Toledo E, Minagar A. Toxic-metabolic, nutritional, and medicinal-induced disorders of cerebellum. Neurol Clin. 2014;32(4):901–11. https://doi.org/10.1016/j.ncl.2014.07.001.
9. Dalmau J, Rosenfeld MR. Paraneoplastic syndromes of the CNS. Lancet Neurol. 2008;7(4):327–40. https://doi.org/10.1016/S1474-4422(08)70060-7.
10. Vedeler CA, Antoine JC, Giometto B, Graus F, Grisold W, Hart IK, Honnorat J, Sillevis Smitt PA, Verschuuren JJ, Voltz R. Management of paraneoplastic neurological syndromes: report of an EFNS Task Force. Eur J Neurol. 2006;13:682–90.
11. Briani C, Samaroo D, Alaedini A. Celiac disease: from gluten to autoimmunity. Autoimmun Rev. 2008;7(8):644–50. https://doi.org/10.1016/j.autrev.2008.05.006.
12. Bataller L, Valero C, Díaz R, Froufe A, Garcia-Zarza A, Ribalta T, Vilchez JJ, Saiz A. Cerebellar ataxia associated with neuroendocrine thymic carcinoma and GAD antibodies. J Neurol Neurosurg Psychiatry. 2009;80(6):696–7. https://doi.org/10.1136/jnnp.2008.161042.
13. Castillo P, Woodruff B, Caselli R, Vernino S, Lucchinetti C, Swanson J, Noseworthy J, Aksamit A, Carter J, Sirven J, Hunder G, Fatourechi V, Mokri B, Drubach D, Pittock S, Lennon V, Boeve B. Steroid-responsive encephalopathy associated with autoimmune thyroiditis. Arch Neurol. 2006;63(2):197–202.
14. Graus F, Ribalta T, Abos J, Alom J, Cruz-Sanchez F, Mallolas J, Miro JM, Cardesa A, Tolosa E. Subacute cerebellar syndrome as the first manifestation of AIDS dementia complex. Acta Neurol Scand. 1990;81(2):118–20.
15. Zerr I, Kallenberg K, Summers DM, Romero C, Taratuto A, Heinemann U, Breithaupt M, Varges D, Meissner B, Ladogana A, Schuur M, Haik S, Collins SJ, Jansen GH, Stokin GB, Pimentel J, Hewer E, Collie D, Smith P, Roberts H, Brandel JP, van Duijn C, Pocchiari M, Begue C, Cras P, Will RG, Sanchez-Juan P. Updated clinical diagnostic criteria for sporadic Creutzfeldt-Jakob disease. Brain. 2009;132(Pt 10):2659–68. https://doi.org/10.1093/brain/awp191.
16. Klockgether T. The clinical diagnosis of autosomal dominant spinocerebellar ataxias. Cerebellum. 2008;7:101–5. https://doi.org/10.1007/s12311-008-0023-2.
17. Fogel BL, Perlman S. Clinical features and molecular genetics of autosomal recessive cerebellar ataxias. Lancet Neurol. 2007;6(3):245–57.

Functional Vestibular Disorders

There are circumstances in which vestibular symptoms, including unsteadiness, dizziness, and vertigo, may occur in persons that have normal vestibular systems. These are functional disorders, but they may eventually evolve to true vestibular diseases.

Usually the symptoms result from lack of blood supply to the vestibular organs, or toxic effects from different substances, or changes in the density of endolymph.

Medications for Hypertension

The use of diuretics and beta-blockers to control blood pressure may cause central vestibular disturbances due to reduced cerebral blood flow. All medications for hypertension cause some reduction of the cerebral blood flow [1], but diuretics and beta-blockers are the ones most frequently associated with orthostatic hypotension, unsteadiness, and vertigo in elderly patients. In approximately 10% of 43 elderly patients with central vestibular disorders, these were caused by diuretics [2]. This rarely occurs in young populations.

It must be taken in consideration the fact that many elderly patients present vascular problems, so that probably the reduction of cerebral vascular flow would not be alone responsible for the vestibular symptoms.

Alcohol

Alcohol can affect a person's balance via poisoning brain receptors, especially in the cerebellum, as well as altering the density of fluids within the inner ear [3].

P. L. M. Albernaz et al., *The New Neurotology*,
https://doi.org/10.1007/978-3-030-11283-7_14

Increased alcohol blood levels reduce the density of blood and rapidly diffuse into the cupulae of the semicircular canals, causing an imbalance called *positional alcohol nystagmus type I (PAN I)*.

Gradually the alcohol diffuses into the endolymph. When the density of the cupula and that of the endolymph are the same, the symptoms disappear.

As the blood alcohol levels start to fall, the reverse situation occurs. The cupula becomes denser than the endolymph, causing a *positional alcohol nystagmus type II (PAN II)*.

The overstimulation of the inner ear during PAN I and PAN II is associated with unsteadiness, nausea, and vertigo. PAN I is more associated with postural problems (e.g., standing and walking), while PAN II has been more associated with the feelings of a hangover. There is a brief symptomless interval between PAN I and PAN II.

Toxic Substances

Cases of vertigo have been described in patients whose houses were painted, caused by volatile organic compounds in paint, particularly toluene. At present there are many paints that use water as solvent, so that this type of toxicity is infrequent.

Metabolic and Endocrinal Disorders

Metabolic disorders are a consequence of abnormal chemical reactions in the body that may have different causes. Some endocrinal disorders are intimately associated with metabolic problems.

Carbohydrate metabolism disorders are common and may affect the vestibular system. Diabetes mellitus is a common disorder that presently behaves like an epidemic disease. The estimate is that approximately 380 million world inhabitants are affected by this disease, and this number will increase to approximately 470 million in year 2035.

Vascular disorders are common as diabetes progresses, and patients may become susceptible to vascular vestibular disorders. But there are also vestibular disorders related to the use of medications employed to control diabetes.

Inner ear homeostasis is very sensitive to changes in carbohydrate metabolism. This is an extensive subject and will be discussed in a separate chapter (see Chapter 15).

Thyroid malfunction may cause cochlear and vestibular symptoms, as demonstrated clinically and in research [4, 5]. From a clinical point of view, these symptoms are usually related to serious thyroid disorders, like myxedema or Hashimoto's autoimmune thyroid disease. Milder degrees of thyroid hormonal changes are rarely related to auditory or vestibular symptoms.

Other Medications

There are many medications that may induce vestibular symptoms, such as amphetamines, barbiturates, benzodiazepines, ketamine, lithium, several anticonvulsants and sedatives, serotonin inhibitors, and salicylates.

The use of cinnarizine and flunarizine in patients with metabolic disorders usually blocks the symptoms but aggravates the disease, often leading patients to a prolonged use of the medication that may lead to an eventual return of the symptoms or to side effects, including extrapyramidal disorders [6].

References

1. Fagan SC, Ewing JR, Levine SR, Tietjen GE, Ramadan NM, Welch MA. Assessing the effects of antihypertensive medication on cerebral blood flow: demonstrations in internal carotid artery occlusion. DICP A. 1991;25(12):1299–301.
2. Mangabeira-Albernaz PL. Vertigo in elderly patients: a review of 164 cases in Brazil. Ear Nose Throat J. 2014;93(8):322–30.
3. Aschan G, Bergstedt M. Positional alcoholic nystagmus (PAN) in man following repeated alcohol doses. Acta Otolaryngol Suppl. 1975;330:15–29.
4. Rybak LP. Metabolic disorders of the vestibular system. Otolaryngol Head Neck Surg. 1995;112(1):128–32.
5. Meza G, Acuña D, Escobar C. Development of vestibular and auditory function: effects of hypothyroidism and thyroxine replacement therapy on nystagmus and auditory evoked potentials in the pigmented rat. Int J Dev Neurosci. 1996;14(4):515–22.
6. Mangabeira-Albernaz PL. Calcium antagonists as a peripherally acting labyrinthine suppressant in humans. Acta Otolaryngol Suppl. 1988;460:99–103.

Glucose, Insulin, and Inner Ear Pathology

The inner ear is a highly complex organ with similarly complex metabolic mechanisms. This chapter is a study of the interrelation between carbohydrate metabolism and inner ear physiology that has been well established by experimental and clinical research.

Biochemical investigations in laboratory animals have demonstrated the intense metabolic activity of the inner ear [1–3] and its dependence on oxygen supply [4, 5]. The importance of glucose concentration required by the labyrinth for the maintenance of the endocochlear potential has also been demonstrated [6–8]. A common conclusion of these studies was that the inner ear has high metabolic activity but little stored energy that makes it sensitive to metabolic changes.

The stria vascularis is the essential metabolic center of the inner ear (Fig. 1). It is responsible for the endocochlear potential and the maintenance of the chemical structure of endolymph, removing its sodium and controlling the high concentration of potassium. This is accomplished by an enzyme well distributed in the organism and present in the stria in high concentration, {Na^+-K^+} ATPase, commonly called the sodium-potassium pump [9].

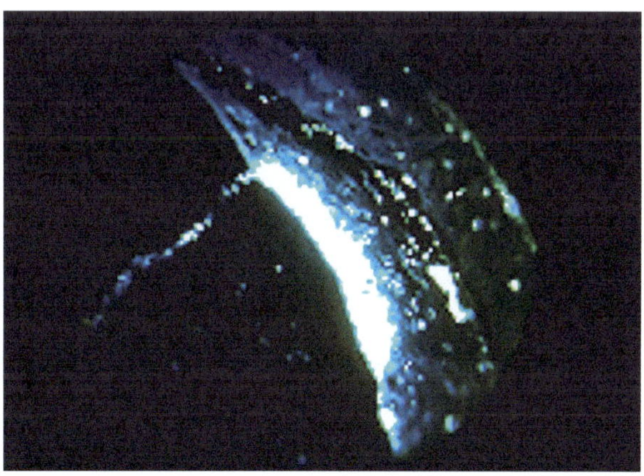

Fig. 1 A photomicrograph of the stria vascularis with a histochemical stain to show intense metabolic activity. (Mangabeira-Albernaz, 1962 [1])

P. L. M. Albernaz et al., *The New Neurotology*,
https://doi.org/10.1007/978-3-030-11283-7_15

Koide et al. [10], in 1960, studied the action of insulin in the inner ear of guinea pigs and noticed that a reduction of cochlear microphonics occurred 3 hours after the administration of 80 μUI of insulin per kg of body weight. This reduction lasted for approximately 80 minutes. The administration of glucose or other Krebs cycle substrates resulted in a partial recovery.

Mendelsohn and Roderique [7], in 1972, administered insulin to guinea pigs and reported changes in the chemical composition of endolymph: progressive reduction of the potassium concentration and progressive increase in sodium concentration. Three hours after insulin administration, the potassium concentration varied from 147.8 mEq/l to 57.1 mEq/l, and the sodium concentration increased from 5.85 mEq/l to 96.4 mEq/l. There was a simultaneous reduction of the endocochlear potential and also of cochlear microphonics.

It is well known that glucose and oxygen are essential nutrients to the sodium-potassium pump, but glucose transport mechanisms in the cochlea are not well known. There are studies showing that glucose transport is accomplished through communication junctions (nexus) with the help of a transporter (GLUT1), the presence of which has been demonstrated in the basal cells of the stria vascularis in mice. Immunochemical tests have shown that GLUT1, occludin (a protein that closes the nexus), and proteins connexin 26 and connexin 30 were also demonstrated in the basal cells of the stria, also in mice [11].

The +80 mV endocochlear potential is essential for normal hearing and is intimately related to the mechanisms for potassium transportation [11, 12]. Sodium is also metabolized by the stria vascularis by means of selective channels [13].

Changes in glucose and insulin blood concentration affect cochlear homeostasis by changing the chemical structure of endolymph. The increase in sodium concentration and the reduction of potassium increase the osmotic pressure, demanding more water into the endolymphatic space. This volume increase causes a certain degree of endolymphatic hydrops. It is known that endolymphatic hydrops is the substrate of Menière's disease, but it is also known that hydrops occurs in other inner ear disorders, such as Mondini dysplasia and syphilis. On the other hand, hydrops may not be related to changes in the chemical composition of endolymph; it may also derive from lack of absorption of endolymph, and this mechanism is not related to metabolic disorders. The hydropic changes in Menière's disease are probably much more intense than those observed in typical metabolic problems.

A clinical relation between hearing loss and diabetes was first reported by Abel Jordão in 1864 [14]. The loss of hearing in diabetic patients is most probably of vascular origin, due to atherosclerosis. Rust et al. [15], however, demonstrated a loss of external hair cells in diabetic rats, more intense for the animals that ingested rapidly absorbable sugars. It is quite possible that these changes can also happen in diabetic patients.

Hypoglycemia, however, affects the inner ear by means of strictly metabolic mechanisms. Harril [16], in 1951, described hypoglycemia as a cause of migraine and vertigo. Tintera and Goldman [17], in 1956; Goldman [18], in 1962; and Powers [19], in 1972, analyzed patients with vestibular symptoms associated with hypoglycemia.

Updegraff [20], in 1977, proposed routine insulin titration for the investigation of patients with auditory and/or vestibular disorders that presented a clinical possibility of altered carbohydrate metabolism.

Updegraff's proposal was based on the observations of Joseph R. Kraft [21], who published in 1975 his data based on 3000 glucose tolerance tests including simultaneous insulin titration and demonstrated that glucose levels alone were insufficient to accurately diagnose carbohydrate metabolism disorders. He introduced the concept of diabetes in situ, or occult diabetes, to describe types of changes that would evolve gradually to clinical diabetes. In his book published in 2008 [22], he concluded, based on more than 14,000 tests, that his original observations were correct.

The interpretation of the insulin curves, as proposed by Kraft, is essential to the clinical evaluation of the changes in the inner ear induced by disorders of carbohydrate metabolism. He classified the insulin curves into five different categories that will be briefly explained.

Kraft's type I curve represents the normal pattern of insulin release. The normal fast levels are 5–30 μUI/ml, and the peak values occur either at 30 or at 60 minutes. The maximum value for the sample obtained at 120 minutes is 50 μUI/ml, and the sum of the value for 120 and 180 minutes shall not exceed 60 μUI/ml.

In Kraft's type II curve, the peak levels also occur at 30 or 60 minutes, but the values at 120 and 180 minutes are higher, characterizing a *normal peak and slow recovery*.

In Kraft's type III curve, the peak is delayed. The peak may occur at 120 minutes – subtype IIIa – or at 180 minutes, subtype IIIB.

Kraft's type IV curve is characterized by high fast values of insulin (50 μUI/ml or more) and are seen in diabetic patients.

Kraft's type V curve shows low values of insulin at all times (flat curve).

Based on his findings, Kraft demonstrated that the patients with insulin curves of the types II and III had a significant chance of becoming diabetic.

Fukuda [23], in 1982, and Mangabeira-Albernaz and Fukuda [24], in 1984, using Kraft's method, analyzed a group of patients with metabolic problems and inner ear disorders and concluded that hyperinsulinemia was often a cause of hearing loss and/or dizziness. They also confirmed that insulin levels were more sensitive indicators of carbohydrate metabolism changes than glucose levels.

This study led to the observation that patients with type V insulin curves often presented symptoms similar to the ones with curves II, III, and IV. Many of these patients were found to present gastrointestinal problems, and in 1985, Mangabeira-Albernaz, Fukuda, Vilela, and Miszputen [25] described inner ear disorders caused by defective enzyme mechanisms of the small intestine (brush border membrane disease). In patients with these disorders, the high concentrations of lactose and saccharose in the small intestine create an osmotic unbalance that results in transposition of blood glucose to the intestine, producing hypoglycemia. The unabsorbed sugars proceed to the colon and are digested by intestinal bacteria, resulting in abdominal distension and often gases and diarrhea. This subject was reviewed by Mangabeira-Albernaz and Miszputen in 2014 [26].

Kazmierczak and Doroszewska [27], in 2001, studied a group of patients with impaired carbohydrate metabolism who presented vertigo, tinnitus, and hearing loss.

Mangabeira-Albernaz, in 2005, presented a long-term follow-up on patients with hyperinsulinemia and brush border membrane disease, based on 891 patients [28].

D'Avila and Lavinsky, in 2005, studied the glucose and insulin profiles in patients with Menière's disease [29], and Zuma e Maia and Lavinsky, in 2006, studied otoacoustic emissions in an animal model of induced hyperinsulinemia [30].

Selcuk et al., in 2014, described cochlear damage as a result of gestational diabetes [31].

Mangabeira-Albernaz, in 2016, published extensive data on 376 additional patients [32].

Symptoms

Clinical History Approximately 50% of the patients with disorders of carbohydrate metabolism present vestibular symptoms; cochlear symptoms alone are observed in approximately 30%. Cochlear and vestibular symptoms occur in approximately 20%. Some patients with Menière's disease may present metabolic problems, but there are no positive indications of a clinical relationship.

Tinnitus occurs in approximately 30% of the patients; 10% present episodes of metabolic migraine, caused by excessive accumulation of sodium in the brain cells.

Drop attacks and panic syndrome may be occasionally found.

The most common cochlear symptom is discomfort with loud sounds. Some patients complain of hearing fluctuation, often mistaken for auditory tube disorders.

The most common vestibular symptom is the sensation of floating, like walking on a soft rubber foam floor. Many patients present typical vertiginous episodes.

A common symptom is the sudden need to ingest foods rich in sugar, which coincide with peaks of hypoglycemia. A family history of type II diabetes is not uncommon.

Some patients present digestive problems such as constipation, diarrhea, and abdominal distention, which are suggestive of brush border membrane disease.

Episodes of severe hypoglycemia, due to dumping, are frequent in patients submitted to gastrectomy or bariatric surgery.

A few patients refer episodes of blurred vision which results from loss of glycogen in the lens in moments of intense hypoglycemia. This is recognized as a cause of cataracts in young persons.

All of the patients' symptoms are aggravated by stress and tension.

Table 1 shows the approximate frequency of the patients' symptoms.

Table 1 Approximate frequency of patients' symptoms

Symptoms	Frequency (%)
Vestibular symptoms	50
Cochlear symptoms	30
Tinnitus	30
Migraine	8
Aural pressure	4
Panic syndrome	3
Drop attacks	2

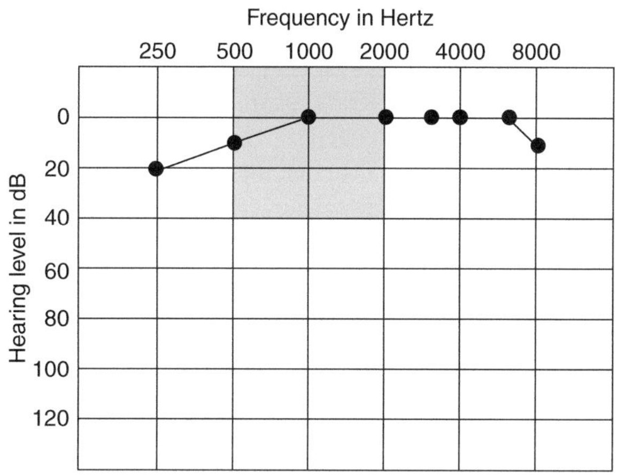

Fig. 2 Audiogram most commonly seen in patients with metabolic disorders

Findings

Audiological Tests

Figure 2 shows the most common audiometric curve observed in these patients. Speech discrimination is usually normal. It should be noted that if these hearing level thresholds are converted to sound pressure or intensity levels, they will show a flat curve, characteristic of the reduction of the endocochlear potential.

Immittance tests are also usually normal. Electrocochleography may show changes in the relation of the summation and action potentials in some cases, but it is mostly normal.

Vestibular Examination

Vestibular hyperreflexia was the most characteristic finding in the vestibular evaluation of these patients. It can be seen in rotational tests and in video head impulse tests. Caloric tests should be avoided in these patients, for they often have nausea and vomits during the stimulation. It is most frequently symmetrical, related to unsteadiness and floating sensation; asymmetrical responses may be observed, particularly in patients with episodes of vertigo.

Glucose and Insulin Assays

The percentage of abnormal glucose and insulin curves in the author's patients is of approximately 90%, demonstrating the significance of the clinical histories in the evaluation of metabolic disorders.

Figure 3 shows the average glucose curves in a group of 376 patients, according to the corresponding Kraft insulin curves. Figure 4 shows the average insulin levels for the different Kraft curves.

It is interesting to note that the glucose curves maintain a positive correlation to the insulin curves.

Figure 5 shows a comparison of the mean glucose levels in patients with hyperinsulinemia – including Kraft curves II, IIIA, IIIB, and IV – and brush border membrane disease, curve V.

Figure 6 shows the comparison of the mean insulin levels in patients with hyperinsulinemia and brush border membrane.

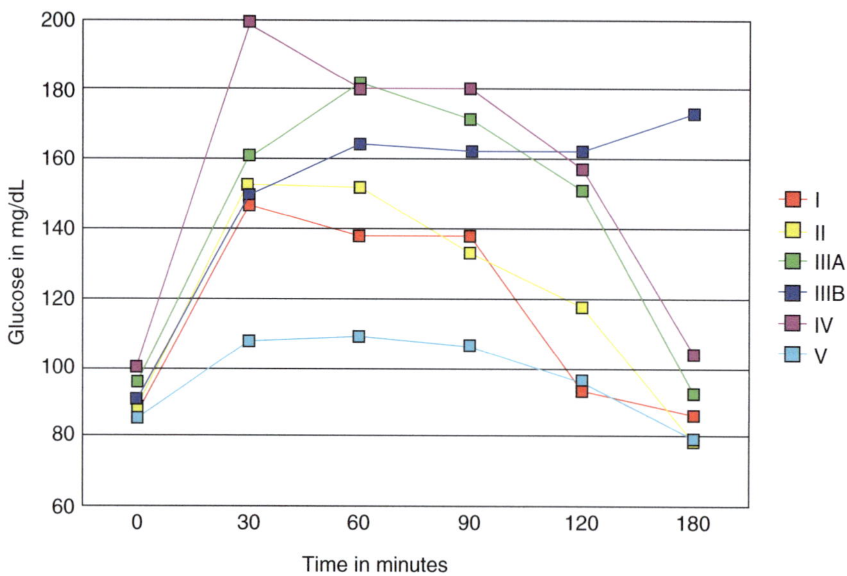

Fig. 3 Glucose levels in a group of patients, classified according to the Kraft insulin curves

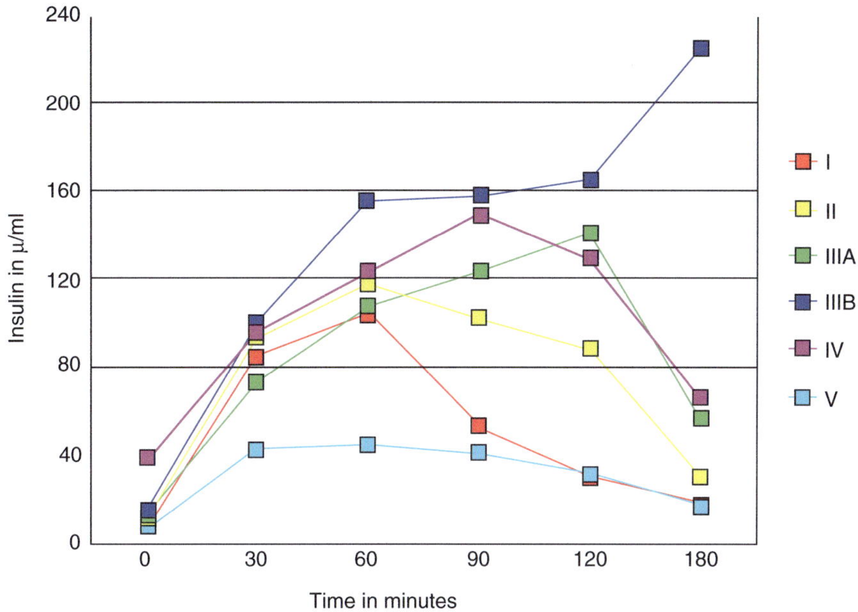

Fig. 4 Average insulin levels for the different Kraft curves

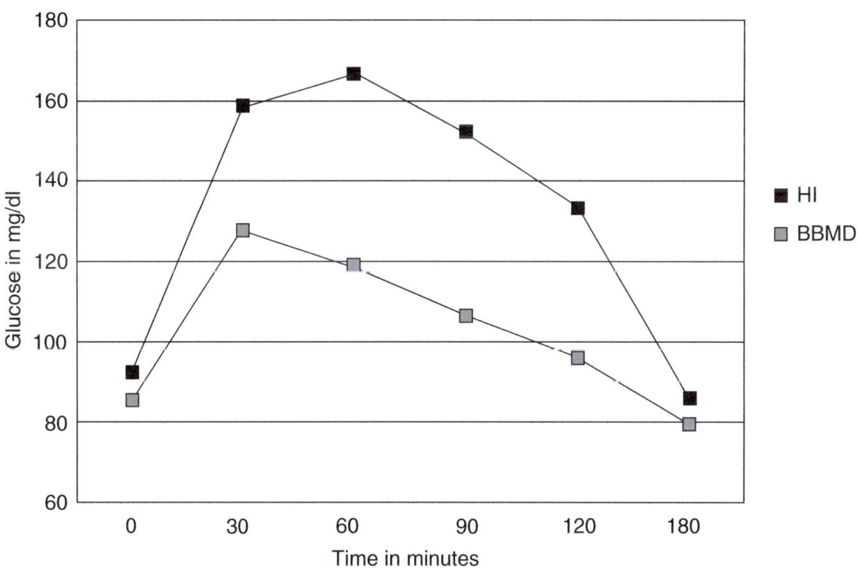

Fig. 5 Mean glucose levels in patients with hyperinsulinemia (HI) and brush border membrane disease (BBMD)

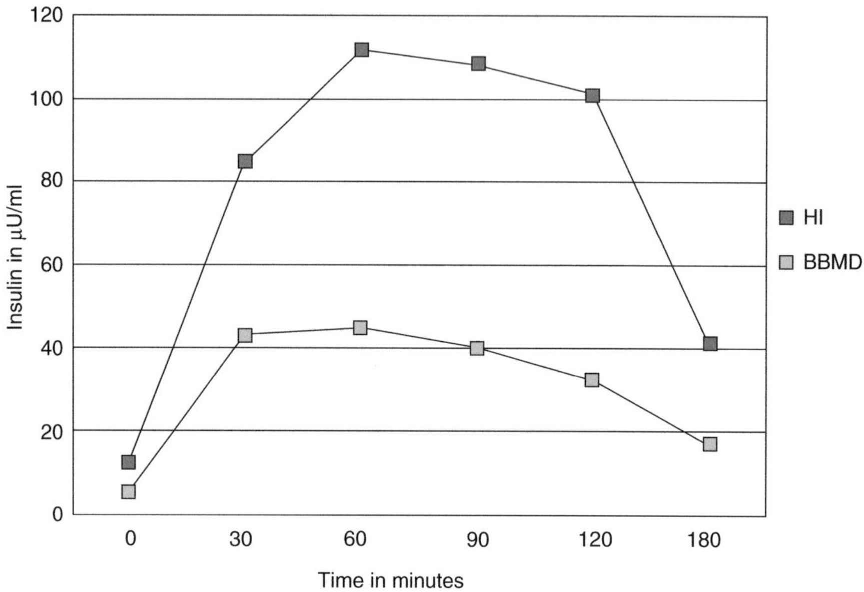

Fig. 6 Mean insulin levels in patients with hyperinsulinemia (HI) and brush border membrane disease (BBMD)

The homeostatic model assessment (HOMA) is a commonly used method to quantify insulin resistance and beta-cell function. It was first described under the name HOMA by Matthews et al. [33]. Figure 7 shows the percentage of patients who presented a HOMA value above 2.7, which is considered the normal limit.

Menière's Disease and Disorders of Carbohydrate Metabolism

The association of Menière's disease and carbohydrate metabolic disorders is fairly common. In a recently analyzed group of 98 patients, 33 patients had hyperinsulinemia, 24 had brush border membrane disease, and 5 had diabetes mellitus type II; 36 patients did not have metabolic disorders.

The treatment of the metabolic disorder ameliorates the clinical treatment of Menière's disease. It does not, however, preclude the development of the more serious cases of the disease.

Discussion

There are no clear explanations for the fact that some patients have only cochlear symptoms, some have only vestibular symptoms, and some have both cochlear and vestibular symptoms. Since the endolymph in the vestibular portion of the system

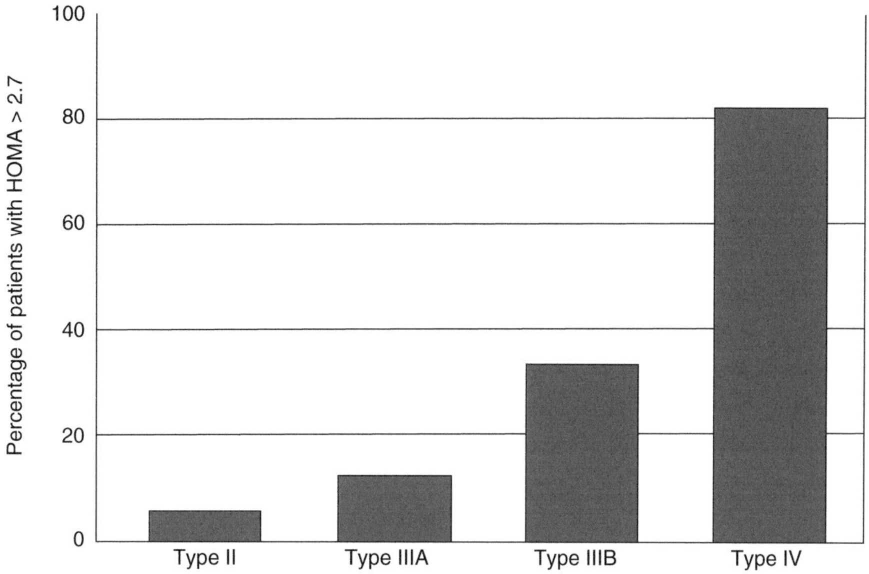

Fig. 7 Percentage of patients with high values of HOMA (≥2.7) in each type of insulin curve

does not have the 80 mV electric charge, it would be reasonable to infer that the cochlea should be more sensitive to the changes in the fluids' chemical composition, but this is not the case. Mention must be made of symptoms not related to the inner ear, such as metabolic migraine, caused by excessive accumulation of sodium in the brain cells, and blurred vision, caused by loss of glycogen in the lens in moments of intense hypoglycemia, recognized as a cause of cataracts in young persons.

Patients with hyperinsulinemia (Kraft's types II, IIIA, IIIB, and IV curves) and patients with brush border membrane disease (Kraft's type V curve) exhibit some clinical differences.

Patients with excessive liberation of insulin have a tendency to present low glucose blood levels in certain hours of the day. The foods that cause excessive insulin liberation in sensitive people are the rapid absorption carbohydrates, such as purified sucrose and fructose.

Overweight patients have high levels of blood insulin caused by the increased peripheral insulin resistance due to blocked receptors. It is interesting to note the effect of bariatric surgery on these patients.

Figure 8 shows the marked differences in glucose and insulin blood levels in a 41-year-old female patient who underwent bariatric surgery. After the operation, her small hearing loss returned to normal, and her vestibular symptoms disappeared.

The glucose preoperative curve shows a high fast blood level that rises to a delayed peak at 120 minutes. The postoperative glucose curve shows a normal fast level, a normal peak at 30 minutes, and reactive hypoglycemia at 120 minutes. This reactive hypoglycemia is common in total or partial gastrectomies due to dumping.

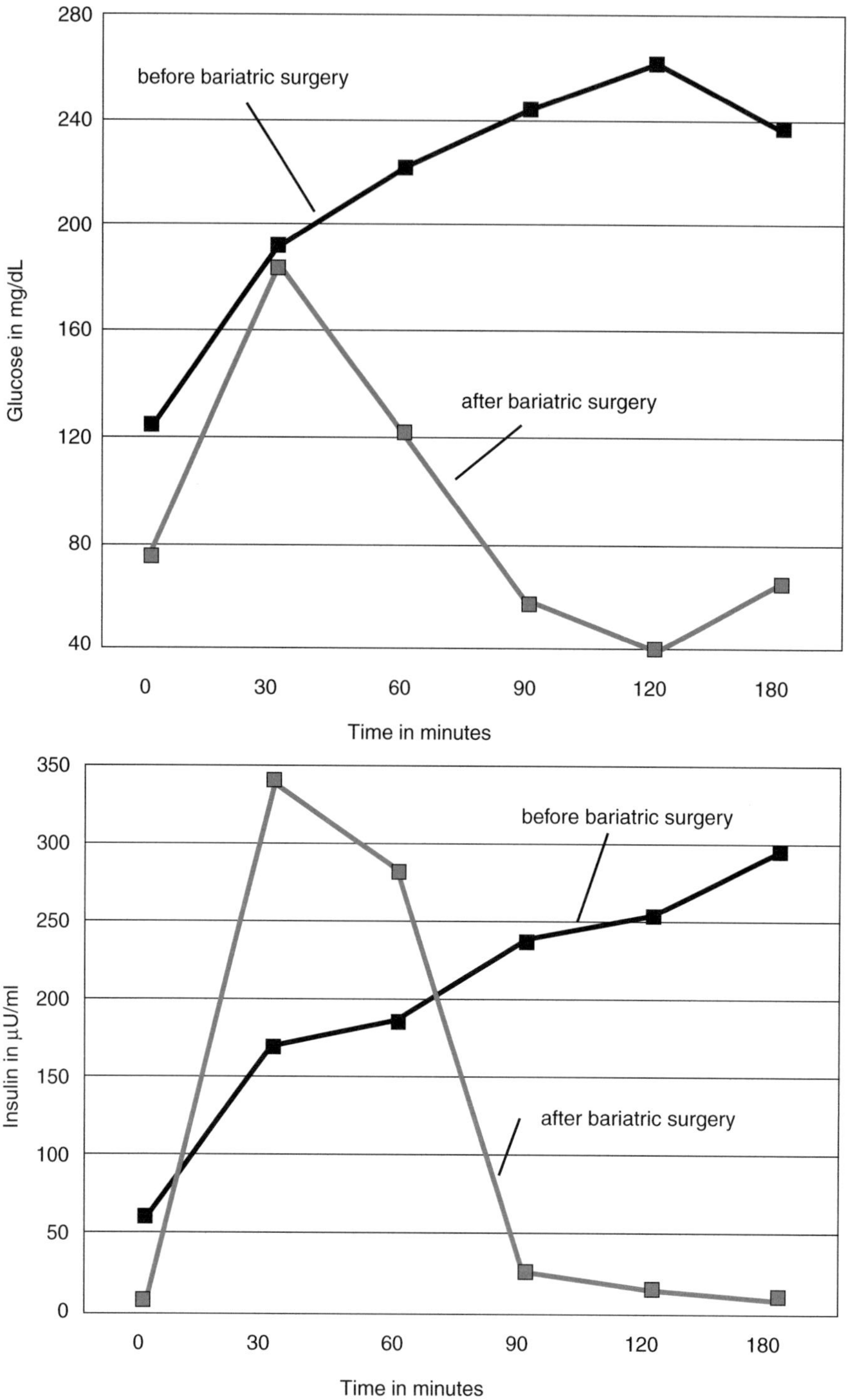

Fig. 8 Glucose (top) and insulin (bottom) blood levels in a patient before and after bariatric surgery

The preoperative insulin curve shows a delayed peak at 180 minutes, showing that the pancreas is unable to react to the sudden increase in the glucose blood level. The postoperative insulin curve is normal.

Brush border membrane disease, on the other hand, causes fluctuations of the glucose level due to osmotic unbalance caused by unabsorbed sugars (mainly lactose) in the small intestine. The limit established by Kraft is 30 μUI/ml, but it was observed that some patients with confirmed disaccharidases had values up to 50 μUI/ml. A double-peaked insulin curve, parallel to the glucose curve, was also found to be common in patients with intestinal carbohydrate malabsorption.

The hypoglycemic peaks for these patients usually occur 1–2 hours after the glucose ingestion, while in patients with hyperinsulinemia, it usually occurs 3 hours or more after the ingestion. In view of fact that the patients with brush border membrane disease have symptoms similar to those with hyperinsulinemia, it is believed that the inner ear symptoms are actually related to hypoglycemia.

The involvement of the transport proteins that carry the monosaccharides into the blood stream, after the enzymatic breakup of the disaccharides, is usually affected by the disorder, so sucrose must also be restricted to a certain extent. Maltase production is very rarely affected; it was only seen in rare cases of marathon runners, who eat only carbohydrates for long periods of time. Contrary to patients with hyperinsulinemia, patients with brush border membrane disease do not become diabetic.

In our original study [12], biopsies of the jejunal mucosa of the patients with suspected brush border membrane disease were obtained, and the reduction or absence of lactase was confirmed by microchemical assay. This was performed in order to exclude other types of intestinal disorders that could eventually produce similar symptoms. This turned out to be an unnecessary procedure, and it was no longer used.

The hearing loss presented by each of these categories of patients is usually mild. Most of the time, the hearing thresholds for the low and high tones show some fluctuation. As a rule, there is no complaint of hearing loss, since the thresholds for the speech frequencies are almost always within the normal social range, but they often report the sensation of intermittent blocking that they compare with what they experience in a descending airplane and may be compared to auditory tube obstruction. Many patients, when interrogated, refer a sensitivity, or discomfort, in relation to loud noises.

The fluctuant hearing loss and the sensitivity to noise are usually reversible with treatment. In some untreated cases, however, the hearing losses may become socially significant.

The episodic sensation of floating, or walking over foam, is the most frequent vestibular symptom, but many patients refer episodes of vertigo. Vestibular hyperreflexia is the most common finding in vestibular examination and is probably related to the changes in the density of endolymph caused by the increased sodium concentration and the accumulation of water to correct the osmotic changes.

Tension and stress often aggravate the symptoms by increasing the consumption of glucose by central nervous system cells.

The diagnosis of altered carbohydrate metabolism is confirmed by the oral glucose tolerance test with simultaneous insulin titration. Most clinicians rely only on the glucose fast levels for the investigation of carbohydrate metabolism disorders, but this is a test of low sensitivity, even when interpreted together with the glycated hemoglobin test. In this series of 376 patients, only 56 (14.89%) had glucose fast levels of 100 mg/dL or more. HOMA IR was abnormal (2.7 or greater) only in 25 patients (6.72%), suggesting that the majority of the patients in this study have intolerance to rapidly absorbable carbohydrates and do not show resistance to insulin.

The insulin curves were found to be twice as sensitive as the glucose curves for the diagnoses of carbohydrate metabolism impairment [11]. Furthermore, in a group of 376 patients [31], the diagnosis of previously non-identified cases of diabetes mellitus type II was established in 39 patients, confirming the sensitivity of the inner ear to this disorder.

It is interesting to note that there is a reluctance, on the part of many clinicians and endocrinologists, to accept the predictions based on Kraft's classification, in spite of the clinical and experimental data available [9, 11, 18, 19, 26]. Our findings confirm Kraft's observations that the insulin curves do allow for the prediction of future diabetes [8, 9].

On the other hand, only approximately 8% of the patients presented a normal (Kraft type I) insulin curve, indicating the value of the clinical history and neurotological evaluation as a basis for the diagnosis of impaired carbohydrate metabolism.

The hearing losses that result from impaired carbohydrate metabolism are among the few sensorineural hearing problems that can be adequately treated and that can return to normal. The same can be said about the vestibular symptoms that disappear in most patients. In fact, the control of the glucose blood levels and the amount of insulin liberation by the pancreas are effective not only to control the inner ear symptoms but also to identify the patients who are prone to become diabetic and delay the onset of the disease.

These patients must reduce the intake of quickly absorbable sugars and must also reduce the intervals between their meals, eating every 3 hours during the day. The ideal food for the intermediate meals are fruits; the fructose in the fruit is not rapidly absorbed, being attached to the pulp of the fruit. As an alternative, unsweetened cereal bars or crackers can be used or a light yogurt. Large molecule carbohydrates (bread, pasta, rice, beans, etc.) may be consumed up to 100 g per day. Obese patients are strongly advised to lose weight in order to reduce the effect of insulin resistance due to the blocking of insulin receptors. An alternative is bariatric surgery, when indicated.

In patients with brush border membrane disease, only milk products without lactose must be consumed. Commercially available lactase may also be used to help digest milk and derivatives.

In view of the frequent involvement of the transport proteins that carry monosaccharides into the blood stream, sucrose must also be restricted. The amount of sugar intake must be determined by each patient using a trial-and-error approach. These diets usually take 45–90 days to regulate the patient's glucose levels. If they suffer from severe vestibular disorders, they are given medications for a small period of time, until the audiological tests show that the hearing has been stabilized. Many vasodilator drugs increase the glucose consumption by the central nervous system cells; these medications must be avoided.

The follow-up of patients with carbohydrate metabolism disorders of the inner ear is quite complex. Many patients do not return for tests. Occasionally patients' friends, or patients referred by them, relate that they are well. Some patients who abandoned their diets occasionally return when their symptoms get worse; most of them have been found to be diabetic [26].

The identification of these problems, however, is very important for the patients. It provides them with a better quality of life, correcting their inner ear symptoms and preventing, or at least postponing for many years, the occurrence of clinical diabetes.

Conclusions

The inner ears are very sensitive organs and in many patients are the first to show signs of carbohydrate metabolism disorders. The cochlear and vestibular symptoms resulting from these disorders are very common, can be diagnosed and treated, and are often reversible.

On the other hand, carbohydrate metabolism problems are not routinely checked by otologists or neurotologists. It is quite possible that the complaints of these patients can be suppressed by symptomatic treatment, but etiologic treatment is always the best treatment, and, additionally, it will help in the prevention of the progression of these disorders.

References

1. Mangabeira-Albernaz PL, Covell WP. Acoustic trauma lesions by fluorescence microscopy. Laryngoscope. 1962;72:1278–96.
2. Thalmann R, Matschinsky FM, Thalmann R. Quantitative study of selected enzymes involved in energy metabolism of the cochlear duct. Ann Otol Rhinol Laryngol. 1970;79:12–29.
3. Degerman E, Rauch U, Lindberg S, Caye-Thomasen P, Hultgårdh A, Magnusson M. Expression of insulin signalling components in the sensory epithelium of the human saccule. Cell Tissue Res. 2013;352(3):469–78. https://doi.org/10.1007/s00441-013-1614-x.
4. Fernandez C. The effect of oxygen lack on cochlear potentials. Ann Otol Rhinol Laryngol. 1955;64:1193–203.
5. Tsunoo M, Perlman HB. Respiration of the cochlea and function. Acta Otolaryngol. 1969;67:17–23.

6. Wing KG. The experimental use of hypoglycemia to show whether glucose is a major fuel for the cochlear response, and further remarks concerning the lability of the vascular bed supplying the cochlear partition. Acta Otolaryngol. 1959;Suppl 148:87–93.
7. Mendelsohn M, Roderique J. Cationic changes in endolymph during hypoglycemia. Laryngoscope. 1972;82:1533–40.
8. Thalmann R, Miyoshi T, Kusakari J, Ise I. Normal and abnormal energy metabolism of the inner ear. Otolaryngol Clin N Am. 1975;8:313–33.
9. Kuijpers W, Bonting SL. Localization and properties of ATPase in the inner ear of the guinea pig. Biochim Biophys Acta. 1969;173:477–85.
10. Koide Y, Tajima S, Yoshida M, Konno M. Biochemical changes in the inner ear induced by insulin, in relation to cochlear microphonics. Ann Otol Rhinol Laryngol. 1960;69:1083–97.
11. Suzuki T, Matsunami T, Hisa Y, Takata K, Takamatsu T, Oyamada M. Roles of gap junctions in glucose transport from glucose transporter 1-positive to -negative cells in the lateral wall of the rat cochlea. Histochem Cell Biol. 2009;131(1):89–102.
12. Nin F, Hibino H, Doi K, Suzuki T, Hisa Y, Kurachi Y. The endocochlear potential depends on two K+ diffusion potentials and an electrical barrier in the stria vascularis of the inner ear. Proc Natl Acad Sci U S A. 2008;105(5):1751–6.
13. Quraishi IH, Raphael RM. Generation of the endocochlear potential: a biophysical model. Biophys J. 2008;94(8):L64–6.
14. Jordão A. Estudos sobre a Diabete. Lisboa: Typographia da Academia; 1864.
15. Rust KR, Prazma J, Triana RJ, Michaelis OE 4th, Pillsbury HC. Inner ear damage secondary to diabetes mellitus. II. Changes in aging SHR/N-cp rats. Arch Otolaryngol Head Neck Surg. 1992;118(4):397–400.
16. Harril JA. Headache and vertigo associated with hypoglycemia tendency. Laryngoscope. 1951;61:138–45.
17. Tintera JW, Goldman HB. Hypoadrenocorticism in otolaryngological surgical procedures. N Y St J Med. 1956;56:872–7.
18. Goldman HB. Hypoadrenocorticism and endocrinologic treatment of Meniere's disease. N Y St J Med. 1962;62:377–82.
19. Powers WH. Metabolic aspects of Meniere's disease. Laryngoscope. 1972;82:1176–85.
20. Updegraff WR. Impaired carbohydrate metabolism and idiopathic Meniere's disease. Ear Nose Throat J. 1977;56(4):160–3.
21. Kraft JR. Detection of diabetes mellitus in situ (occult diabetes). Lab Med. 1976;6:10–22.
22. Kraft JR. Diabetes epidemic and you: Trafford Publishing; 2008.
23. Fukuda Y. Glicemia, Insulinemia e Patologia da Orelha Interna. 1982, Ph.D. thesis. Escola Paulista de Medicina.
24. Mangabeira Albernaz PL, Fukuda Y. Glucose, insulin and inner ear pathology. Acta Otolaryngol (Stockh). 1984;97:496–501.
25. Mangabeira-Albernaz PL, Fukuda Y, Vilela MP, Miszputen SJ. Vestibular disorders caused by defective enzyme mechanisms in the small intestine. Acta Otolaryngol (Stockh). 1985;99:330–5.
26. Mangabeira-Albernaz PL, Miszputen SJ. Vertigem e enzimas digestivas. In: Zuma e Maia FC, Mangabeira Albernaz PL, Carmona PL, editors. Otoneurologia Atual. Rio de Janeiro: Revinter; 2014. p. 365–79.
27. Kazmierczak H, Doroszewska G. Metabolic disorders in vertigo, tinnitus, and hearing loss. Int Tinnitus J. 2001;7(1):54–8.
28. Mangabeira-Albernaz PL. Inner ear disorders induced by impaired carbohydrate metabolism – a long term follow up. In: Lim DJ, editor. Meniere's disease & inner ear homeostasis disorders – proceedings of the 5th international symposium. Los Angeles: House Ear Institute; 2005. p. 326–7.

29. D'Avila C, Lavinsky L. Glucose and insulin profiles and their correlations in Ménière's disease. Int Tinnitus J. 2005;11:170–6.
30. Zuma e Maia FC, Lavinsky L. Distortion product otoacoustic emissions in an animal model of induced hyperinsulinemia. Int Tinnitus J. 2006;12:133–9.
31. Selcuk A, Terzi H, Turkay U, Kale A, Genc S. Does gestational diabetes result in cochlear damage? J Laryngol Otol. 2014;128:961–5.
32. Mangabeira-Albernaz PL. Hearing loss, dizziness, and carbohydrate metabolism. Int Arch Otorhinolaryngol. 2016;20(3):261–70. https://doi.org/10.1055/s-0035-1558450.
33. Matthews DR, Hosker JP, Rudenski AS, Naylor BA, Treacher DF, Turner RC. Homeostasis model assessment: insulin resistance and beta-cell function from fasting plasma glucose and insulin concentrations in man. Diabetologia. 1985;28:412–9.

Surgical Treatment of Vestibular Disorders

Vertigo can be a severely incapacitating symptom, and there are patients in whom all attempts of clinical treatment result in failure. For these disabled patients, surgical treatment is recommended.

The extent of the disability has to be judged for each particular patient. It will depend on his profession, his level of activity, and his own perception of his degree of social or professional incapacitation.

This chapter reviews the types of procedures that can be employed for the treatment of incapacitating vertigo and their indications. It will not deal with details of the surgical techniques that are not a subject of this book.

Surgery for Menière's Disease

Approximately 95% of the patients with Menière's disease respond to different kinds of medical treatment. Surgical procedures may be needed for the remaining 5% of the patients.

Labyrinthectomy

The surgical destruction of the labyrinth was the first operation indicated as a treatment for Menière's disease.

Labyrinthectomy has been performed in four different ways:

1. Through the ear canal, removing the stapes, joining the vestibular and cochlear windows, and filling the vestibule with streptomycin or gentamicin. This simpler technique is usually indicated for elderly patients with severe or profound unilateral hearing loss. It was proposed by Schuknecht in 1957 [1].

P. L. M. Albernaz et al., *The New Neurotology*,
https://doi.org/10.1007/978-3-030-11283-7_16

2. Through the mastoid, opening the lateral semicircular canal and extracting the membranous labyrinth. This technique was proposed by Cawthorne in 1947 [2].
3. Through the mastoid, opening the three semicircular canals. This is a more thorough procedure that can be used for patients of all age groups.
4. Through a translabyrinthine approach, destroying the three semicircular canals and sectioning the vestibular nerves. This technique was proposed as an attempt to obtain better vestibular compensation, which did not occur; for this reason it has been mostly abandoned. It has been suggested that the cochlear nerve should not be sectioned, so that the patient can eventually be submitted to a cochlear implant.

In the 1950s, there was a general belief that Menière's disease was usually a unilateral disease and that the uncommonly seen bilateral cases were bilateral from the onset. This reasoning was a justification for the use of labyrinthectomy in unilateral cases.

This concept, however, turned out to be totally untrue. Many patients develop the disease in the opposite ear, usually after a variable period of time. One can imagine the difficult situations of patients who were submitted to a labyrinthectomy and, years later, developed Menière's disease in the non-operated ear. Therefore, labyrinthectomy for Menière's disease was totally abandoned, except for patients with no degree of socially useful hearing in the ear to be operated.

Today labyrinthectomy is indicated mainly in cases of ipsilateral delayed endolymphatic hydrops. Patients with this problem have a history of unilateral deafness since childhood and then develop episodic vertigo [3]. For these patients, who have no hearing in the diseased ear, labyrinthectomy is the best treatment. They must be carefully evaluated, however, to ensure that the vertiginous episodes arise from the deaf ear; a differential diagnosis must be established with contralateral delayed endolymphatic hydrops and bilateral delayed endolymphatic hydrops.

Endolymphatic Fistulas

There have been several attempts to create fistulas to release excessive endolymphatic pressures. Fick [4] proposed a saccular decompression through the oval window, making a hole in the stapes footplate, performing the operation as soon as possible after a vertiginous episode. Cody [5] suggested placing a tack through the stapes footplate, causing repeated perforations of the saccular membrane. William House devised an otic-perotic shunt that required placing a small tube through the basilar membrane, operating through the round window; this procedure was later performed by cryosurgery [6, 7].

All of these techniques resulted in a high percentage of severe or profound hearing losses and were, therefore, abandoned.

Endolymphatic Sac Operations

A German ophthalmologist and otologist, Hermann Jacob Knapp, suggested that the symptoms of Menière's disease might be due to an increase in labyrinth pressure and compared it with the glaucoma in the eye [8].

In 1927, following Knapp's suggestion and after making experiments in sharks, George Portmann advocated an opening of the endolymphatic sac in patients with Menière's disease [9]. It is interesting to note that the pathological confirmation of the increased pressure of endolymph – endolymphatic hydrops – was obtained only in 1938 by Hallpike and Cairns, studying two temporal bones of patients who died after a section of the acoustic nerve through the posterior cranial fossa [10].

House, in 1964 [11], proposed an endolymphatic-subarachnoid shunt for Menière's disease, attempting to improve the results of Portmann's operation. He felt that the endolymphatic sac is the vestibular structure that is farthest from the cochlea, therefore reducing the probability of hearing loss as a consequence of the procedure. Different technical variations, from simple sac decompression to mastoid shunts, were eventually suggested by different authors.

The sac operations are the only procedures that attempt to repair the system rather than destroy it in part or totally [12]. On the other hand, there are controversies regarding its effectiveness. Some Danish investigators compared endolymphatic sac surgeries with simple mastoidectomies, and their statistical results were essentially the same [13]. Their studies, however, have also been questioned [14]. In fact, endolymphatic sac surgeries continue to be performed and show a high percentage of good results.

Endolymphatic sac operations have also been performed for endolymphatic hydrops caused by tertiary syphilis and Mondini dysplasia [15, 16]. They have been attempted in cases of enlarged vestibular aqueducts, but most patients had some degree of additional hearing loss after the procedure.

Nerve Sections

Intracranial section of the eighth nerve was advocated by Dandy [17], who reported a series of 401 cases and 1 death. Other neurosurgeons, however, reported on serious damage to the cerebellum and other cranial nerves and 5% of deaths. It should be reminded that endolymphatic hydrops, as the primary pathology of Menière's disease, was established with the temporal bones of two patients who died from this operation [10].

House, in 1960 [18], reported on his attempts to reach the internal acoustic meatus through the cranial middle fossa and translabyrinthine and retrolabyrinth approaches. Each of these accesses offers adequate exposure for the section of the vestibular nerves. Besides, new instrumentation was then available, and the use of the surgical microscope created adequate conditions for the development of these new techniques.

The vestibular nerve section through the middle cranial fossa became a very popular operation for many years. Many otologists, however, prefer the retrolabyrinthine approach, which allows for easy identification of the vestibular nerves and has less risks of damaging the facial nerve [19].

Vestibular nerve section is very efficient for the elimination of the vertiginous episodes. It does not affect, however, the cochlear symptoms of the disease; most patients continue to feel fluctuant hearing, aural pressure, and variable tinnitus. Some patients complain of unsteadiness, due to imperfect vestibular compensation, and need vestibular rehabilitation [20].

The advent of the transtympanic chemical treatments has reduced the number of patients subjected to vestibular nerve sections.

Transtympanic Treatments

Transtympanic administration of gentamicin has been extensively used in the treatment of Menière's disease. There are many different approaches, doses and administration intervals, and conflicting reports on treatment-induced hearing losses in some patients. It is well known that gentamicin is more toxic to the vestibular hair cells than to cochlear hair cells, but the use of higher doses can increase the patients' hearing loss. The clinical reports suggest that the successful treatment is not dependent on a total destruction of the labyrinth [21].

Corticosteroids have also been used transtympanically for Menière's disease, with some good results. It has been primarily indicated, however, in treating autoimmune deafness.

Surgery for Perilymphatic Fistulas

Perilymphatic fistulas of the oval or round windows may appear as a complication of stapedectomies or may be spontaneous [22]. They may be *explosive* or *implosive.*

The explosive type is caused by a sudden episode of spinal fluid hypertension that reaches the cochlea through the internal auditory meatus or through the cochlear aqueduct; these episodes usually result from physical efforts or intense stress.

The implosive type is caused by barotrauma, due to excessive attempts to reinflate the tympanic cavity, that will cause lesions of the oval or round window. Although some cases have been described during flights, the barotraumatic fistulas are more commonly seen in SCUBA divers.

Both the explosive and implosive mechanisms are a cause of sudden or rapidly progressing hearing loss, usually with altered speech discrimination, and often accompanied by vertigo. The surgeon uses a transmeatal approach to examine both windows, and, if the fistula is found, it is blocked with a fragment of adipose tissue from the earlobe and stabilized with biological glue.

There are many controversies regarding the existence of spontaneous perilymphatic fistulas [23]. One of us feels that these fistulas do exist and that they occur in persons with especially sensitive ears, since they often result from traumatic events that usually do not cause any harm to the inner ear of other persons [24, 25]. It is quite possible that the same sort of thing happens in the cases of delayed endolymphatic hydrops, since very few of the patients with unilateral hearing loss in childhood, due to epidemic parotiditis, develop late hydrops [3].

The diagnosis of perilymphatic fistula is difficult. In some patients there is a clear mention of a short, sharp, explosive sound that precedes the hearing loss, but this does not happen in every case. The history of intense physical effort or stress is also suggestive, as well as the absence of recent viral infections. Hearing losses in young people without a history of vascular problems are also significant.

Approximately one half of the patients will present a positive Tullio and/or Hennebert sign.

The amount of hearing loss is probably dependent on the inner ear trauma determined at the moment of the fistula formation. The surgical closure of the fistula helps the healing process, but undoubtedly the best surgical results are the ones obtained in patients with smaller degrees of hearing loss. In patients with profound hearing loss, the operation must be performed as soon as possible. In operations performed more than 3 weeks after the hearing loss, the results obtained are seldom satisfactory. In relation to vertigo, however, the results are usually good, regardless of the time lapse. Approximately 60% of the operations result in some useful hearing improvement.

Surgery for Benign Paroxysmal Positional Vertigo

With the advent of different diagnostic and therapeutic maneuvers, and more precise determination of the semicircular canal with cupulolithiasis or canalolithiasis, the surgical treatment of BPPV is now rarely indicated. Surgery will be restricted to the cases of intractable disease, non-responsive to all medications and all physical therapy. The involved canal and side must be clearly determined, and the operation will not be performed in an only hearing ear. Special attention should be given to exclude the possibility of central paroxysmal vertigo.

Gacek [26, 27], in 1978, proposed the section of the singular nerve, the nerve fibers that arise from the posterior semicircular canal and join the inferior vestibular nerve. This operation was indicated only for cases of BPPV arising from the posterior semicircular canal.

A different approach is the plugging of the semicircular canal that has been performed in many patients, with good results [28]. According to the established diagnosis, any of the semicircular canals can be plugged.

The Perilymphatic Hypertension Syndrome

This is a congenital disorder related to structural changes in the cochlear modiolus or enlarged cochlear aqueducts, resulting in an excessive amount of spinal fluid in the inner ear. These patients present mixed hearing losses, but the tympanic reflexes are normal, in spite of the air-bone gap [29]. There are mild cases that show fluctuant hearing but do not present progression of their hearing losses, and there are cases that are accompanied by episodes of cerebrospinal otorrhea, often related to recurrent otic meningitis [30]. Attempts to perform stapedectomies in these patients resulted in stapes gushers – a large flow of cerebrospinal fluid fills the operating field when the stapes is punctured or removed [31]. The hearing results of these procedures may show some temporary gains, but they do not persist, as the perilymphatic hypertension will, after a short time, exert itself again. Procedures to block the cochlear aqueduct have also failed to achieve hearing improvements and did not prevent the progression of the hearing loss in the more serious cases.

Perilymphatic hypertension is rare and should not receive surgical treatment, except in the cases of recurring meningitis.

Surgery for Dehiscence of the Superior Semicircular Canal

Minor et al., in 1998, reported on patients that presented positive Tullio and Hennebert signs, related to bone dehiscence of the superior semicircular canal [32]. It is interesting to note that Tullio's phenomenon – vertigo induced by loud sounds – was described in 1929 and Hennebert' sign, later regarded as a fistula test, was described in 1911 in patients with tertiary syphilis involving the inner ear.

This report led to better evaluation of the superior semicircular canal in computerized tomography scans of the temporal bones, showing that this condition, although not frequent, was not uncommon. The openings at the canal represent a "third" inner ear window, which induces many changes in the mechanics of the cochlea and vestibule.

Patients with dehiscent superior canals may present the following symptoms:

Common complaints Autophony, tinnitus, dizziness, and occasional episodes of oscillopsia, usually pulse-synchronous, related to intense sounds or changes in intracranial pressure.

Auditory symptoms Mild mixed hearing loss, less intense than that observed in the perilymphatic hypertension syndrome, and small air-bone gap. They also present normal tympanic reflexes.

Vestibular symptoms Dizziness, unsteadiness, and occasional episodes of vertigo. Altered results are obtained in both cervical and ocular vestibular myogenic electric responses (cVEMP and oVEMP). These are most probably the most sensitive tests for this disorder. The results of the vHIT tests are variable.

Imaging The temporal bone computerized tomographic scans are important in the diagnosis of superior canal dehiscence. Reconstructions using the Pöschl and Stenvers positions are particularly useful. It should be mentioned, however, that the images alone do not constitute a proof that there is an opening in the canal, demanding a verification by functional tests (vHIT and VEMP).

Superior canal dehiscence is most probably a congenital defect, but the symptoms are seldom seen in a young population. Most of the diagnosed patients have 40 or more years of age, and the reason why they become symptomatic after a long period of time is unknown. Furthermore, many patients have mild symptoms and may be simply followed. For those with more intense disabilities, the surgical obliteration of the third window is recommended.

The middle fossa approach provides the best approach to the tip of the superior semicircular canal. Some surgeons prefer a transmastoid approach, but the available space is limited and makes it more difficult to achieve an adequate obliteration.

Vascular Loops

In 1975 Jannetta described a clinical entity, characterized by a compression of a cranial nerve by a vascular loop [33]. He was also the first to perform microvascular decompression for intractable positional vertigo [34]. Magnan [35] and Ricci et al. [36] have used an endoscope-assisted retrosigmoid approach to treat hemifacial spasms and in rare cases of tinnitus caused by vascular loops.

Vascular loops around AICA or PICA or their branches are relatively common, but many of them are observed in asymptomatic patients. It is difficult to decide which of these loops are actually causing a vascular compression syndrome. There are many controversies in the literature in relation to the precise determination of the vascular loops that demand surgical treatment [37–41].

Vestibular Schwannomas

These benign tumors are the most frequent of the brain tumors and can be diagnosed with great precision by means of magnetic resonance images performed with contrast.

Some tumors grow in the fundus of the internal acoustic meatus and a hearing loss due to compression of the cochlear nerve is apt to occur early in the development of the tumor. Others grow on the medial portion of the meatus and may not produce hearing losses for several years. Tumors that grow in the cisterna of the cerebellopontine angle may attain large sizes before being diagnosed; some of these patients may present normal hearing.

Vertigo is infrequent, as the slow growth of the tumor stimulates simultaneous compensation.

Small tumors totally enclosed in the internal acoustic meatus should be followed by periodic magnetic resonance, for some of them grow very slowly and may not require surgery. When surgery becomes necessary, they may be removed through a middle fossa operation or by a retrolabyrinthine approach. Larger tumors may be removed by a translabyrinthine or suboccipital approach.

Some good results have been obtained with radiosurgery. It should not be performed in young patients, however, for the risk of changing the tumor into a malignant schwannoma.

Neurofibromatosis type II, which results from a defect on chromosome 22, frequently gives origin to bilateral vestibular schwannomas and other brain tumors, particularly meningiomas. When the patient has good hearing, it is customary to operate on the larger tumor and follow the other tumor as long as possible, without endangering the patient's life. Cochlear implants have been advised to some patients to make them hear better until the tumor is operated.

For patients with bilateral profound hearing loss, the auditory brainstem implant (ABI) has been employed. Its results are inferior to those of the cochlear implants, but they definitely give to the patient's a better quality of life.

Vestibular Implants

These experimental procedures [42–45] are being tried in people with total bilateral loss of vestibular function, which is a severely incapacitating disease. The results are promising.

Final Comments

Surgical treatment of vestibular disorders is restricted to patients with very severe problems. In the last few years, the number of patients that demand surgery is gradually becoming smaller, due to better possibilities of clinical diagnosis and treatment and better techniques in vestibular rehabilitation.

The availability of these operations, however, is very important, as they offer a better quality of life to the patients for whom they are indicated.

References

1. Schuknecht HF. Ablation therapy in Meniere's disease. Acta Otolaryngol (Stockh). 1957;Suppl 132:1.
2. Cawthorne TE. Meniere's disease. 1947. Quoted by Shambaugh GE, Jr. Surgery of the Ear. Philadelphia: Saunders; 1959.
3. Mangabeira-Albernaz PL. Unusual cases of delayed endolymphatic hydrops. Acta Otolaryngol. 2007;127(4):355–9.
4. van Fick IA. Symposium: management of Ménière's disease. VI Sacculotomy for hydrops. Laryngoscope. 1965;75(10):1539–46.
5. Cody DT. The tack operation for endolymphatic hydrops. Laryngoscope. 1969;79(10):1737–44.
6. House WF. Shunt and other operations for hydrops. Arch Otolaryngol. 1969;89(1):104–7.
7. Belal A Jr, House WF, Antunez JC. Histopathology of cryosurgery for Meniere's disease. Am J Otol. 1980;1(3):147–50.
8. Knapp HJ. A clinical analysis of the inflammatory affections of the inner ear. 1871. Quoted by Shambaugh GE, Jr. Surgery of the Ear. Philadelphia: Saunders; 1959.
9. Portmann G. The saccus endolymphaticus and an operation for draining the same for the relief of vertigo. Proc R Soc Med. 1927;20(12):1862–7.
10. Hallpike CS, Cairns H. Observations on the pathology of Ménière's syndrome: (section of otology). Proc R Soc Med. 1938;31(11):1317–36.
11. House WF. Subarachnoid shunt for drainage of hydrops. A report of 63 cases. Arch Otolaryngol. 1964;79:338–54.
12. Portmann G, Shambaugh GE Jr, Arenberg IK, Arenberg CR. The first inner ear surgery to conserve or improve a sensory hearing loss: a candid discussion of the first 50 years of endolymphatic sac surgery for hydrops with its innovator. Rev Laryngol Otol Rhinol (Bord). 1978;99(5–6):277–98.
13. Bretlau P, Thomsen J, Tos M, Johnsen NJ. Placebo effect in surgery for Menière's disease. A double-blind placebo-controlled study on endolymphatic sac shunt surgery. Adv Otorhinolaryngol. 1982;28:139–46.
14. Pillsbury HC 3rd, Arenberg IK, Ferraro J, Ackley RS. Endolymphatic sac surgery. The Danish sham surgery study: an alternative analysis. Otolaryngol Clin N Am. 1983;16(1):123–7.
15. Mangabeira-Albernaz PL, Fukuda Y, Chammas F, Ganança MM. The Mondini dysplasia – a clinical study. ORL (Basel). 1981;43:131–52.
16. Mangabeira-Albernaz PL. The Mondini dysplasia – from early diagnosis to cochlear implant. Acta Otolaryngol. 1983;95:627–31.
17. Dandy WE. The surgical treatment of Menière's disease. 1941. Quoted by Shambaugh GE, Jr. Surgery of the Ear. Philadelphia: Saunders; 1959.
18. House WF. VIII nerve and cochlear surgery in advanced otosclerosis: a preliminary report. In: Schuknecht HF, editor. Otosclerosis. Henry Ford Hospital International Symposium. Boston: Little, Brown; 1962. p. 371–89.
19. Miyazaki H, Nomura Y, Mardassi A, Deveze A, Miura M, Jike M, Magnan J. How minimally invasive vestibular neurotomy for incapacitating Meniere's disease improves dizziness and anxiety. Acta Otolaryngol. 2017;137(7):707–11. https://doi.org/10.1080/00016489.2017.1278790.
20. Devèze A, Montava M, Lopez C, Lacour M, Magnan J, Borel L. Vestibular compensation following vestibular neurotomy. Eur Ann Otorhinolaryngol Head Neck Dis. 2015;132(4):197–203. https://doi.org/10.1016/j.anorl.2015.04.003.
21. Lavinsky L, Lavinsky J. Tratamento cirúrgico do paciente vertiginoso. In Maia FCZ, Mangabeira-Albernaz PL, Carmona S, Otoneurologia atual 2014, Rio de Janeiro, Revinter, p 479–499.
22. Goodhill V. Sudden deafness and round window rupture. Laryngoscope. 1971;81(9):1462–74.
23. Hornibrook J. Perilymph fistula: fifty years of controversy. ISRN Otolaryngol. 2012;2012:281248. https://doi.org/10.5402/2012/281248.

24. Mangabeira-Albernaz PL. Fístula perilinfática espontânea. In: Lopes Filho O, editor. Temas de Otorrinolaringologia, vol. 2. São Paulo: Manole; 1978. p. 165–72.
25. Caldas NCR, Mangabeira-Albernaz PL. Fístula perilinfática. In: Mangabeira-Albernaz PL, Ganança MM, House WF, editors. Surdez neuro-sensorial. São Paulo: Moderna; 1978. p. 135–51.
26. Gacek RR. Posterior ampullary nerve transection for benign paroxysmal positional vertigo. Trans Pa Acad Ophthalmol Otolaryngol. 1978;31(2):190–3.
27. Gacek RR, Gacek MR. Singular neurectomy in the management of paroxysmal positional vertigo. Otolaryngol Clin N Am. 1994;27(2):363–79.
28. Suzuki M. Surgery. In: Suzuki M, editor. Basic and clinical approach to BPPV based on model experiment results. Tokio: SPIO; 2012. p. 119–24.
29. Mangabeira-Albernaz PL, Hidal LBT, Iorio MCM. The Perilymphatic hypertension syndrome. Acta Otolaryngol. 1992;112:306–10.
30. Brown Farrior J, Endicott JN. Congenital mixed deafness: cerebrospinal fluid otorrhea. Ablation of the aqueduct of the cochlea. Laryngoscope. 1971;81:684–99.
31. Glasscock ME III. The stapes gusher. Arch Otolaryngol. 1973;98:82–91.
32. Minor LB, Solomon D, Zinreich J, Zee DS. Sound and/or pressure-induced vertigo due to bone dehiscence of the superior semicircular canal. Arch Otolaryngol Head Neck Surg. 1998;124:249–58.
33. Janetta PJ. Neurovascular cross-compression in patients with hyperactive dysfunction of the eighth cranial nerve. Surg Forum. 1975;26:467–9.
34. Janetta PJ, Moller MB, Mollar AR. Disabling positional vertigo. N Engl J Med. 1984;310:1700–5.
35. Magnan J. Endoscope-assisted decompression of facial nerve for treatment of hemifacial spasm. Neurochirurgie. 2018;64(2):144–52. pii: S0028-3770(18)30036-5. https://doi.org/10.1016/j.neuchi.2018.01.007.
36. Ricci G, Di Stadio A, D'Ascanio L, La Penna R, Trabalzini F, Della Volpe A, Magnan J. Endoscope-assisted retrosigmoid approach in hemifacial spasm: our experience. Braz J Otorhinolaryngol 2018. pii: S1808-8694(18)30179-4. https://doi.org/10.1016/j.bjorl.2018.03.015.
37. Gultekin S, Celik H, Akpek S, Oner Y, Gumus T, Tokgoz N. Vascular loops at the cerebellopontine angle: is there a correlation with tinnitus? Am J Neuroradiol. 2008;29(9):1746–9. https://doi.org/10.3174/ajnr.A1212.
38. Gorrie A, Warren FM 3rd, de la Garza AN, Shelton C, Wiggins RH 3rd. Is there a correlation between vascular loops in the cerebellopontine angle and unexplained unilateral hearing loss? Otol Neurotol 2010;31(1):48–52. https://doi.org/10.1097/MAO.0b013e3181c0e63a.
39. Hitchon PW, Zanaty M, Moritani T, Uc E, Pieper CL, He W, Noeller J. Microvascular decompression and MRI findings in trigeminal neuralgia and hemifacial spasm. A single center experience. Clin Neurol Neurosurg. 2015;139:216–20. https://doi.org/10.1016/j.clineuro.2015.10.012.
40. Ezerarslan H, Sanhal EO, Kurukahvecioglu S, Ataç GK, Kocatürk S. Presence of vascular loops entering internal acoustic channel may increase risk of sudden sensorineural hearing loss and reduce recovery of these patients. Laryngoscope. 2016;127:210. https://doi.org/10.1002/lary.26054.
41. Abreu Junior L, Kuniyoshi CH, Wolosker AB, Borri ML, Antunes A, Ota VK, Uchida D. Vascular loops in the anterior inferior cerebellar artery, as identified by magnetic resonance imaging, and their relationship with otologic symptoms. Radiol Bras. 2016;49(5):300–4.
42. Guinand N, Van de Berg R, Ranieri M, Cavuscens S, DiGiovanna J, Nguyen TA, Micera S, Stokroos R, Kingma H, Guyot JP, Pérez Fornos A. Vestibular implants: hope for improving the quality of life of patients with bilateral vestibular loss. Conf Proc IEEE Eng Med Biol Soc. 2015;2015:7192–5. https://doi.org/10.1109/EMBC.2015.7320051.

43. Della Santina CC, Migliaccio AA, Patel AH. A multi-channel semicircular canal neural prosthesis using electrical stimulation to restore 3-D vestibular sensation. IEEE Trans Biomed Eng. 2007;54:1016–30.
44. Guinand N, Van de Berg R, Cavuscens S, Stokroos R, Ranieri M, Pelizzone M, Kingma H, Guyot JP, Pérez Fornos A. Restoring visual acuity in dynamic conditions with a vestibular implant. Front Neurosci, 2016;10. https://doi.org/10.3389/fnins.2016.00577.
45. van de Berg R, Lucieer F, Guinand N, van Tongeren J, George E, Guyot J-F, Kingma H, van Hoof M, Temel Y, van Overbeeke J, Perez-Fornos A, Stokroos R. The vestibular implant: hearing preservation during Intralabyrinthine electrode insertion—a case report. Front Neurol 2017;8. doi https://doi.org/10.3389/fneur.2017.00137.

Index

A
ABR, 99–100
Action potentials, 6
Acute vestibular syndromes, 121–127
Air conduction, 91–92
Alcoholic Cerebellar Degeneration, 185–186
Ampulla, 5
Anterior canal BPPV, 168–169
Anteroinferior cerebellar artery (AICA) syndrome, 117
Apogeotropic posterior canal BPPV, 158–159
Arnold-Chiari malformation, 49
Ataxia, 181
  age of onset, 186
  autoimmune, 187
  due to mitochondrial diseases, 190
  due to Vitamin Deficiency, 188–189
  etiology, 187
  related to anti-GAD antibodies, 187
  related to Hashimoto's encefalopathy, 188
  toxic, 187
Atypical paroxysmal positional vertigo, 169–172
Auditory adaptation, 95
Auditory brainstem responses, 99–100
Auditory evoked responses, 101, 102
Auditory thresholds, 90–93
Autoimmune ataxia, 187
Autosomal recessive ataxia, 190

B
Bacterial brainstem encephalitis, 123
Barbecue rotation techniques, 164
Basilar membrane, 5
Bedside tests, 49
Benign paroxysmal positional vertigo (BPPV), 46, 151–172
  classification, 153
  surgery, 213
Benign paroxysmal torticollis of childhood, 147–148
Benign paroxysmal vertigo of childhood, 147–149
Bilateral peripheral acute vestibular syndrome, 122
Bilateral peripheral vestibular syndrome, 127–128
Bilateral vestibulopathy, 175–179
Bone conduction, 91–92, 109
BPPV, *see* Benign paroxysmal positional vertigo
Brainstem evoked response audiometry (BERA), 99
Brain tumors, 124
Brush border membrane disease, 199

C
Caloric tests, 7–73
Canalolithiasis, 46
Central acute vestibular syndromes, 122–124
Central paroxysmal positional vertigo (CPPV), 120
Cerebellar ataxia, 182–183
Cerebellar transient ischemic attacks, 116–118
Cerebellum, 33–34
Cerebral vascular accident (CVA), 123
Cervical vestibular evoked myogenic potentials (cVEMP), 46, 73
Chronic vestibular syndromes, 127–129
Cochlea, 4

P. L. M. Albernaz et al., *The New Neurotology*,
https://doi.org/10.1007/978-3-030-11283-7

Cochlear duct, 4
Cochlear Menière's disease, 136
Cochlear microphonics, 6
Cochleo-vestibular dissociation, 103
Coriolis effect, 43
Cortical electrical response audiometry, 101
Cover test, 55
Cranial trauma, 125
Cupula ampullaris, 7
Cupulolithiasis, 47, 152
cVEMP, *see* Cervical vestibular evoked myogenic potentials

D
Deadly D's, 117
Débarquement syndrome, 43
Definite Menière's disease, 134
Definite Vestibular Migraine, 143
Dizziness, 39, 43
Ductolithiasis, 46
Dynamic Visual Acuity, 60

E
Electrical response audiometry, 96–102
Electrocochleography (ECochG), 97–99
Electronystagmography, 66
Endocochlear potential, 6
Endolymph, 5
Endolymphatic duct, 12
Endolymphatic hydrops, 12
Endolymphatic sac, 12
Episodic ataxia, 189
Episodic ataxia type 2, 123
Episodic positional syndromes, 119–120
Episodic vestibular syndromes, 115
Epley's maneuver, 156–157
Eye movements, 19
Eye muscles, 28

F
Functional vestibular disorders, 193–195

G
Gaze nystagmus, 67–68
Gufoni's maneuver, 167

H
Hair cells, 2
Head impulse test, 61
Head shaking nystagmus (HSN), 59
Head shaking tilt suppression (HSTS), 59
Head tilt, 54
Helicotrema, 4
HINTS, 61–62
Horizontal saccades, 21, 57
Hypermetric saccades, 57
Hyperventilation nystagmus, 59
Hypoglycemia, 198
Hypometric saccades, 57

I
Idiopathic late onset cerebellar ataxia (ILOCA), 189
Imbalance, 39, 40
Immittance tests, 95–96
Infectious ataxia, 189–190
Inferior vestibular nerve, 13
Inner ear mechanical hearing loss, 103
Internuclear Ophthalmoplegia, 69

K
Kinocilia, 2
Kraft insulin curves, 201

L
Labyrinthectomy, 209–210
Lateral canal BPPV, 170–171
Lermoyez syndrome, 137
Lindsay-Hemenway syndrome, 45

M
Maculae, 11
Mechanical hearing loss, 92
Medial longitudinal fasciculus, 13
Menière's disease, 44, 116, 133–141
  surgery, 209–212
Metabolic hearing loss, 105
Middle ear hearing loss, 103
Middle latency responses (MLR), 100–101
Mixed hearing loss, 109
Modiolus, 4
Mondini dysplasia, 44
Motion sickness, 148–149
Multiple sclerosis, 124
Multiple System Atrophy (MSA), 188

N
Nystagmus, 21–22

O
Ocular counterroll (OCR), 20
Ocular vestibular evoked myogenic potentials (oVEMP), 46, 73, 74
Optokinetic nystagmus (OKN), 58
Optokinetic system, 30
Optokinetic test, 69
Organ of Corti, 5
Orthostatic hypotension, 119
Oscillopsia, 39, 43
Otic capsule, 4
Otoacoustic emissions, 96
Otoconia, 11
Otolithic membrane, 11
Otoliths, 2–4, 11
Ototoxicity, 124
oVEMP, *see* Ocular vestibular evoked myogenic potentials

P
P300, 101–102
Paraneoplastic cerebellar degeneration, 187
Perilymph, 4
Perilymphatic fistula, 44, 212–213
Perilymphatic hypertension, 44
Persistent postural-perceptual dizziness (PPPD), 128–129
PICA syndrome, 117
Posterior canal BPPV, 171
Presbyastasis, 46
Probable Menière's disease, 134
Probable vestibular migraine, 143
Progressive sensorineural hearing loss, 104–109

R
Recruitment of loudness, 94–95
Reissner's membrane, 4
Reticular formation, 13
Rotatory chairs, 70–71

S
Saccades, 57
  tests, 68–69
Saccule, 4, 10–12
Scala media, 4
Scala tympani, 4
Scala vestibuli, 4
Semicircular canals, 4, 7–10
Semicircular ducts, 5
Semont's maneuver, 157–158
Sensorial convergence, 34–35
Sensorineural hearing loss, 92
Sensory ataxia, 183
SHIMP test, 86
Smooth pursuit, 19–20, 31, 57
SO STONED, 40
Speech discrimination, 93
Spinocerebellar Ataxia, 190
Spiral ligament, 5
Spontaneous nystagmus, 54, 67
Statocyst, 2, 3
Stereocilia, 2
Stria vascularis, 5
Striola, 11
Subjective visual vertical (SVV), 54
Sudden hearing loss, 104
Summating potentials (SP), 6
Superior canal dehiscence, 215
Superior vestibular nerve, 13

T
Timing, Triggers, And Target Examination (TiTrATE), 53, 115
Toxic ataxia, 187
Transtympanic treatments, 212
Truncal ataxia in acute vestibular syndrome, 125–127
Tullio's phenomenon, 15, 60
Tunnel of Corti, 6
Type I cells, 9
Type II cells, 9

U
Unilateral peripheral acute vestibular syndrome, 121–122
Unsteadiness, 39, 43
Usher syndrome, 45
Utricle, 4, 10–12

V
Valsalva induced nystagmus, 59–60
Vannucchi-Asprella's maneuver, 166
Vannucchi forced prolonged position, 166–167
Vascularization, inner ear, 25–26

Vascular loops, 215
VEMPs, *see* Vestibular-evoked myogenic potentials
Vergence, 58
Vertical saccades, 21, 57
Vertigo, 39, 43
  and alcohol, 193–194
  and beta-blockers, 193
  and diuretics, 193
  and hearing loss, 103
  and metabolic disorders, 194
  and toxic substances, 194
Vestibular compensation, 121
Vestibular-evoked myogenic potentials (VEMPs), 46, 73–75
Vestibular implants, 216
Vestibular migraine, 116, 143–149
Vestibular neuritis, 45
Vestibular paroxysmia, 128
Vestibular schwannomas, 215–216
Vestibulo-ocular reflex (VOR), 16, 50–52, 80–81
Vestibulo-ocular reflex suppression (VORS), 61
Vibration induced nystagmus, 4, 9
Video head impulse test (vHIT), 73, 79–86
  artifacts, 85
  and caloric tests, 84
  indications, 84
  parameters, 83–84
Videonystagmography, 66
Viral encephalitis, 122–123
Visually enhanced vestibular ocular reflex (VVOR), 60
Von Hippel–Lindau disease, 45
VOR, *see* Vestibulo-ocular reflex

W

Wernicke's encephalopathy, 125

MIX
Papier aus verantwortungsvollen Quellen
Paper from responsible sources
FSC® C105338

If you have any concerns about our products,
you can contact us on
ProductSafety@springernature.com

In case Publisher is established outside the EU,
the EU authorized representative is:
Springer Nature Customer Service Center GmbH
Europaplatz 3, 69115 Heidelberg, Germany

Printed by Libri Plureos GmbH
in Hamburg, Germany